Dental Office *Administration*

Dental Office *Administration*

GERALDINE IRLBACHER-GIRTEL, BScN, RN, MEd

GUY S. GIRTEL, DDS

Wolters Kluwer | Lippincott Williams & Wilkins
Health

Philadelphia • Baltimore • New York • London
Buenos Aires • Hong Kong • Sydney • Tokyo

Acquisitions Editor: Peter Sabatini
Product Director: Eric Branger
Development Editor/Product Manager: David R. Payne
Marketing Manager: Christen Murphy
Design Coordinator: Doug Smock
Compositor: Aptara Inc.

351 West Camden Street
Baltimore, Maryland 21201

530 Walnut Street
Philadelphia, Pennsylvania 19106

Printed in China

Library of Congress Cataloging-in-Publication Data

Irlbacher-Girtel, Geraldine.
Dental office administration / Geraldine Irlbacher-Girtel, Guy S. Girtel.
p. ; cm.
ISBN 978-0-7817-9160-1
1. Dental offices—Management. 2. Dental office managers. I. Girtel, Guy S. II. Title.
[DNLM: 1. Dental Offices—organization & administration. 2. Accounting—methods. 3. Office Management—organization & administration. 4. Personnel Management—methods. WU 77 I69d 2009]
RK58.I75 2009
617.60068—dc22

2009021969

---

1 2 3 4 5 6 7 8 9 10

CCS0809

For Everett and Simon

Preface

Advancements in the field of dentistry are constant. As clinical advancements grow, there is an increasing need for educated professionals in the administrative area of the dental field. The oral health of the public is much too important to be left up to personnel who are not formally trained in the dental field. Dental office administrators are dental professionals who receive the formal training required. The formally trained dental administrative assistant has become a critical component in the delivery of quality oral health care. As an administrative member of the dental profession, you are embarking on an exciting and challenging career.

OBJECTIVE

The primary objective of this text is to make available a comprehensive resource on dental office administration to the dental profession and the administrative and clinical staff who affect the success of a dental office. As you progress through the chapters, you will find that all the information reflects current information and developments in the dental industry.

ORGANIZATION

This textbook is organized into five parts.

Part 1 provides an introduction to the dental administration profession by providing insight into the dental office from the business perspective. This section explores the characteristics of a successful dental administrator. A thorough definition of the role of the dental administrator and explanation of the importance of the position give the reader a complete understanding of the qualifications and expectations of the position. A comprehensive review of the components of a successful dental office, such as office layout, team members and their roles, and the specialties found in the dental profession, provides students with the knowledge required for success in the profession. This section also covers the ethical and legal knowledge necessary for dental administrators and further outlines the responsibilities that they have to patients in the dental practice as mandated by HIPAA in the United States and PIPEDA in Canada. Section 1 is rounded out with the importance of asepsis in the clinical and administrative dental environment and the responsibilities of the dental administrator in this regard.

Part 2 begins with a dental terminology section as a necessary resource for the reader to ensure correct pronunciation and usage of dental terminology in the industry. The main focus in the section is on communication in the dental office and the importance of correct and accurate communication. Emphasis is on the development of successful verbal and nonverbal communication skills and their effect on patient relationship development. Effective telephone and written communication skills are brought together in this section to emphasize this very important area of the dental administrator role.

Part 3 introduces the critical features of the role of the dental office administrator: patient record management, patient development and maintenance, appointment management, office policies and procedures, filing procedures, inventory, and technology. For success in the dental practice to occur, the dental office administrator must grasp the fundamental skills of establishing and maintaining patient relationships. The reader will become well-versed in methods used in the dental office to achieve a balanced patient flow such as recall systems, telephone reminders, and written reminders.

Appointment management is introduced, and readers are given real-life scenarios to challenge them. Providing insight into how to deal with late patients, no-shows, walk-ins, and emergencies will enhance the confidence to effectively deal with patients for any reader new to the dental industry. An understanding of dental office policies and the role they play in the development of a successful practice outlines other management responsibilities that dental office administrators must be familiar with. This section ends with a look at dental office filing and inventory procedures, and an in-depth look at computerized practice management. An overview of a computerized practice management program is given with applications for the reader to get a feel for the real thing.

Part 4 addresses the financial management aspects to dental office administration. Patient billing and payment is a large part of dental administration. One chapter is devoted to the collection of funds from patient by various means, with the bulk of the attention being given to insurance companies and the forms required for filing a dental claim, as well as the different types of dental plans available. Accounts receivable and accounts payable are both given equal time to provide a comprehensive lesson in collecting monies and paying expenses in the dental office. Banking procedures and payroll functions are outlined in the final two chapters of this section. In smaller dental clinics, the dental office administrator becomes the one staff member who is responsible for the financial aspects of the practice. A full overview of these procedures provides the reader with essential knowledge for management of a dental office.

Part 5 is devoted to the career considerations of the dental office administrator. As students begin the transition from student to employee, tips for making that transition as smooth and successful as possible are provided.

FINAL NOTE

In all chapters, Web sites and references used are current. These are included to substantiate the content and to encourage self-study by the reader. Self-education is essential for professional growth in the dental industry, especially if your career has just begun!

It is hoped that this book will facilitate the learning and knowledge necessary for success in the role of the dental office administrator. As the program you are in prepares you to be a respected professional of the dental industry, the knowledge this book provides will stay with you as you enter the world of dentistry and enhance the face of dental office administration.

Geraldine Irlbacher-Girtel, BScN, RN, MEd
Guy S. Girtel, DDS

User's Guide

This User's Guide helps you take full advantage of the *Dental Office Administrationtal* Office Administration text. Each chapter offers helpful features that enable you to quickly master new concepts and put your new skills into practice.

A number of features are included in this text to facilitate learning.

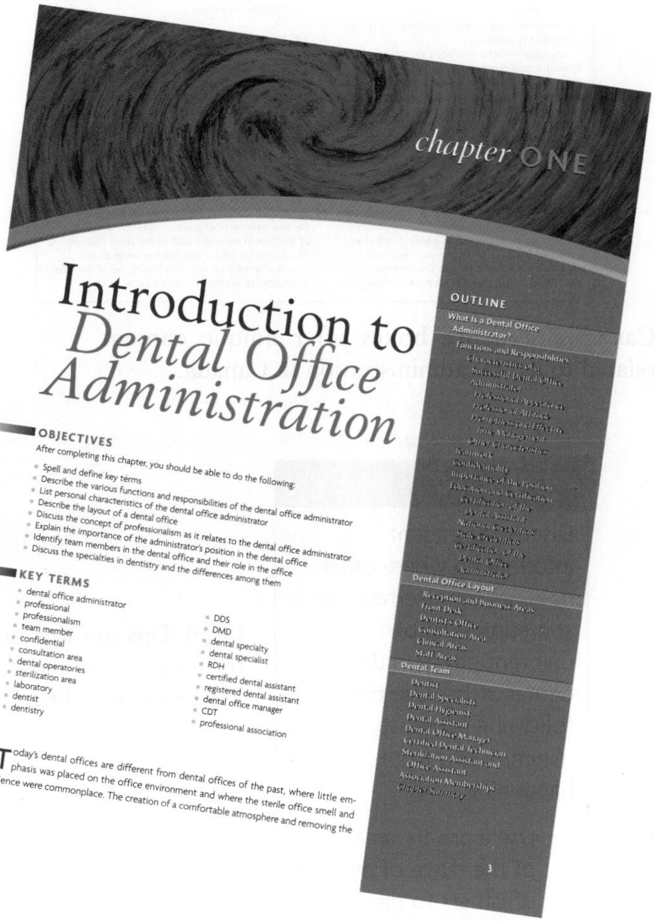

chapter ONE

Introduction to *Dental Office Administration*

OUTLINE

What Is a Dental Office Administrator?
Functions and Responsibilities
Characteristics of a Successful Dental Office Administrator
Professional Appearance
Professional Attitude
Promptness and Effective Time Management
Other Characteristics
Teamwork
Confidentiality
Importance of the Position
Education and Certification
Certification of the Dental Assistant
National Credentials
State Credentials
Certification of the Dental Office Administrator
Dental Office Layout
Reception and Business Areas
Front Desk
Dentist's Office
Consultation Area
Clinical Areas
Staff Areas
Dental Team
Dentist
Dental Specialists
Dental Hygienist
Dental Assistant
Dental Office Manager
Certified Dental Technician
Sterilization Assistant and Office Assistant
Association Memberships
Chapter Summary

OBJECTIVES

After completing this chapter, you should be able to do the following:

- Spell and define key terms
- Describe the various functions and responsibilities of the dental office administrator
- List personal characteristics of the dental office administrator
- Describe the layout of a dental office
- Discuss the concept of professionalism as it relates to the dental office administrator
- Explain the importance of the administrator's position in the dental office
- Identify team members in the dental office and their role in the office
- Discuss the specialties in dentistry and the differences among them

KEY TERMS

- dental office administrator
- professional
- professionalism
- team member
- confidential
- consultation area
- dental operatories
- sterilization area
- laboratory
- dentist
- dentistry
- DDS
- DMD
- dental specialty
- dental specialist
- RDH
- certified dental assistant
- registered dental assistant
- dental office manager
- CDT
- professional association

Today's dental offices are different from dental offices of the past, where little emphasis was placed on the office environment and where the sterile office smell and silence were commonplace. The creation of a comfortable atmosphere and removing the

3

Learning Objectives provide clear goals to ensure mastery of the content presented in the chapter, and **Key Terms** are listed at the beginning of each chapter and are boldfaced at first use within each chapter to introduce the student to the basic vocabulary of dental office administration. These key words are also listed and defined in the glossary at the back of the book.

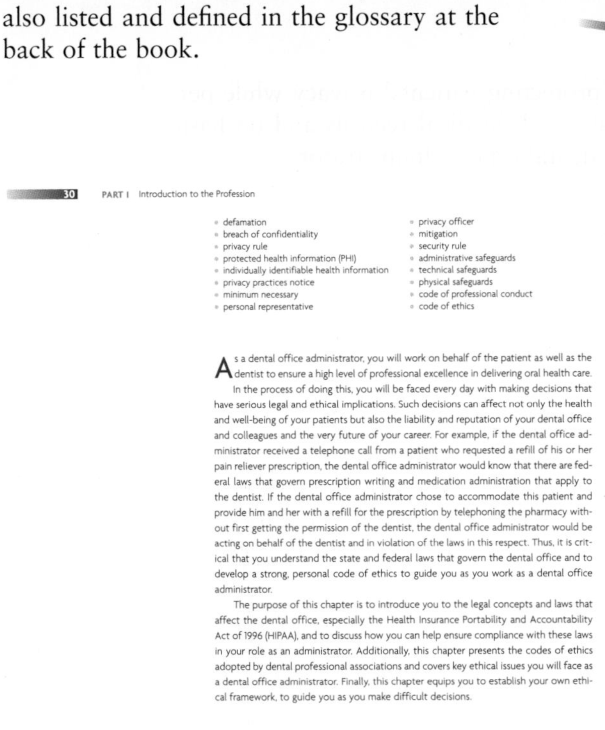

30 PART I Introduction to the Profession

- defamation
- breach of confidentiality
- privacy rule
- protected health information (PHI)
- individually identifiable health information
- privacy practices notice
- minimum necessary
- personal representative
- privacy officer
- mitigation
- security rule
- administrative safeguards
- technical safeguards
- physical safeguards
- code of professional conduct
- code of ethics

As a dental office administrator, you will work on behalf of the patient as well as the dentist to ensure a high level of professional excellence in delivering oral health care.

In the process of doing this, you will be faced every day with making decisions that have serious legal and ethical implications. Such decisions can affect not only the health and well-being of your patients but also the liability and reputation of your dental office and colleagues and the very future of your career. For example, if the dental office administrator received a telephone call from a patient who requested a refill of his or her pain reliever prescription, the dental office administrator would know that there are federal laws that govern prescription writing and medication administration that apply to the dentist. If the dental office administrator chose to accommodate this patient and provide him and her with a refill for the prescription by telephoning the pharmacy without first getting the permission of the dentist, the dental office administrator would be acting on behalf of the dentist and in violation of the laws in this respect. Thus, it is critical that you understand the state and federal laws that govern the dental office and to develop a strong, personal code of ethics to guide you as you work as a dental office administrator.

The purpose of this chapter is to introduce you to the legal concepts and laws that affect the dental office, especially the Health Insurance Portability and Accountability Act of 1996 (HIPAA), and to discuss how you can help ensure compliance with these laws in your role as an administrator. Additionally, this chapter presents the codes of ethics adopted by dental professional associations and covers key ethical issues you will face as a dental office administrator. Finally, this chapter equips you to establish your own ethical framework, to guide you as you make difficult decisions.

Chapter Introductions lay out the topics that will be covered in each chapter.

CANADIAN PRACTICE: WORKPLACE HAZARDOUS MATERIALS INFORMATION SYSTEM

The **Workplace Hazardous Materials Information System (WHMIS)** is a classification system established by the Canadian Center for Occupational Health and Safety (http:// www.ccohs.ca/oshanswers/legisl/intro_whmis.html) that groups chemicals that have similar properties. In the dental office, there are many materials you may come across through stocking, disposing, ordering, or using that fall under any one of the categories outlined by the WHMIS. There are six classes of hazardous materials in this system, some of which subdivide to include other classes.

The figure shows each of the six classes and the symbol associated with each. The symbol for each class is the symbol that can be found on the container of the material. For example, cleaning supplies, dental x-ray developer, mercury amalgam waste containers, and sharps disposal containers will all have one of the symbols you see in the figure on the outside of the container. The purpose of the symbol is to aid in the identification of the hazardous material.

The six classes are as follows: compressed gas, flammable and combustible material, oxidizing material, poisonous and infectious material, corrosive material, and dangerously reactive material. One of the regulations concerning these materials is that they are considered dangerous goods and, as such, are not able to be transported without an MSDS, discussed later in this chapter.

Although you may not come across every one of these hazardous materials in the dental office, it is useful to study these symbols so that you will recognize any hazardous materials that are in the dental office.

Compressed Gas

The compressed gas symbol is a picture of a cylinder surrounded by a circle.

Any material that is normally a gas and contained in a cylinder is considered compressed gas. Compressed gas is considered dangerous because it is under pressure. If the cylinder is broken by misuse and handling, it can become a projectile, which could cause damage to an object or a person nearby. Also, if a cylinder of compressed gas is heated, it will explode. In the dental office, you may see a cylinder of oxygen or nitrous oxide for sedation purposes.

Flammable and Combustible Material

Flammable means that the material will burn or catch fire easily at normal temperatures. Reactive flammable materials are those that may suddenly start burning when they touch air or water or may react with air or water to make a flammable gas. The material may be a solid, liquid, or gas. Combustible materials usually have to be heated before they catch fire. In the dental office, you may see butanes or solvents with the symbol of a flame inside a circle, which indicates that the material is flammable or combustible.

Oxidizing Material

The symbol for this class of materials is an "o" with flames on top of it. Oxidizers are materials that assist in the fire process by providing oxygen. An oxidizer can be a gas, a liquid, or a solid.

Poisonous and Infectious Material

These materials can cause serious harm to a person. There are three subdivisions of materials in this class, all of which are found in the dental office, so they will receive our attention.

1. *Division 1*: Materials causing immediate toxic effects, such as poisons, cleaning supplies, or dental x-ray developer, make up this division. These materials are identified by the "skull and cross-bones" symbol.
2. *Division 2*: Materials causing other toxic effects, such as cancer, allergies, or reproductive changes, are part of this division. The symbol is a "T" with an exclamation point at the bottom. Materials such as mercury and benzene, which are found in the dental office, fall into this category.
3. *Division 3*: Biohazardous infectious waste refers to the organisms that can be produced from infectious waste and cause diseases. In the dental office, sharps are the most common form of biohazardous waste. The symbol looks like three "c's" joined together in a circle.

Corrosive Material

Corrosive material can cause severe burns if it comes in contact with skin or other human tissue and can usually burn through clothing and other material as well. The damage is permanent. The symbol for this class of materials is two test tubes pouring material, one onto a hand, the other onto a bar, and showing the items being affected. This type of material would more likely be found in a dental laboratory than in the dental office.

Dangerously Reactive Material

Most of materials classified as dangerously reactive are extremely hazardous if they are not handled properly because they can react quickly and easily. An example of this type of material would be aluminum chloride. The symbol for dangerously reactive materials is a picture of a test tube with lines coming out of the tube surrounded by a letter "R" inside a circle.

Canadian Practice boxes offer unique content related to dental administration in Canada.

what IF ?

A patient has arrived for an appointment and has expressed concern to you about the dental assistant wearing gloves during treatment. The patient feels that this is offensive since she does not have any diseases that the dental assistant should be concerned with contracting. How do you respond?

It is important to educate the patient on the meaning of "standard precautions" and what is involved with this process, particularly, how these precautions protect the dental patient and staff members. The patient needs to be aware that every patient is treated the same; that is, all members of the clinical staff wear gloves for each treatment performed on each patient.

What If boxes are hypothetical scenarios in the dental office that require the reader to apply knowledge to resolve a realistic issue or problem.

legal TIP

Discussing patient information where other patients can overhear can sometimes happen unintentionally in the dental office. Use the following points to minimize this from happening:

- Use a private area out of the range of hearing of others to discuss patient information.
- Use a low voice when speaking with patients in public areas.
- Never address a patient by his or her full first and last name.
- Never discuss patients outside of the dental office with other people.

Legal Tips are tips on protecting patients' privacy while performing day-to-day tasks with medical records and on basic legal responsibilities of dental office administrators.

Administrative Tips are tips on how to perform some administrative task in the dental office.

Administrative TIP

When a new patient telephones the dental office to schedule an appointment, there is specific information that is necessary to obtain from the patient to establish a patient record before setting an appointment. Some dental offices may require only name and contact phone number as the information necessary for scheduling the appointment. Other offices may require more information to establish a patient record. A new patient telephone call information sheet is a very useful tool in establishing a patient record. This is a form that is kept in an accessible place to collect the necessary patient information, such as name, address, phone number, date of birth, and insurance information. Having this information prior to the patient appointment allows you to mail the proper forms to the patient for completion prior to the appointment and verify insurance information. The form can also be used to collect information such as the referral source of the patient. If a current patient has referred a new patient, this is an opportunity to send a thank you card or other acknowledgment to the referring patient. Finally, documenting when the new patient demographic and health history forms were sent can also be verified on this form. When the patient arrives for the scheduled appointment, the form can then be filed in the patient chart, as it is written documentation of the initial contact with the patient. Figure 8-7 is an example of what the new patient telephone call information sheet may look like. This form can be modified to fit the requirements of the dental office.

Tips From the Dentist are tips from the perspective of the dentist regarding optimal practices for dental administrators.

Tip FROM THE DENTIST

One of the most distressing things that I see when I am leading my team to provide a caring, safe, and stressfree environment for our patients is when members of the team don't understand or appreciate their role in maintaining the flow in the dental office. For instance, if the dental office administrator fails to be ready and able to work at the opening of the office, someone must take the place of that individual to answer the phone and greet patients as they arrive. If the person filling in is the dental assistant, then he or she is no longer available to help the dentist or attend to patients' needs in the operatory. The responsibility of every employee in the dental office is not to the dentist or patient alone but to every member of the dental team.

Each member of the team must understand and appreciate the role of all team members and how each person is integral in maintaining an efficiently run office. Just as important, team members must be aware of how their actions affect the team.

Team members may appear disorganized and incompetent when they are trying to fill in where they don't feel comfortable; this creates a pressure-filled environment that patients can sense.

PROCEDURE 3-1 *Hand Washing*

The following steps outline a correct hand-washing procedure.

1. Remove all jewelry (rings, watches, bracelets).
2. Turn on the tap and run cool water at a medium stream. Use antimicrobial soap.
3. Lather hands, wrists, and forearms. Rub all surfaces using light pressure. Fingers should interlace. Wash each finger individually, rubbing with a back-and-forth motion with light pressure.
4. Rinse thoroughly under the running water, starting from the forearms to the fingertips.
5. Repeat the process.
6. Use a paper towel to dry your hands and forearms.
7. Use a paper towel to turn off the tap. Do not use hands to turn off the tap as the risk of recontamination to hands is greater.

Procedure boxes provide step-by-step directions on performing common office management tasks.

checkPOINT

2. Describe five personal characteristics of the dental office administrator.
3. Why is it important for the dental office administrator to think and act calmly in emergency situations?

Checkpoint Questions are review questions interspersed throughout each chapter that allow students to check their recall of the content presented in the section just read.

Chapter Summary

Dentistry is constantly evolving. The formally trained dental office administrator will be a part of one of the most exciting times in dentistry, as new advances in dentistry appear everyday. The dental team members can make a dental practice very successful when they work together to deliver high-quality dentistry. As a dental office assistant, the value you add to the dental office by embracing the responsibilities and challenges that present themselves every day is an important resource to the dental office. The dental office needs a dental office administrator to create a smoothly run environment. As you grow professionally, your career as a dental office assistant will prove to be as exciting and steadfast as the advancements you'll encounter in the dental profession.

Chapter Summaries offer a brief review of the content covered in the chapter.

Review Questions

1. In addition to the qualities touched on in this chapter, discuss some personal qualities that you think a dental office administrator should possess and why they would be important in the dental office.
2. Describe some of your personal experiences as a patient in the dental office and think about what could have been done to make the experience different or better. If your experience was a positive one, what were the things that made it so? If your experience was negative, what could have been done differently to prevent it?
3. Review the list of dental specialists and think about which of them you would like to work for. Are there any specialists in the geographic area in which you live? If they have a Web site, can you get any more information on their office? Prepare a written response to these questions.

Multiple Choice

1. **Time management is**
   a. the utilization of processes that increase a person's time efficiency.
   b. a process that occurs naturally over time.
   c. the biggest challenge faced by administrators in dental offices today.
   d. an evolving method of scheduling proficiency.
2. **A common time waster in the dental office is**
   a. a patient who consistently arrives late.
   b. staff who discuss personal issues during lunch hour.
   c. lengthy important telephone calls to patients.
   d. reading personal e-mails during office hours.
3. **Which of the following does not contribute to professional appearance?**
   a. Long curly hair tied back
   b. Finger nails cut to a short, active length
   c. Shoes that are scuffed from overwear
   d. Clean, pressed uniform
4. **A main concern for the dental office administrator should be**
   a. building relationships with all employees.
   b. caring for patients and their welfare.
   c. being available for weekend work.
   d. ensuring that all employees receive their paychecks.
5. **Which of the following credentials applies to dentists?**
   a. RDH
   b. CDT
   c. DMD
   d. RDA
6. **The reception area of the dental office**
   a. should be updated regularly.
   b. is the main "hub" of the office.
   c. should accommodate the patient.
   d. is maintained by the office assistant.
7. **Procedures a dental assistant may perform**
   a. vary depending on the state in which the dental assistant works.
   b. are based on the requirements of the dentist and office needs.
   c. vary depending on the number of dental assistants in the office.
   d. are all the same, regardless of certification and training.
8. **The duties of an office manager include all of the following except**
   a. interviewing job applicants.
   b. performing dental procedures.
   c. maintaining accurate financial records.
   d. managing payroll.
9. **The purpose of dental professional associations is to**
   a. produce CE courses for ongoing learning.
   b. keep all members in contact with one another.
   c. provide support, recruitment, and retention for dental professionals.
   d. none of the above.
10. **Which of the following is not a responsibility of dental office administrators?**
    a. Greeting patients as they enter the office
    b. Ensuring correct treatment performed
    c. Scheduling appointments for patients
    d. Collecting payment on accounts

Web Sites

American Dental Association
http://www.ada.org/

American Dental Hygienists Association
http://www.adha.org/

American Dental Assistants Association
http://www.dentalassistant.org/

Chapter Review Questions are multiple-choice questions appearing at the end of the chapter that help the student review the chapter material.

76 PART I Introduction to the Profession

Review Questions

Multiple Choice

Select the best response for each question.

1. **The spread of disease through contact with contaminated surfaces such as instruments, countertops, and handles is referred to as**
   a. cross-contamination.
   b. parenteral.
   c. airborne transmission.
   d. infectious waste.
2. **A pathogen is**
   a. a disease caused by a biological agent such as a parasite or bacterium.
   b. waste capable of causing or transmitting an infectious disease.
   c. a virus or microorganism that causes disease.
   d. the contact with infectious material as a result of an employee's duties.
3. **Sharps are infectious materials to be disposed of in a**
   a. dental material garbage can.
   b. sharps container.
   c. sterilized waste container.
   d. regulated waste container.
4. **The transmission of infectious diseases from body fluids contaminated with blood is called**
   a. airborne transmission.
   b. bloodborne transmission.
   c. cross-contamination.
   d. occupational exposure.
5. **Biohazardous waste refers to waste such as**
   a. items contaminated with saliva only.
   b. items contaminated with blood only.
   c. items contaminated with blood and saliva.
   d. all items used in the dental office.
6. **The following are all examples of personal protective equipment, except**
   a. glasses.
   b. masks.
   c. shoes.
   d. lab coat.

Critical Thinking

1. One of the team members in the dental office continually brings patients' charts to the front desk while still wearing gloves worn during treatment and has on occasion used pens and left them on the desk when finished. Is there anything wrong with this, and, if so, how would you deal with it?
2. As a dental office administrator, you will spend most of your time in the administrative areas of the dental office, so why do you need to understand asepsis procedures and controls?
3. How do you think a malpractice lawsuit might occur as a result of improper infection control techniques?
4. Why do you think it would be beneficial to patients if you were to educate them regarding infection control procedures in the dental office?
5. How is learning about hazardous materials useful to your role as a dental office administrator?

Critical Thinking Questions help the student process and apply the chapter material through a number of thought-provoking questions.

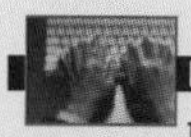

HANDS-ON ACTIVITY

1. Design a fax cover page for the office you are working in.
2. Write a letter to a new patient, thanking him or her for the referral to the practice. Use the semi-block format.
3. Prepare a letter for an insurance company of your choice, asking it to send payment for a claim that you are attaching. Prepare the letter for folding into an envelope by showing marks on the letter to indicate the folds, and address the proper size envelopes for mailing.

Hands-On Activities require the student to practice a common task, such as dental charting, writing a memo, or conducting a mock telephone call with another student.

ADDITIONAL RESOURCES

Additional resources for both instructors and students are available on the book's companion Web site at thePoint.lww.com/Girtel1e and on a disk at the back of this book. These resources include the following:

For faculty (on Web site)

- test generator
- image bank
- PowerPoint lecture slides

For students (on disk at the back of book and on Web site [note: DENTRIX G4 practice management software available on the CD only])

- Educational version of DENTRIX G4 practice management software (DENTRIX G4 software courtesy of Henry Schein Practice Solutions, American Fork, UT)
- DENTRIX G4 learning activities
- DENTRIX G4 practice management User's Guide
- DENTRIX G4 practice management Installation Guide
- Quiz bank

Acknowledgments

This book was born out of a passion to teach and assist in the evolution of the dental health profession. Many people have offered encouragement, support, and ideas throughout the development of this book and contributed to it by showing their commitment to and concern for its realization. We wish to thank, in particular, those who have made exceptional contributions.

First and foremost, we would like to thank David Payne, the managing editor of this project, who provided invaluable insight and patience when necessary for the development of this textbook. His expertise and dedication were a contributing force to the completion of this book. In addition, the staff at LWW who were involved in the book development provided the support and resources necessary to generate the textbook: John Goucher, Executive Acquisitions Editor, for his enthusiasm for the book and assistance with proposal development, and Eric Branger, Managing Editor, for his assistance in the development process.

Finally, we wish to acknowledge our immediate and extended family members who all played a role with their encouragement and love during challenging times that arose during the book writing process. We wish to thank Ryan Girtel for the patience and youthful enthusiasm he displayed as the book unfolded as well as Lili, our constant writing companion. We consider our family to include the staff members of the dental office who have grown with us as we developed this book and our dental practice and evolved along with the dental profession. Most notably, we would like to thank Mrs. Nicole Paranica, who has been an unwavering friend and who believed in us and the necessity of this textbook for the dental profession.

Geraldine Irlbacher-Girtel, BScN, RN, MEd
Guy S. Girtel, DDS

Reviewers

TAMARA J. ERICKSON, BA
Director of Dental Assisting
Herzing College, Lakeland Academy Division
Crystal, MN

MARI FROHN, AS, BS
Professor
Tri-County Regional Vocational Technical High School
Franklin, MA

KRISTYN HAWKINS, LDH, BGS
Clinical Instructor
Indiana University, South Bend
South Bend, IN

TONI HOFFA, BS
Instructor
Lakeland Academy Division of Herzing College
Crystal, MN

STELLA LOVATO, CDA, MSHP, MA
Chair of Allied Health
San Antonio College
San Antonio, TX

MARTHA MCCASLIN, BSBM
Dental Assisting Program Director
Dona Ana Branch Community College
Las Cruces, NM

RITA OHRDORF, MA
Instructor
University of Northern Colorado
Pueblo, CO

SUE RAFFEE, RDH, EFDA, MSA
Sinclair Community College
Dayton, OH

SHEILA SEMLER, Phd
Instructor
Lansing Community College
Lansing, MI

DIANA SULLIVAN, ME
Dental Department Chair
Dakota County Technical College
Rosemount, MN

JO SZABO, CDA, CDR, BED
Coordinator
Niagara College
Welland, ON

MARY CLARE SZABO, CDA, CDR
Professor
George Brown College
Toronto, Ontario, Canada

MARK THORESON, DDS
The Academy of Dental Assisting
Redmond, OR

Contents

part ONE

Introduction to *the Profession*

chapter ONE

Introduction to *Dental Office Administration*

OUTLINE

OBJECTIVES

After completing this chapter, you should be able to do the following:

- Spell and define key terms
- Describe the various functions and responsibilities of the dental office administrator
- List personal characteristics of the dental office administrator
- Describe the layout of a dental office
- Discuss the concept of professionalism as it relates to the dental office administrator
- Explain the importance of the administrator's position in the dental office
- Identify team members in the dental office and their role in the office
- Discuss the specialties in dentistry and the differences among them

KEY TERMS

- dental office administrator
- professional
- professionalism
- team member
- confidential
- consultation area
- dental operatories
- sterilization area
- laboratory
- dentist
- dentistry
- DDS
- DMD
- dental specialty
- dental specialist
- RDH
- certified dental assistant
- registered dental assistant
- dental office manager
- CDT
- professional association

Today's dental offices are different from dental offices of the past, where little emphasis was placed on the office environment and where the sterile office smell and silence were commonplace. The creation of a comfortable atmosphere and removing the anxiety caused by experiences have become important in the dental industry. Sophisticated machines and technology make many of the dental procedures performed less painful and more pleasant than in the past.

Dental offices have also grown in size and complexity. No longer just one- or two-dentist operations, many large group practices are available. Some dental offices now have the capability to maintain a patient's record without the use of paper. With technology in the dental industry constantly evolving, so too must the dental office employees who contribute to its success. Every employee must be computer literate and have an understanding of the dental insurance plans available for patients. The dental office employee who is trained in his or her area of expertise through a formal education will better keep up with the changes and regulations related to the dental profession.

The goal of this book, therefore, is to prepare dental office administrators in order to successfully work in the modern dental office. This chapter first introduces the role of the dental office administrator, presenting responsibilities and personal qualities required for success in this position. Next, the layout of the dental office is presented. Finally, the chapter ends with an introduction to the various roles that make up the complete dental team.

WHAT IS A DENTAL OFFICE ADMINISTRATOR?

Also known as the dental receptionist, the dental business assistant, or the dental administrator, the **dental office administrator** is the individual who manages the daily flow of the dental office through control and maintenance of the front office and administrative functions in the dental office. The dental office administrator is a member of the dental team who performs administrative procedures in the dental office.

The dental office administrator holds one of the most important positions in the dental office. Below are described in detail the duties, responsibilities, and expectations of this position. As the book progresses, you will begin to realize the comprehensiveness of this very important position.

Functions and Responsibilities

The precise functions and responsibilities of a dental office administrator can vary widely, depending on several factors, such as practice setting. Dental office administrators are employed in general dentist practices, specialty practices, dental hospital environments, and dental claims departments of insurance companies. Each office or dental environment will have various versions of the job description shown in Figure 1-1 to fit its office philosophy and image.

Likewise, the rate of pay, number of hours worked, and benefits provided also vary. For example, work experience, size of the practice, and the state in which the practice is located all contribute to the differences found among dental administrator positions. However, the primary responsibilities of the dental office administrator include carrying out tasks that are directly related to business functions in the dental office. The duties of the administrator can vary in their complexity from greeting patients to bookkeeping responsibilities. Following is a list of some of the duties dental administrators perform in their work environment:

- Maintaining the reception area
- Answering incoming telephone calls
- Greeting patients
- Ensuring patient chart completeness
- Scheduling appointments
- Collecting payment

Position overview

The dental office administrator will maintain the everyday activities in the business area of the dental office. This person will be responsible for maintaining patient records, accounts receivable, accounts payable, and other duties that provide support to the dental team. These duties include the following:

Specific duties

Appointment scheduling and confirmation
- Schedules and confirms patients for their dental and hygiene appointments

Patient reception
- Answers the telephone
- Greets patients as they arrive
- Discusses financial and treatment options with the patient
- Organizes incoming and outgoing mails
- Maintains positive front office appearance

Patient records management
- Maintains correct and up-to-date patient charts
- Oversees re-care/recall system and patient care quality control
- Maintains patient referral programs

Business records management
- Maintains accurate accounts receivable and accounts payable records
- Maintains company financial records
- Performs daily, weekly, and monthly billing procedures

Clinic support
- Inventory control
- Internal and External Marketing
- Patient education

Qualifications
- Certificate or Diploma from a recognized Dental Administration program
- Excellent keyboarding skills – 35 words per minute
- Familiarity with Microsoft Word and other computer programs
- Ability to relate positively with the public
- Being a team player
- Professional appearance

FIGURE 1-1 Job description of a dental office administrator.

- Filing insurance claim forms
- Maintaining company financial records
- Processing payroll
- Sorting mails
- Arranging patient referrals
- Managing office assistants
- Educating patients in dental treatment follow-through
- Managing accounts receivable
- Coordinating dentist and hygiene schedules
- Cultivating patient relationships

Often the dental office administrator is responsible for the management duties in the dental practice. This is usually the case in smaller dental offices. As offices grow to accommodate increasing numbers of patients and employees, job duties generally become more specific as new positions are created to adapt to the demands of the practice. In a large practice, for example, the office manager would maintain control of the bookkeeping duties, the dental administrator would focus on reception duties, and the general clerk, or office assistant, would assist the dental office administrator with various tasks.

To summarize, the dental office administrator can be responsible for tasks that range from patient relations to staff relations, as well as records management and correspondence maintenance. The focus for the dental office administrator, however, will always be on business activities in the dental office.

checkPOINT

1. Name and explain five duties of a dental office administrator.

Characteristics of a Successful Dental Office Administrator

Making the decision to enter the dental profession means that you have decided to enter one of the most challenging and exciting professions. Becoming a dental administrator means becoming a **professional** in the dental industry.

How you dress, talk, act, and work determines whether you are a professional. In the dental profession, there is great emphasis on the importance of **professionalism.** Your overall attitude toward yourself and the work that you do represents your level of professionalism. When you demonstrate professionalism, you treat patients and colleagues with respect at all times and show pride in the work that you do by arriving promptly every day and by doing your absolute best work every day. Your coworkers and the patients will show their appreciation for this professional attitude, and you will become a valued member of the dental team. Your role as a dental administrator is key in the development and maintenance of the image of the dental office you work in.

Professional Appearance

To begin with, a neat and well-groomed appearance is essential in the dental industry. The clothes you wear should be clean and pressed. Keep a sweater or spare shirt in your car or office should you soil the one you are wearing at lunch, to ensure a neat appearance at all times. Your footwear should be free of scuffs and dirt. Your hair should be neat and clean and kept off your face. Makeup should be simple, jewelry should be kept to a minimum, and your fingernails should be kept clean. In the dental environment, consideration must be given to patients and employees who may have allergies to strong scents. Perfume and strong scented hand creams should not be used in the dental office to avoid allergic reactions by patients and other employees.

Professional Attitude

Besides your appearance, your attitude is also important in developing the image of the dental practice. As you meet patients and develop friendships with colleagues and other dental professionals, your circle of associates in the dental industry will widen. It is important to remember that your professional attitude should not remain at work. You may encounter patients and dental colleagues outside of work. As you shop at the grocery store, walk your dog around the neighborhood, or go out for an evening on the town, there is always a chance you may see or will be seen by a patient or colleague. Maintaining a positive and professional attitude at all times while in public places is important.

Promptness and Effective Time Management

Time is of the essence in the dental office. For this reason, the nature of the dental administrator position requires an individual who is dependable and arrives on time

Tip FROM THE DENTIST

One of the most distressing things that I see when I am leading my team to provide a caring, safe, and stressfree environment for our patients is when members of the team don't understand or appreciate their role in maintaining the flow in the dental office. For instance, if the dental office administrator fails to be ready and able to work at the opening of the office, someone must take the place of that individual to answer the phone and greet patients as they arrive. If the person filling in is the dental assistant, then he or she is no longer available to help the dentist or attend to patients' needs in the operatory. The responsibility of every employee in the dental office is not to the dentist or patient alone but to every member of the dental team.

Each member of the team must understand and appreciate the role of all team members and how each person is integral in maintaining an efficiently run office. Just as important, team members must be aware of how their actions affect the team.

Team members may appear disorganized and incompetent when they are trying to fill in where they don't feel comfortable; this creates a pressure-filled environment that patients can sense.

for work. Often, the dental administrator is the first to arrive at the dental office in order to open the office for the day before the first patient arrives. Tardiness and regular absences are not acceptable. Lateness is costly to everyone who is affected by it, namely, the person who is late, the other members of the dental team, and the patient. Unexcused time off means another team member must vacate his or her position to fill in for you.

Time management is the utilization of processes and tools that increase a person's or business' time efficiency. The basis of good personal and professional habits is effective time management. In your role as a dental office administrator, you are expected to successfully accomplish many tasks throughout the course of the day that demand an effective time management plan. To do this, you must be able to prioritize tasks by determining which tasks must be completed first, which tasks require the greatest amount of time, and which tasks require a particular environment such as a quiet area. Developing effective time management skills evolves as your efficiency on the job increases.

Time management is a skill that few people master and one that many people need. There are many ways to determine whether you are managing your time efficiently. One of these ways is to analyze your personal work habits. Analyzing the time you spend on certain activities over a specific period of time, usually 1–2 weeks, will identify areas where too much time or not enough time is spent completing tasks. Analyzing areas where time is wasted or used efficiently helps identify which tools are most useful in developing efficiency. Common time wasters in an office environment include the following:

- **Telephone calls.** Calls in the dental office should be kept on topic and dealt with quickly. Using the telephone to catch up on gossip or to chit-chat is an ineffective use of time. The phone should be used for business purposes with personal calls kept to a minimum and completed out of view of patients. Personal calls should be limited to emergency and urgent calls during office hours.
- **E-mail and Internet use.** Some patients will contact the dental office through e-mail, as will dental supply companies. Office memos may be sent to all employees using e-mail as a source of contact. Create separate e-mail addresses for work and personal use. Use your personal time outside of office hours for reading and replying to personal e-mails. Avoid using the Internet for personal use during office hours.
- **Conversations with coworkers.** Keep conversations with coworkers professional by reserving personal conversations for the lunch room. Having a lengthy personal conversation is not an effective use of time in a work environment.

The quickest way to develop effective time management is to develop a schedule for yourself that lists all the tasks to be accomplished within 1 day and a specific amount of time in which they are to be accomplished. It is important to set reasonable limits on the amount of time for each task in order to avoid frustration. Box 1-1 outlines tips on time management that are useful in your role as a dental office administrator.

BOX 1-1
Tips for Developing Effective Time Management

- Use an appointment schedule book that provides a 1-week view of the tasks to be completed each day. Record everything you need to accomplish and check them off as they are completed.
- Prioritize your tasks into your schedule on the basis of their urgency. For example, a bill that must be paid by a certain date to avoid interest charges would have to be completed by a certain date. Reorganizing the inventory cupboard would not be given the same priority.
- If you find that you are not getting all of the tasks you schedule for yourself completed in the day allotted, try allowing yourself more time to complete fewer tasks or analyze which tasks you can delegate to others.
- Accepting tasks that have been assigned to you or that you have agreed to take on may cause you to feel overwhelmed if you are unable to accomplish all of them in the time requested. Being honest with coworkers and informing them that you do not have the time to complete the task will be appreciated more than not completing it.
- Set goals for yourself. If your goal is to collect a certain amount of patient receivables, meeting that goal will let you know that you have succeeded. Not meeting the goal tells you that you need to set new goals.
- Procrastinating regarding a particular task could tell you a lot about yourself and your time management. If you find you are procrastinating, ask yourself how the task makes you feel. Does you feel a sense of dread or boredom, or are you overwhelmed? Identify the reason to overcome your procrastination.
- Perform an occasional analysis of your time management effectiveness. This will help you identify not only what you are spending your time on but what areas require changes.

Other Characteristics

In addition to being a professional, the dental administrator must also possess qualities of an individual who is sensitive to patients' needs and is sincere in his or her communications with them. Building rapport and trust with the patients is a large part of what the dental administrator is responsible for.

Other personal characteristics fundamental for success in the dental industry are as follows:

- **Effectiveness in oral and written communication with dental professionals and patients**
- **The ability to act calmly and precisely in stressful and emergency situations**
- **Attention to detail,** with both the information recorded in the patient chart and the services billed to patients and their insurance company. Inaccuracy can create a lack of trust between yourself and the patient.
- **Honesty at all times with patients and coworkers.** Being dishonest is not acceptable in a dental office. Placing blame on others or covering up errors should never be done.
- **Respect for patient confidentiality.** Divulging patient information can leave you without a job and permanently damage your career.
- **Commitment to a common goal.** As a member of the dental team, you must work toward achieving the common goal: high-quality, optimal dental health for the patient.
- **High moral and ethical standards.** Having high standards will ensure you gain trust from those around you and the confidence you need to be successful in the profession.
- **Care for patients.** Caring for patients and their welfare while in the dental office should be a main concern of the dental office administrator. Showing empathy to the patient is important for cultivating relationships.
- **Positive attitude.** Your confidence and attitude about yourself and your abilities will be obvious to those you communicate with everyday. Always have a positive attitude.

- **Courtesy, respect, and manners with coworkers and patients.** Treat everyone with respect.
- **Personal responsibility.** Take responsibility for your duties and position in the dental office; never assume someone else will "do it for you" or make excuses as to why it is not done.

As evident by this list, the characteristics and skills required for the position are diverse. Your knowledge of the dental environment and effective management of the flow of patients on a daily basis greatly contribute to the success of the dental team. Moreover, the dynamic nature of the dental profession—with each day bringing exciting new challenges—helps sharpen your skills as you develop your career in the industry.

> **checkPOINT**
>
> 2. Describe five personal characteristics of the dental office administrator.
> 3. Why is it important for the dental office administrator to think and act calmly in emergency situations?

Teamwork

Being a member of a dental office means living the belief that "there is no 'I' in team." In order for the practice to be successful, everyone must work together to achieve success. If you think of a rowing team and visualize how hard every member on the boat works in unison to reach the finish line with determination and precision, you have a good idea of how a successful dental office operates. Each member of the dental team must be on board with the goals of the practice and dedicate himself or herself to achieve those goals. If one person chooses not to row the boat, the momentum changes and the team will have trouble reaching its goals. A dental office administrator who can adapt to many personalities and work as a **team member** by assisting his or her colleagues when required is a team player and a valuable resource to the dental office. A more in-depth discussion on teamwork is available in Chapter 11.

Confidentiality

As a member of the healthcare profession, the dental office administrator has the responsibility to keep **confidential** all patient information in the dental office. Discussing patients outside of the dental office is a breach of confidentiality and could have legal implications. What happens in the dental office must remain confidential. Chapter 2 addresses the importance of confidentiality and the prominent role that patient privacy plays in the job function of the dental office administrator.

Importance of the Position

One of the most important positions to hold in the dental office is that of a dental office administrator. This is the person who is at the head of the ship, steering it to success through sometimes-murky waters. This is a position of great responsibility. As a member of the dental team, the dental administrator's main duty is to cultivate and maintain the patient relationship. Without patients, there is no work to do. The dental office administrator is the first and last contact the patient has with the dental office. Whether the patient telephones the office or decides to come in and schedule an appointment, the impression that the dental office administrator makes on the patient is one that can make or break the relationship. A pleasant, positive attitude toward patients as they enter and leave the dental clinic adds to the positive dental experience and can contribute to relationships that last many years.

If you look again at Figure 1-1 and review the duties and responsibilities of the dental office administrator, you may begin to see that the many and varied tasks outlined can create a very busy day in the dental office! As you read through this text, you will begin to see why this is such an important position as the many aspects that make up this position come together to form a whole.

> **checkPOINT**
>
> 4. Why is the dental office administrator an important position in the dental office?

Education and Certification

Given the importance of the position, formal education and certification are needed to properly prepare dental office administrators. The most common educational routes for dental office administrators are dental assisting programs offered at community colleges and technical schools and through online programs. The duration of most programs is 4 months up to 1 year. Upon completion of the program, a diploma or certificate is awarded to the student. Dental office administration programs generally focus on the management of the office workflow in a dental practice with some focus on the clinical aspects. Dental assisting programs not only focus on the administrative functions in the dental office but also spend a great deal of time expanding on the clinical skills of the certified dental assistant (CDA). The certification process and pathways for certification for the dental assistant and dental office administrator are discussed in the following section.

Certification of the Dental Assistant

Becoming a CDA assures the public that the dental assistant is committed to excellence and prepared to assist competently in delivering oral health care. Possessing the credentials of the state and national authorities demonstrates professional growth of the dental assistant and the commitment to the profession, which further enhances the professional image of the dental team. Currently there are two classifications of examinations that the dental assistant may be eligible to write in order to obtain the required credentials. There is a state examination, which is regulated by the state board of dentistry or the Dental Assisting National Board (DANB) examination.

Dental assistants become certified by passing a state or national examination that evaluates their knowledge of dental assisting. The dental assistant certification examination itself is approximately 4 hours long and consists of 320 test questions. The national test is broken down into three parts: (1) general chairside, (2) radiation health and safety, and (3) infection control. Most dental assistants who choose to become nationally certified take the CDA examination offered by the DANB.

Academic dental assisting programs can take from 9 months to 2 years to complete and are offered at community colleges and technical institutes on a full- or part-time basis, with some schools offering distance and online courses. A graduate of a dental assisting program usually receives a certificate.

National Credentials

National certification of dental assistants is mandated by the DANB. Obtaining a passing grade on the DANB examination allows the dental assistant to use the credential CDA. There are three pathways a dental assistant can consider in preparation for the DANB examination for certification. Dental assistants are eligible to take the CDA examination offered by the DANB if they have completed a dental assisting program accredited by the Commission on Dental Accreditation. Potential candidates who have been trained on the job or have graduated from non-accredited programs are eligible to take the national certification examination if they have completed 2 years of full-time work experience as dental assistants. In addition, those candidates who have held a previous certification with the DANB and certification has lapsed more than 18 months, can reactivate their certification through the examination process.

Dental assistants who wish to achieve national credentials in other areas of dental assisting can also write specialty examinations offered through the DANB, such as dental practice management, oral and maxillofacial surgery, and orthodontics.

State Credentials

Some states may grant a license, registration, or certificate for dental assistants in the state. The educational and examination requirements are different among states and should be investigated by the dental assistant to ensure that the credential

TABLE 1-1 Dental Assistant Certification Through the Dental Assisting National Board Examination

Pathway I	Pathway II	Pathway III
Graduate of a dental assisting or dental hygiene program accredited by the American Dental Association Current CPR certification earned within 2 years prior to examination date	High school graduate (or equivalent) Two years of full-time employment (or 3500 hours over 2 years) as a dental assistant verified by dentist-employer Current CPR certification earned within 2 years prior to examination date	Meet one of the following three requirements: Current or former DANB certified dental assistant Graduate of an accredited dental school (DDS/DMD) Graduate of a foreign dental degree program Current CPR certification earned within 2 years prior to examination date

CPR, cardiopulmonary resuscitation; DANB, Dental Assisting National Board; DDS, doctor of dental surgery; DMD, doctor of dental medicine.

process is followed. Some states also recognize passage of components of the CDA examination, such as the Radiation Health and Safety examination, or the Infection Control examination, for licensing and regulatory purposes. State regulations vary among states, and some states offer registration or licensure in addition to the national certification program.

There are many benefits of certification. The dental assistant, the employer, and the patient all derive benefits from a certification held by the dental assistant. The dental assistant derives benefit by enhancing career mobility, which means that the certification recognized by many states provides opportunities for employment throughout the country. A dental assistant's credentials are a representation of the expertise in the area of dental assisting to potential employers and a source of personal accomplishment and pride for the dental assistant. Dental assistants who are nationally certified are recognized as having a commitment to competence and professionalism that is an asset recognized by many dental office employers. In addition, the patient can be assured that the knowledge and skills held by the dental assistant enable competency of practice in the provision of dental care. The patient can further be assured that the delivery of care by the dental assistant is achieved by focusing on the goal of delivering safe care to all patients.

Certification of the Dental Office Administrator

Dental office managers and administrators can become certified by the DANB for many reasons. The DANB is the only national certification agency for dental assistants recognized by the American Dental Association (ADA) and it maintains the responsibility of promoting standards of professionalism and competency through testing and certification. Upon successful completion of an accredited dental administration program, students will be prepared to take the Dental Practice management component or the National Dental Assisting Certification examination administered by the DANB.

Dental office personnel who earn the national DANB Certified Dental Practice Management Administrator (CDPMA) credential demonstrate their motivation to show the public and their employers that they are assets to the entire professional team.

Certification is a recognition of the professional skills you bring to the dental team. The DANB CDPMA is a national credential that is available for dental office professionals who take pride in their participation in the delivery of oral health care through office and clinical procedures. The DANB CDPMA examination is

TABLE 1-2 Certified Dental Practice Management Administrator Level 1: Certification Through the Dental Assisting National Board Examination

Pathway I	Pathway II	Pathway III
Status as a current DANB CDA, COA, or COMSA	Status as a current DANB CDA, COA, or COMSA	Status as a current or previous DANB CDPMA *or* graduation from an accredited DDS/DMD program
Work experience in a dental practice setting verified by dentist-employer	Completion of a practice management course from an accredited program *or* employment as an educator-director of an accredited dental program	Current CPR certification earned within 2 years prior to examination date
Current CPR certification earned within 2 years prior to examination date	Current CPR certification earned within 2 years prior to examination date	

CDA, certified dental assistant; CDPMA, certified dental practice management administrator; COA, certified orthodontic assistant; COMSA, certified oral and maxillofacial surgery assistant; CPR, cardiopulmonary resuscitation; DANB, Dental Assisting National Board; DDS, doctor of dental surgery; DMD, doctor of dental medicine.

developed and administered by the DANB. There are two versions of the CDPMA examination. The CDPMA-1 examination is a 100-question examination completed in 1 hour and 15 minutes and is available for individuals who are current DANB certified assistants (CDA, certified orthodontic assistants, and certified oral and maxillofacial surgery assistants) or former CDPMAs. The CDPMA-2 examination is a 150-question examination completed in 2 hours and is available for non-DANB certified assistants and office personnel. The multiple-choice examination is given in a computerized format at national computerized test centers, or it is offered three times a year as a written examination at selected locations. Table 1-2 and Box 1-2 outline the pathways for achieving the CDPMA-1 and CDPMA-2 certification.

To continue to use and maintain the CDPMA certification once it is earned, DANB Recertification Requirements must be met. These requirements include attending at least 12 hours of DANB-accepted continuing dental education courses, maintaining a current certification in cardiopulmonary resuscitation, and paying an annual renewal fee. Access to continuing education (CE) courses to maintain certification as a CDPMA can be gained through professional associations for dental assistants and dental office personnel. Box 1-3 lists some of these resources.

Whether a DANB-certified assistant is looking to expand recognition of his or her current skills and competencies or a non–DANB-certified assistant or office administrator is looking for professional recognition, CDPMA certification is both a personal and professional achievement. DANB-certified assistants and office personnel

BOX 1-2
Certified Dental Practice Management Administrator Level 2: Certification Through the Dental Assisting National Board Examination

High school graduation or equivalent
AND
Minimum 1 year and maximum 2 years of full-time or part-time work experience of 1750 hours as a dental assistant/office personnel verified by dentist/employer

Current cardiopulmonary resuscitation certification earned within 2 years prior to examination date

BOX 1-3
Resources for Accreditation and Certification

The following agencies are helpful resources for finding accreditation and certification information:

American Dental Assistants Association (ADAA)

The ADAA is a national professional organization for dental assistants.
203 North LaSalle Street, Suite 1320
Chicago, IL 60601-1225
Tel: (312) 541-1550
Fax: (312) 541-1496

Dental Assisting National Board, Inc. (DANB)

The DANB is a nationally recognized premier certification and credentialing agency for dental assistants.
444 N. Michigan Avenue, Suite 900
Chicago, IL 60611-3985
Tel: (312) 642-3368
Fax: (312) 642-1475
Toll-free number: 1-800-FOR-DANB

Commission on Dental Accreditation

The Commission on Dental Accreditation is the accrediting body under the American Dental Association that establishes accreditation standards by which to evaluate dental programs.
203 North LaSalle Street, Suite 1320
Chicago, IL 60601-1225
Tel: (312) 541-1550
Fax: (312) 541-1496

American Association of Dental Office Managers (AADOM)

The AADOM is a professional association for dental administrative personnel.
125 Half Mile Road, Suite 200
Red Bank, NJ 07701
Tel: (732) 842-9977
Fax: (732) 842-0085
www.dentalmanagers.com

are viewed by employers and peers as committed to excellence in oral health care and service. As a dental administrator, you are accountable not only to the dentist and your team but also to the patients being treated in the office. A determined professional who is committed to upholding high practice standards is a valuable asset in any dental office.

DENTAL OFFICE LAYOUT

Once the patient enters the dental office, his or her impression of the office and the dental team is already forming. The dental reception and business areas are usually the first areas of the dental office that patients see. If this area is kept neat and tidy and has a welcoming feel to it, the patient will likely have a positive initial impression of the office. Patients often relate the appearance of the business area to the quality of dental care they will be receiving. Organization, cleanliness, and professionalism in all areas of the dental office are necessary for a positive patient impression. Figure 1-2 shows a sample dental office layout.

Reception and Business Areas

The reception area of the dental office should accommodate the patient (Fig. 1-3). It must be clean and free of debris, with the furniture arranged to allow for free space to walk and children to enter easily. A coat rack should be available as well as an area where patients may remove soiled shoes or boots if necessary. It is important that restrooms are easily accessible for the patient, even if there is not one available in the dental office, but in a public area close by. The dental office should also be accessible to physically challenged people. The Americans with Disabilities

CANADIAN PRACTICE: EDUCATION AND CERTIFICATION

Dental Assisting Certification

Dental assistants in Canada are recognized as CDA in some provinces and as registered dental assistants (RDA) in others. The registration varies among provinces. There are two categories of dental assistants recognized for practice as dental assistants in Canada: (1) Dental Assistant, Level I; and (2) Dental Assistant, Level II. A Level I dental assistant is an individual who has passed an examination approved by the provincial regulatory body and may provide basic supportive dental services. A Level II dental assistant is an RDA who has graduated from an approved dental assisting program and passed the examinations required by the provincial regulatory body and may provide, in addition to the services of an RDA level I, under the supervision of a dentist who is present on the premises, intraoral dental services.

Dental assistant certificate or diploma programs in Canada consist of chairside and intraoral training; alternatively, an individual employed in a dental office may enroll in a chairside assisting correspondence course followed by an intraoral program in a college. Training programs may vary and are usually the equivalent of 10–12 months in duration. The training institution must be recognized by the governing provincial association. Training programs should also be accredited by the Commission on Dental Accreditation of Canada.

In addition to regular course examinations given as part of the required academic program, the applicant must satisfactorily complete the National Dental Assisting Examining Board (NDAEB). This examination is taken, once all educational requirements have been met, and is required for licensure as a dental assistant in most Canadian provinces. Professional development is ongoing and necessary for relicensure.

Applicants who have not graduated from a CDAC-accredited educational program but request to write the NDAEB examination on the basis of extensive working knowledge of the practice of dental assisting must also satisfactorily complete a clinical practice evaluation.

Level II dental assisting is considered to be a restricted healthcare occupation. In the provinces of Alberta and Saskatchewan, the profession of dental assisting is self-regulated. In the provinces of British Columbia, Manitoba, New Brunswick, Nova Scotia, Prince Edward Island, and Newfoundland, Level II Dental Assisting licensure is maintained under either the provincial Health Professions Act or Dental Act. In Ontario, certification is required in order for members to hold the title CDA or CDA II. The scope of practice for dental assistants varies among provinces based on the level of certification attained by the dental assistant. Dental assistants can take courses offered by educational institutions to expand their scope of duties.

The NDAEB

The NDAEB is not a regulatory body. Each provincial association regulates the certification and licensure of its members. Some provincial dental assisting regulatory authorities may require all members to obtain the NDAEB certificate in order to become licensed as a dental assistant. All candidates applying to write the NDAEB must be aware of the regulatory requirements in their province before submitting their applications. The registration and licensure requirements, as well as scope of practice, vary between provinces, therefore contacting the provincial professional body regarding regulatory issues in the province of registration or practice is encouraged.

The purpose of the NDAEB is to ensure that individuals entering the practice of dental assisting have met a national standard regarding the knowledge and skills necessary to practice as dental assistants. The NDAEB provides assistance for the provincial professional association in the licensure or registration of individuals in the province. A dental assistant with the NDAEB certificate can find employment opportunities within provinces, which aids in labor mobility for the dental assisting profession in Canada.

Dental Administrator Certification

Dental administration educational programs in Canada are similar to those offered in the United States. Educational institutions such as community colleges and technical schools, as well as online programs, are available. Upon successful completion of the program, a certificate is awarded. The duration of the programs is from 4 months to 1 year. The focus is on the administrative duties in the role of the dental office administrator with some recognition given to clinical areas. The dental administration programs are separate and distinct from dental assisting programs. Some institutional programs offer a pathway toward becoming a Level I dental assistant in Canada through distance education routes. These distance programs often focus on the theoretical aspects of clinical practice of the dental assistant and require little clinical practice to be performed at an educational facility. To become a Level II dental assistant would require a greater amount of clinical practice at the educational facility.

Dental administrators in Canada are eligible to obtain associate membership through their local provincial dental assistants association or a local city dental assistant association. However, the same pathway available to office personnel in the United States for obtaining the DANB CDPMA certification is available for Canadian personnel. Although DANB CDPMA certification is not officially recognized in Canada, dental office personnel are provided with an opportunity and the resources to continue learning and educating themselves of the advancements of the dental industry through their professional associations.

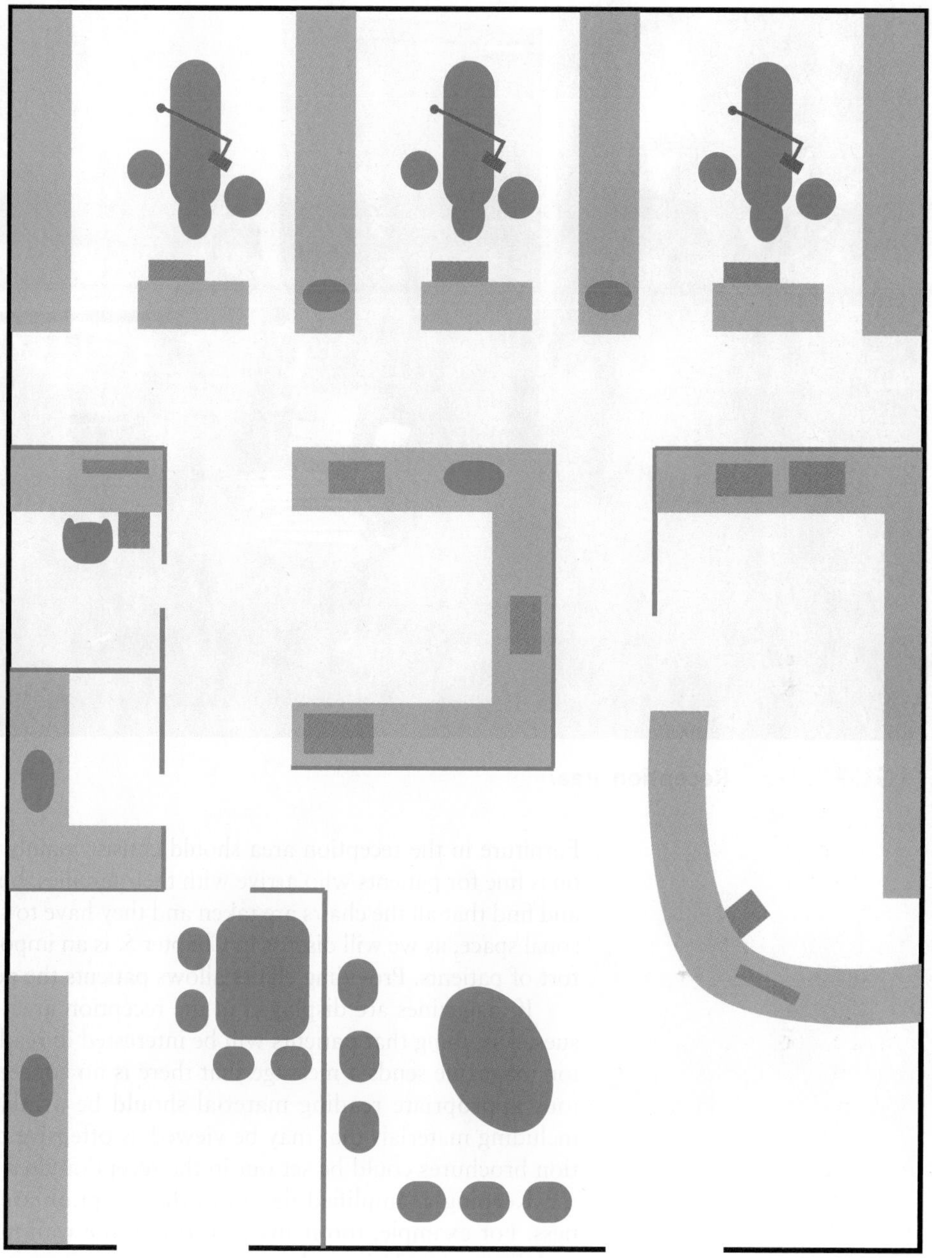

FIGURE 1-2 Dental office layout.

Act, outlined in Chapter 2, requires that all public buildings be accessible to persons with disabilities. Some of the ways the dental office can ensure compliance with the Americans with Disabilities Act are to provide entrance ramps, widen doorways and restroom facilities to ensure wheelchair access, provide Braille signs, and subscribe to specialized telephone services that allow for communication with hearing-impaired patients.

The temperature of the reception area should be kept at a level that is ideal for patient comfort. This is usually 72°F. Keeping the reception area at a cool temperature creates an uncomfortable environment for patients. This is particularly so for those who are waiting for family members receiving treatment and small children and the elderly, who may not tolerate cool temperatures easily.

The reception areas should be well-lit. Lighting should enhance the décor of the office and complement the comfortable surroundings. Decorative lighting is usually used in this area in combination with a softer light.

In addition to lighting and temperature, the use of calming, relaxing colors on the walls, and the furniture adds to the low-stress feel that a reception area should have.

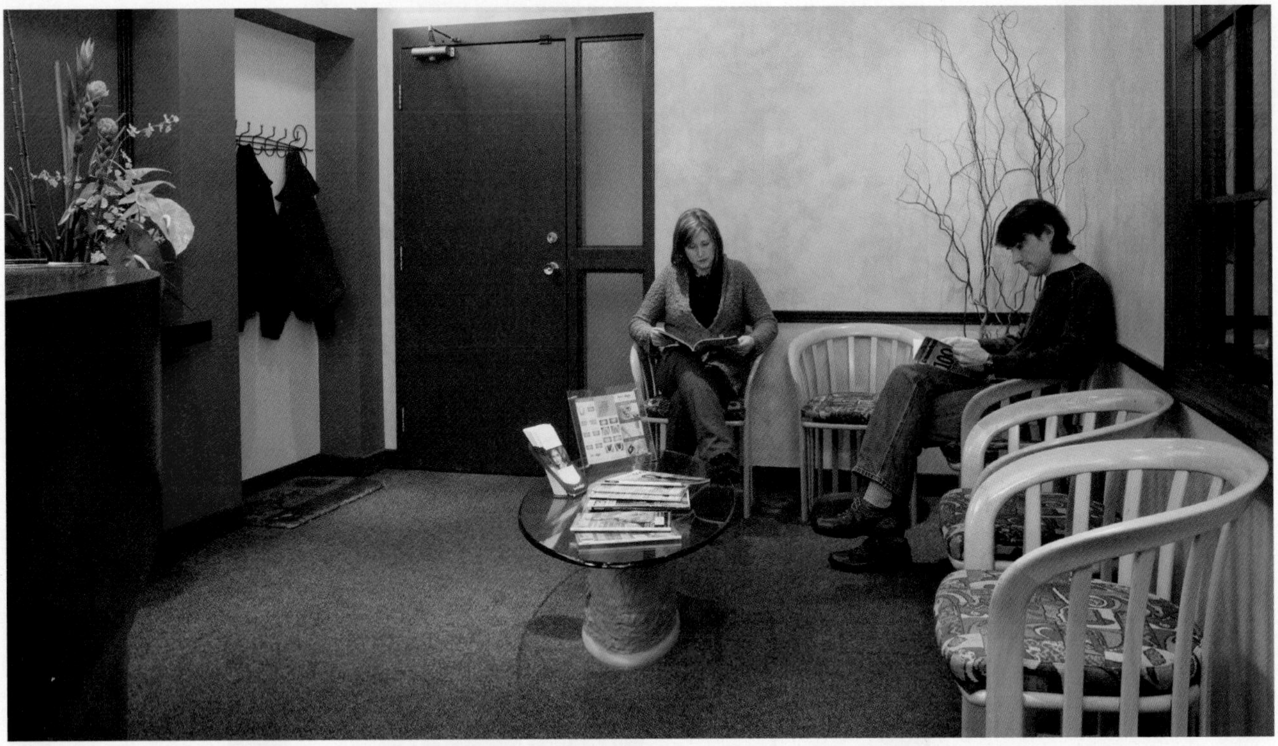

FIGURE 1-3 Reception area.

Furniture in the reception area should consist mainly of chairs. Providing sofas to sit on is fine for patients who arrive with their families, but not for those who arrive alone and find that all the chairs are taken and they have to share a sofa with a stranger! Personal space, as we will discuss in Chapter 5, is an important consideration for the comfort of patients. Providing chairs allows patients the personal space they require.

If magazines are displayed in the reception area, they should include current issues. Assuming that patients will be interested in reading a 5-year-old copy of a fashion magazine sends a message that there is no concern for upkeep in the office. Various appropriate reading material should be available for patients. Refrain from including materials that may be viewed as offensive to some patients. Patient education brochures could be set out in the reception area as additional reading material.

Keeping a simplified design to the reception area helps create a sense of calmness. For example, too many pictures on the wall may make the area seem "busy" and distracting. Using colors such as bright yellow and primary red may increase the anxiety of an already-anxious patient. Above all, consider the clientele that attend the office. If most of the patients in the clinic are families with young children, create an environment appropriate for them. For example, having children's reading material and coloring books available or a separate play area for children would assist parents in keeping their children occupied while waiting. If the clinic is located in an office tower in the business sector of the city and has a large portion of businesspeople as patients, providing amenities such as wireless Internet or a private area where business calls can be made may help create a desirable environment. As a dental office administrator, you should try to identify and provide amenities that patients may require to make their visit an enjoyable one.

checkPOINT

5. Describe three components of the dental reception area that create a welcoming environment for patients.

Front Desk

As a dental office administrator, making an impression on the patient on behalf of the dental team begins with you. If the desk that you spend your day at is messy, the patient may assume that the rest of the clinic is the same way (Figs. 1-4 and 1-5).

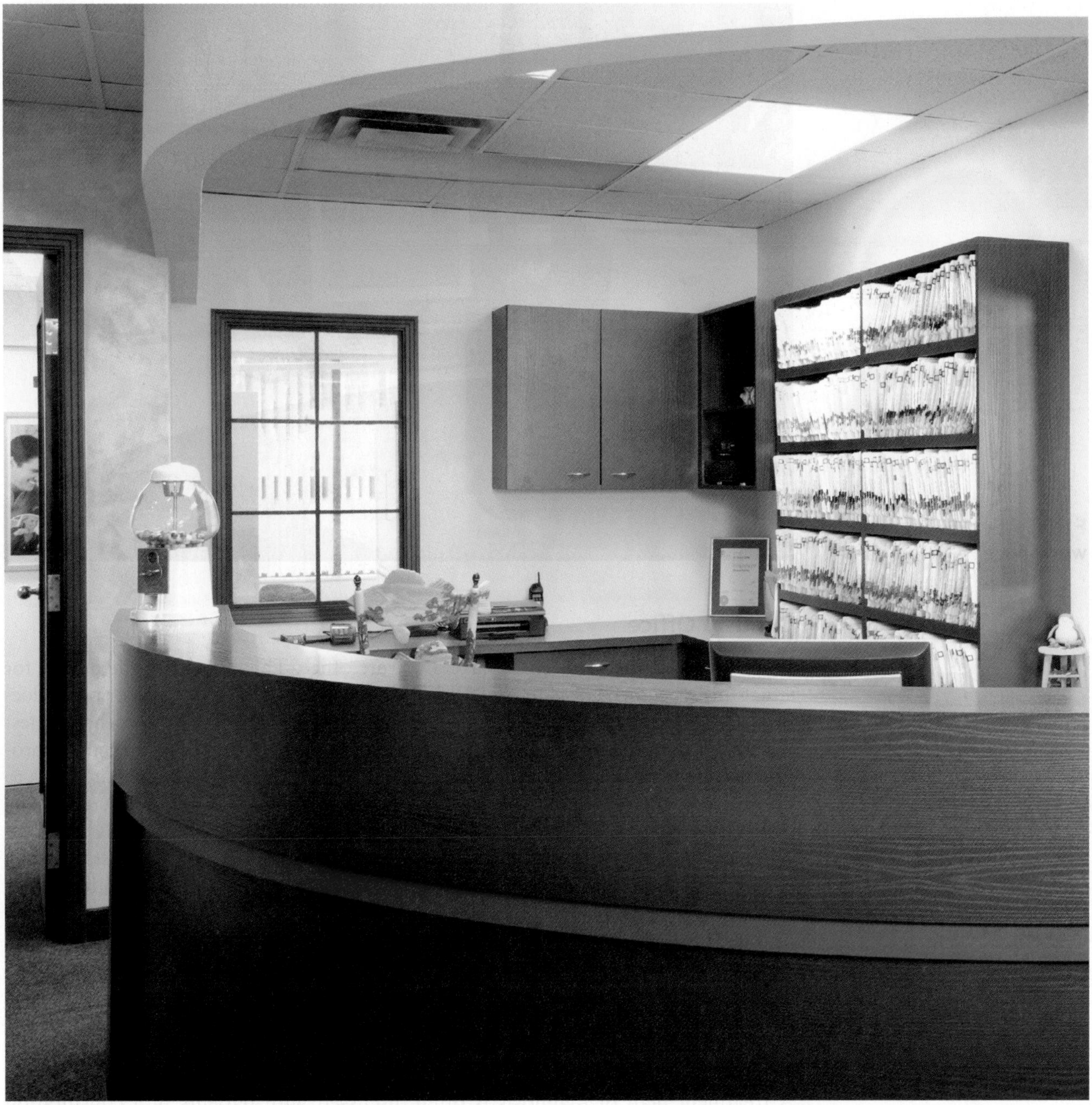

FIGURE 1-4 Front desk.

Furthermore, the patient may be concerned that your disorganization may extend to your management of their services, records, or account. A good rule of thumb in keeping an organized desk is to deal with each item once. Create a single pile of items that require your attention, such as patient charts. Because of the confidentiality of patient records, leaving a chart open on the front desk could create problems for the dental office if it is viewed by other patients. If the phone rings while you are working on a patient chart, close the chart and place it back on top of the "to do" pile. Resume where you left off once you have the opportunity to return to it. Maintaining a neat and orderly front desk gives the impression that the dental office administrator is well organized and capable of providing efficient service to begin or round out the dental appointment. This leaves the patient feeling confident in the quality of dentistry received at the office.

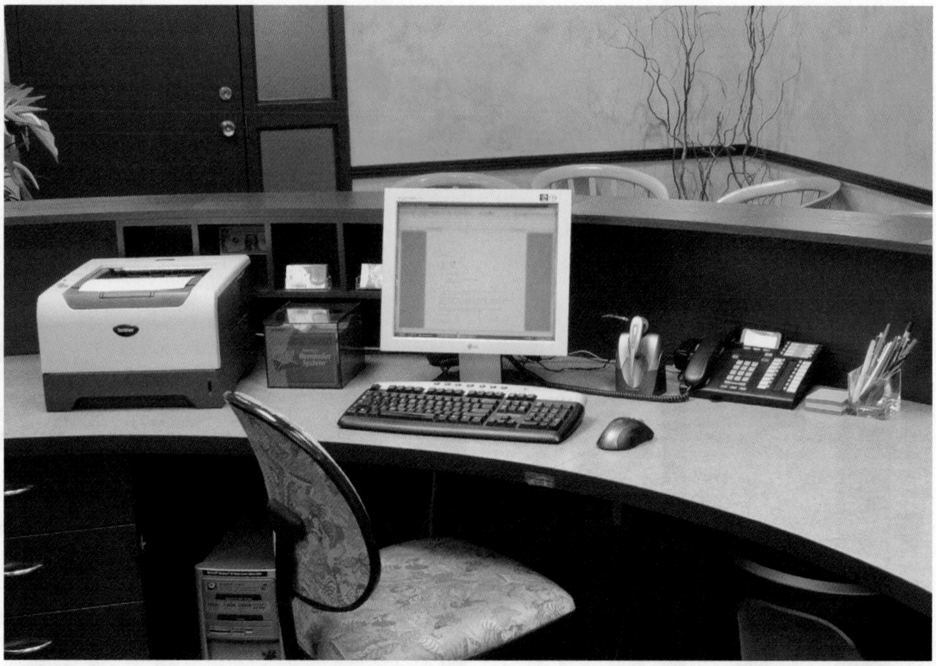

FIGURE 1-5 A neat workspace.

Dentist's Office

✓ checkPOINT

6. How can the dental office administrator give the impression of being organized and competent?

In most offices, the dentist will have a private office. This is used by the dentist for situations when privacy is required such as, telephone calls to patients or other doctors, reviewing charts, writing reports, or meetings with employees or other professionals. A computer with access to the Internet and the practice management program in use should also be located in the dentist's office. This ensures that access to an up-to-date schedule and patient information is available to the dentist. The dentist's office may also be where the security safe is located, which holds confidential financial information such as check books, deposit books, and bank statements. A cash box, used to provide change for patients paying their accounts with cash, or containing the petty cash, is often held in the dentist's private office. The dentist may also use the private office as a place to find time for a short break. This office may be used for private consultations with patients if there is not a **consultation area** available.

Consultation Area

A treatment plan or diagnosis is often discussed with patients in a consultation room to ensure privacy for the patient. A consultation area may be a separate office within the clinic or a table and chairs in an area set apart from public areas of the dental office. When a treatment plan or account discussion is required, use of the consultation area is necessary. This ensures the privacy of the patient and will assist in letting the patient feel relaxed in the discussion. A patient consultation room may also be referred to as a patient conference room.

Clinical Areas

The cleanliness and organization of the clinical areas are the responsibility of the clinical team members. The clinical areas in a dental office include the **dental operatories,** the **sterilization area,** and the **laboratory** (Figs. 1-6 and 1-7).

In general, the environment in the clinical areas of the dental office is somewhat different from that in the reception area. The temperature of the clinical areas is cooler by a few degrees. This is because the proximity between the patient and clinical

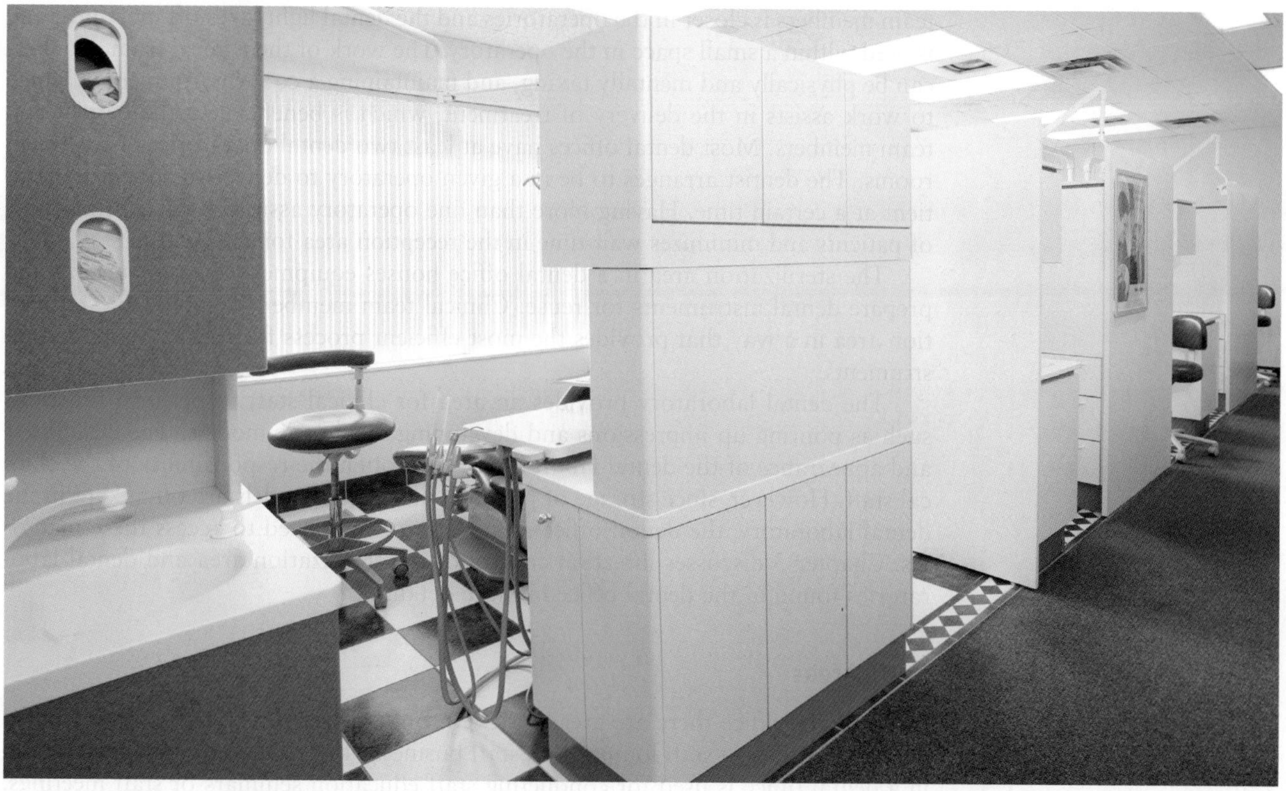

FIGURE 1-6 Clinical area.

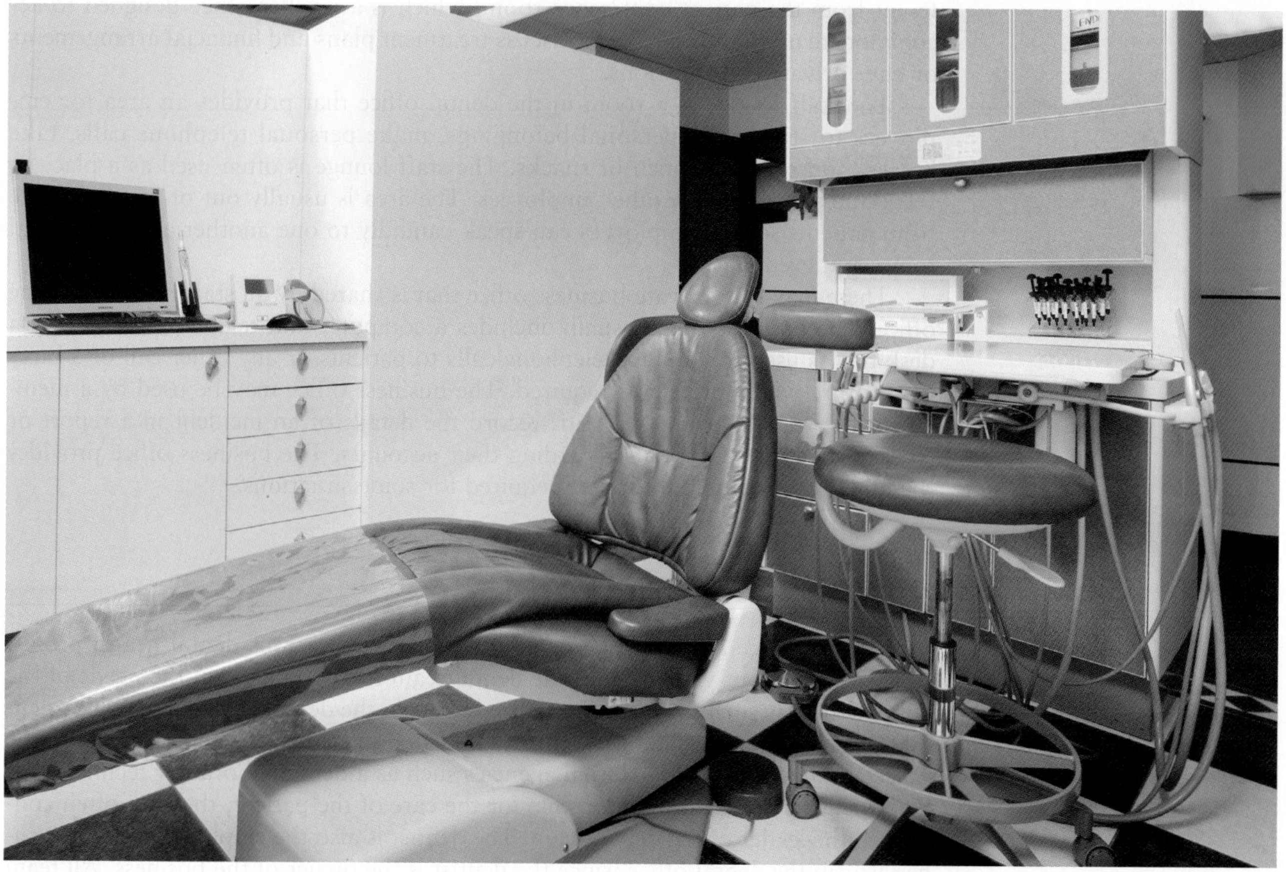

FIGURE 1-7 Dental operatory.

team members is closer in the operatories and the dental light gives off more heat and is used within a small space in the operatory. The work of the clinical team members can be physically and mentally taxing, and maintaining a cool environment in which to work assists in the delivery of treatment, which is beneficial to the patient and team members. Most dental offices have at least two dental operatories or treatment rooms. The dentist arranges to be in a given operatory to deliver treatment to a patient at a certain time. Having more than one operatory assists in the constant flow of patients and minimizes wait time in the reception area for the patient.

The sterilization area in a dental office houses equipment used to sterilize and prepare dental instruments for reuse. Clinical team members organize the sterilization area in a way that provides the most efficient process for sterilizing needed instruments.

The dental laboratory provides an area for clinical staff to perform functions such as pouring up impressions and developing diagnostic models. The cleanliness and appearance of the dental laboratory is also often the responsibility of the clinical staff. However, since storage of patients' diagnostic models are often kept in the dental laboratory, the dental office administrator may need to access these materials. Chapter 3 discusses infection control of the sterilization area and dental laboratories found in the dental office in more detail.

Staff Areas

In the dental office there are areas reserved for staff use. These areas can include a conference room, a staff lounge, or a staff business office. The staff conference room in a dental office is used for conducting staff education seminars or staff meetings. A staff conference room is usually a larger room that can seat all staff members comfortably to have meetings or lunch gatherings. The staff conference room is different from the patient conference room, which is a smaller office designed to accommodate up to four people to discuss treatment plans and financial arrangements or have private conversations.

The staff lounge is a room in the dental office that provides an area for employees to store their personal belongings, make personal telephone calls, take breaks, and eat their lunch or snacks. The staff lounge is often used as a place to relax and socialize with other employees. The area is usually out of hearing range from patients so that employees can speak candidly to one another about personal topics and events.

There may be a private business office that is shared by all staff members in the office. The business office usually includes a computer and telephone as well as a desk that is used to conduct telephone calls to patients or any other call of a business nature where privacy is required. The business office may be used by a member of the team to write a report, record the details of an incident in a report or chart, or telephone patients regarding their accounts. The business office provides the quiet and private atmosphere required for some situations.

DENTAL TEAM

As a dental office administrator, you will work with various dental health professionals throughout your career. The dental team today focuses on the needs of the patient, and, as such, all bring specialized skills to the dental environment. The dental team usually consists of the dentist, the dental hygienist, the dental assistant, the office administrator, and external agencies such as a dental laboratory technologist. Since dentists are legally responsible for the care of the patient, they are often considered the leader of the dental team. The dentist is also the employer and direct supervisor in the dental office, since the dentist is the owner of the business. All team members work in conjunction with each other to meet patient needs.

BOX 1-4
Dental Occupation Credentials

DDS	Doctor of dental surgery	COMSA	Certified oral and maxillofacial surgery assistant
DMD	Doctor of dental medicine	CDPMA	Certified dental practice management administrator
RDH	Registered dental hygienist	CDT	Certified dental laboratory technologist
CDA	Certified dental assistant		
RDA	Registered dental assistant		
COA	Certified orthodontic assistant		

Dentist

A **dentist** is a healthcare professional who practices dentistry. **Dentistry** is the examination, diagnosis, treatment, planning, or care of conditions within the human oral cavity or its adjacent tissues and structures. In most countries, to become a qualified dentist, several years of formal education are required. In most cases, three or more years of undergraduate education followed by 4 years of dental school are required to become a general dentist. Upon receiving the dental degree from a dental school, an individual can then place **DDS** or **DMD** after his or her name. DDS means doctor of dental surgery, and DMD means doctor of dental medicine. There is no difference between these two degrees. The university awarding the degree has the prerogative to choose which degree to award. The state and provincial licensing board accept either of these degrees. To become a dental specialist, such as an orthodontist or oral and maxillofacial surgeon, additional postgraduate training is required. Generally, this takes 2 years to complete. Before they begin the practice of dentistry, all dentists must pass a national board examination. Box 1-4 lists dental occupation credentials.

All dentists must maintain their dental license while they practice dentistry. This is done by the doctor completing CE courses on a regular basis. CE courses are a way for the dentist to learn about advances in the industry and gain new knowledge on various dental topics. The number of hours of CE courses needed to maintain licensure varies from state to state.

Dental Specialists

A **dental specialty** is an area of dentistry that has been recognized by the ADA as meeting the specific requirements for recognition of dental specialties. A **dental specialist** is a dentist who has received additional formal education and postgraduate training in an area of dental specialty.

General dentists are trained to competently perform in all areas of dentistry. However, there may be complex treatment procedures for which the dentist may feel more comfortable referring the patient to a specialist in that area. For example, a patient who requires extraction of a wisdom tooth that is impacted into the bone may be referred by the general dentist to an oral and maxillofacial surgeon for treatment. The patient will return to the general dentist for regular appointments and follow-up care.

Table 1-3 lists the nine dental specialties recognized by the American Dental Association.

checkPOINT

7. What is the name of the specialist who treats children?

Dental Hygienist

The **registered dental hygienist** (**RDH**) is a licensed dental professional who specializes in providing services that focus on the prevention of oral health problems and

TABLE 1-3 Dental Specialties

Specialty	Description
Public health dentistry	This specialty concerns itself with preventing and controlling dental diseases and promoting dental health through organized community efforts. This specialty of dentistry is concerned with the dental health education of the public through dental research. Example: Seniors' dental health and causes of associated oral disease
Endodontics	This area of dentistry is concerned with the morphology, physiology, and pathology of the human dental pulp and the tissues surrounding it. Specialists who practice this form of dentistry focus on the biology of the normal pulp, the etiology, diagnosis, prevention, and treatment of diseases and injuries of the pulp and associated conditions. Example: Root canal therapy
Oral pathology	This specialty of dentistry deals with the nature, identification, and management of diseases affecting the oral and maxillofacial regions. Specialists in this area investigate the causes, processes, and effects of oral diseases using clinical, radiographic, microscopic, biochemical, or other examinations. Example: Cancerous lesion of the mucosa
Oral radiology	A combined specialty of dentistry and discipline of radiology that focuses on the production and interpretation of images and data produced by all modes of radiation that are used for the diagnosis and management of diseases, disorders, and conditions of the oral and maxillofacial region. Example: Radiographs
Oral and maxillofacial surgery	A specialty of dentistry that includes the diagnosis and surgical and adjunctive treatment of diseases, injuries, and defects that involve the functional and esthetic aspects of the hard and soft tissues of the oral and maxillofacial region. Example: Jaw reconstruction
Orthodontics	This area of dentistry includes the diagnosis, prevention, interception, and correction of malocclusion. Orthodontists also treat neuromuscular and skeletal abnormalities of the developing or mature orofacial structures. Example: Braces/full banding
Pediatric dentistry	This is the specialty that provides primary, comprehensive, preventive, and therapeutic oral health care for infants and children through adolescence. This may also include patients with special healthcare needs. Example: Children's dental care
Periodontics	In periodontics, the specialist focuses on the prevention, diagnosis, and treatment of diseases of the supporting and surrounding tissues of the teeth (or their substitutes). This specialty focuses on the maintenance of the health, function, and esthetics of the tooth structures and tissues. Example: Periodontal disease
Prosthodontist	This specialty is concerned with the treatment of patients with missing or deficient teeth, or maxillofacial tissues, where materials that are biocompatible are used to restore function, comfort, and appearance of teeth. Examples: Veneers, crowns, implants

Adapted from the American Dental Association.

disease. Dental hygienists are licensed by each state to provide dental hygiene care or patient education. Once they receive their license, dental hygienists may use "RDH" after their name to denote that they are recognized by their state as an RDH.

The work of a dental hygienist in the dental office setting often involves the planning, assessment, and implementation of oral health care. Some examples of the duties a hygienist can perform in a day include the following:

- Remove deposits and stains from teeth
- Taking radiographs and using intraoral cameras
- Placing pit and fissure sealants on teeth
- Administering local anesthesia for hygiene or dental treatment
- Screening patients for oral cancer
- Providing periodontal care and management
- Performing head, neck, and oral examinations
- Performing scaling or root planing to patients during appointments

Depending on the state in which they practice, dental hygienists can perform a wide range of tasks and oral health care services. They can be employed in private dental practices, hospitals, public health centers, clinics, and various levels of government.

It is usual to hear of a dental hygienist delivering programs outside of the dental office that promote oral health care in the community. Hygienists will provide education in their communities through special interest groups, schools, day care centers, and long-term care facilities. Hygienists are involved in programs on smoking and tobacco cessation, seminars on the necessity of mouth guards for athletes, and well-baby seminars. The dental hygiene profession focuses on preventive healthcare and, as such, is proactive in its educational seminars for patient oral health care.

Generally, hygienists practice under the supervision of a dentist. In some states, however, hygienists are allowed to practice without a dentist's supervision. Furthermore, some states allow hygienists to deliver local anesthesia. This particular duty depends on the regulations set out by the dental hygiene association in their area.

Becoming a dental hygienist requires specialized postsecondary education. Dental hygienists hold a diploma, certificate, or Associate's degree in dental hygiene from a 2-year program or a Bachelor of Science degree with a dental hygiene specialization from a 4-year program. Dental hygienists can also obtain a graduate degree in dental hygiene should they wish to pursue a specialized area of research. Through their studies, dental hygienists acquire theoretical and practical knowledge in anatomy, nutrition, periodontology, pharmacology, materials science, and clinical skills.

checkPOINT

8. What are five responsibilities of a dental hygienist?

Dental hygienists perform many roles in their position in the dental office. They are clinicians, educators, advocates, administrators, and researchers, with public health being the main component of all these roles. The important role the hygienist plays in educating patients on proper oral hygiene and instructing them about the impact of proper nutrition on oral health is invaluable to the dental team.

Dental Assistant

The **CDA** or the **RDA** is a healthcare professional in the dental office whose responsibilities reach beyond the scope of providing assistance to the dentist. Using the designation of RDA or CDA depends on the state in which a dental assistant is certified to practice and what designation is preferred in that jurisdiction. Dental assistants take on a large amount of responsibility for the healthcare team. The efficiency of the dentist and the effective delivery of quality oral health care are increased by the presence of a dental assistant (Fig. 1-8).

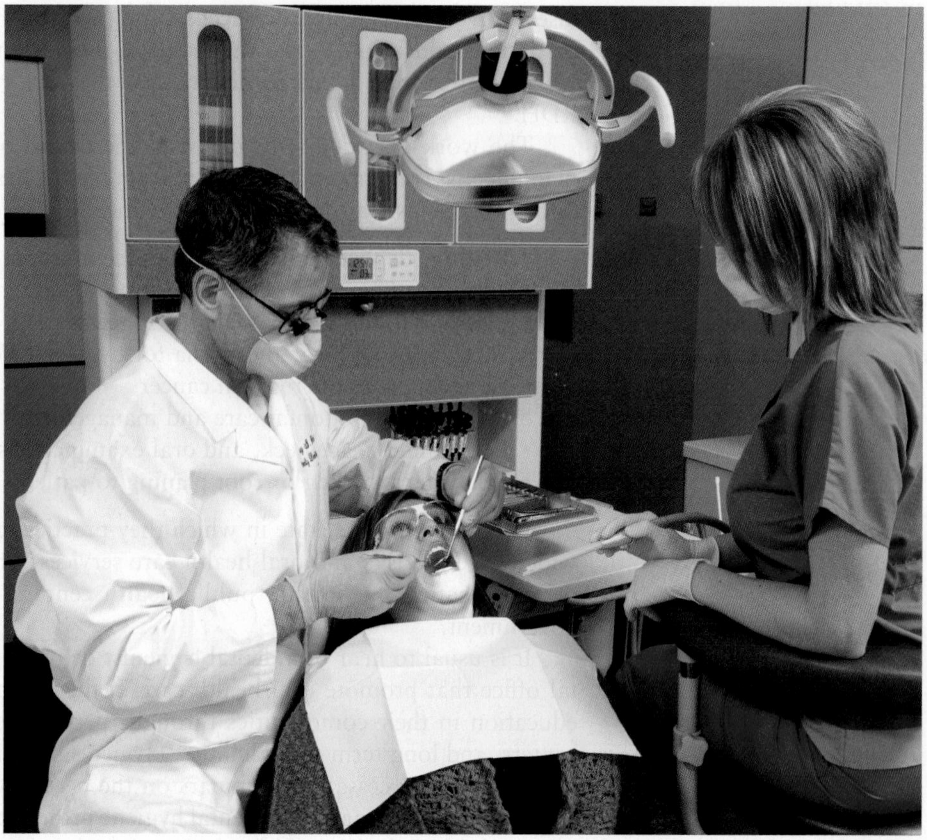

FIGURE 1-8 Dentist and dental assistant in procedure with a patient.

The dental assistant performs many tasks every day. Most of these tasks require both interpersonal and technical skills. The following is a list of duties usually performed by dental assistants:

- Providing assistance to the dentist during treatment
- Taking impressions of patients' teeth for study models
- Taking and developing dental radiographs
- Performing office administration duties
- Providing patient instruction for dental procedures
- Ensuring that infection control and sterilization standards are upheld
- Assisting patients with comfort before, during, and after procedures
- Providing patient care in all areas of dentistry
- Communicating with dental suppliers through the ordering of supplies

Procedures a dental assistant may perform vary depending on the state in which the dental assistant works. The primary tasks performed by all dental assistants in support of the dentist, however, include preparing patients, setting up instruments and equipment for procedures, recording patient information accurately, and providing the assistance to patients for a positive dental experience.

The position of a dental assistant is an interesting and challenging one, whether the assistant prefers to work chairside or in the administrative area of the clinic. In a smaller dental practice, the assistant may work with the dentist as well as manage some of the business aspects of the clinic, such as scheduling, billing, and purchasing. Often, in larger practices, the duties of a dental assistant are more specialized.

The formal education required to become a CDA or an RDA can typically be done in 9 months to 1 year. Details regarding the education and certification needed by dental assistants, which are similar to those for dental office administrators, are covered earlier in the chapter. In the past, dental assistants were not required to

checkPOINT

9. What is the role of the dental assistant in the dental office?

obtain formal educational training for their role. As the profession evolves, more dentists prefer a dental assistant who has completed a training program. This is a result of the dental assistant becoming an increasingly visible member of the dental team. The dental assistant works on behalf of the patient as well as the dental team in helping ensure a high level of professional excellence in the oral health care delivery of the dental office.

Dental Office Manager

The **dental office manager** is the team member who is responsible for the overall smooth operation of the day-to-day business of the dental office. The office manager often works very closely with the dentist to meet the clinic's staffing, equipment, and organizational needs. Duties for an office manager may include the following:

- Interviewing job applicants
- Pricing products from suppliers
- Maintaining accurate financial records
- Managing payroll
- Dealing with insurance companies
- Handling difficult patients
- Managing account concerns
- Motivating employees
- Providing support to employee relationships
- Initiating employee performance appraisals

Time, conflict, and stress management skills, along with effective communication and listening skills, are desired characteristics of a dental office manager. In addition, the dental office manager must exercise sound judgment every day, and any lapse can result in error. Dental office managers are not required to have any specific degree, but most dentists value a college or university degree that emphasizes planning and communication skills. A financial background in the area of accounting and payroll is also recommended.

Certified Dental Technician

The dental laboratory technician or **certified dental technician** (CDT) is not usually found working in the dental office but in a dental laboratory located nearby. The dental laboratory technician makes and repairs dental restorations and appliances on the basis of written instructions from the dentist. This can include dental crowns and bridges, orthodontics appliances, dentures, and other dental appliances. Dental laboratory technologists work with a wide variety of dental materials, including ceramics, precious metal, acrylics, and gypsum. A thorough knowledge of dental anatomy and oral structures is essential, because they examine impressions and models of the teeth.

Dental laboratory technicians usually complete a 2-year training program that qualifies them to take a written examination to become a CDT. Similar to other dental professionals, laboratory technicians are usually members of their respective professional association.

Sterilization Assistant and Office Assistant

checkPOINT

10. What are five ways the office manager can make the office run more smoothly?

In some dental offices, the patient flow can be become very steady and create a busy atmosphere. In the interest of maintaining the effective and efficient service provided to patients, assistants may be required in particular areas of the dental office.

In the sterilization area, a member of the dental team may be assigned to maintain the sterilization area. Responsibilities of this role usually include maintaining equipment, keeping the area clean, and ensuring that all the instruments are sterilized.

This is usually an entry-level position in the dental profession. In smaller offices, these responsibilities belong to the dental assistants. An individual who is developing his or her skills in the clinical area of the dental office may be employed in this role.

The business area of the dental office can also become a hectic environment. An office assistant is an individual who assists in the business area of the dental office. This person typically answers phones, schedules patients, and maintains filing and recare systems for the office manager or dental office administrator. This is usually an entry-level dental office administration position. The office assistant helps maintain the flow of the dental office by assisting in the business areas of the dental office. An individual who performs in the role of office assistant may not have any formal training or education in the dental industry but does have some customer service experience. The office assistant is restricted to performing business tasks in the dental office.

✓ checkPOINT

11. What is the difference between a sterilization assistant and an office assistant?

Association Memberships

The purpose of dental **professional associations** is to provide support, recruitment, and retention for dental professionals. These professional associations are dedicated to the advancement of the profession and the promotion of oral health.

The "Web Sites" list at the end of this chapter includes the Web sites of professional associations relevant to the various dental team members. One such organization, the ADA, is considered the authoritative national voice of dentistry. Although membership in such professional organizations is not required, it does offer many benefits. Some of these are as follows:

- Subscriptions to professional journals and newsletters that keep you apprised of advancements in the industry
- Access to conventions and seminars
- Insurance plan discounts
- Social functions
- Access to CE courses

Dentists and specialists can be members of the ADA. The national professional association for dental hygienists is the American Dental Hygiene Association. The dental assistant also reaps benefits from being a member of a professional association—the American Dental Assistants Association.

The Web sites for each of these associations are listed at the end of the chapter. Talk to your instructor or call your local state dental assisting or hygiene association about the possibility of becoming a student member of one of these associations, as you are quickly becoming a member of the dental profession!

Chapter Summary

Dentistry is constantly evolving. The formally trained dental office administrator will be a part of one of the most exciting times in dentistry, as new advances in dentistry appear everyday. The dental team members can make a dental practice very successful when they work together to deliver high-quality dentistry. As a dental office assistant, the value you add to the dental office by embracing the responsibilities and challenges that present themselves every day is an important resource to the dental office. The dental office needs a dental office administrator to create a smoothly run environment. As you grow professionally, your career as a dental office assistant will prove to be as exciting and steadfast as the advancements you'll encounter in the dental profession.

Review Questions

1. In addition to the qualities touched on in this chapter, discuss some personal qualities that you think a dental office administrator should possess and why they would be important in the dental office.
2. Describe some of your personal experiences as a patient in the dental office and think about what could have been done to make the experience different or better. If your experience was a positive one, what were the things that made it so? If your experience was negative, what could have been done differently to prevent it?
3. Review the list of dental specialists and think about which of them you would like to work for. Are there any specialists in the geographic area in which you live? If they have a Web site, can you get any more information on their office? Prepare a written response to these questions.

Multiple Choice

1. **Time management is**
   a. the utilization of processes that increase a person's time efficiency.
   b. a process that occurs naturally over time.
   c. the biggest challenge faced by administrators in dental offices today.
   d. an evolving method of scheduling proficiency.
2. **A common time waster in the dental office is**
   a. a patient who consistently arrives late.
   b. staff who discuss personal issues during lunch hour.
   c. lengthy important telephone calls to patients.
   d. reading personal e-mails during office hours.
3. **Which of the following does not contribute to professional appearance?**
   a. Long curly hair tied back
   b. Finger nails cut to a short, active length
   c. Shoes that are scuffed from overwear
   d. Clean, pressed uniform
4. **A main concern for the dental office administrator should be**
   a. building relationships with all employees.
   b. caring for patients and their welfare.
   c. being available for weekend work.
   d. ensuring that all employees receive their paychecks.
5. **Which of the following credentials applies to dentists?**
   a. RDH
   b. CDT
   c. DMD
   d. RDA
6. **The reception area of the dental office**
   a. should be updated regularly.
   b. is the main "hub" of the office.
   c. should accommodate the patient.
   d. is maintained by the office assistant.
7. **Procedures a dental assistant may perform**
   a. vary depending on the state in which the dental assistant works.
   b. are based on the requirements of the dentist and office needs.
   c. vary depending on the number of dental assistants in the office.
   d. are all the same, regardless of certification and training.
8. **The duties of an office manager include all of the following except**
   a. interviewing job applicants.
   b. performing dental procedures.
   c. maintaining accurate financial records.
   d. managing payroll.
9. **The purpose of dental professional associations is to**
   a. produce CE courses for ongoing learning.
   b. keep all members in contact with one another.
   c. provide support, recruitment, and retention for dental professionals.
   d. none of the above.
10. **Which of the following is not a responsibility of dental office administrators?**
    a. Greeting patients as they enter the office
    b. Ensuring correct treatment performed
    c. Scheduling appointments for patients
    d. Collecting payment on accounts

Web Sites

American Dental Association
http://www.ada.org/

American Dental Hygienists Association
http://www.adha.org/

American Dental Assistants Association
http://www.dentalassistant.org/

Canadian Practice: Organizational Web Sites

Canadian Dental Association
http://www.cda-adc.ca/

Canadian Dental Hygienists Association
http://www.cdha.ca/

Canadian Dental Assistants Association
http://www.cdaa.ca/

chapter TWO

Legal Responsibilities *and Ethics*

OBJECTIVES

After completing this chapter, you should be able to do the following:

- Spell and define the key terms
- Explain the legal concepts of contracts and consent
- List and explain the laws most applicable to dental professionals
- Identify the Health Insurance Portability and Accountability Act (HIPAA) and its four divisions and discuss how they relate to the dental office
- Discuss the differences between the privacy rule and the security rule and how they are implemented in the dental office
- Describe the eight administrative standards requirements of the privacy rule under HIPAA
- List and explain the three categories of the security rule under HIPAA
- Describe the main principles of the American Dental Association's Code of Ethics and Code of Professional Conduct
- Explain confidentiality in the dental office as it pertains to patient information
- Describe patient rights and responsibilities

KEY TERMS

- law
- statutory law
- civil law
- criminal law
- litigation
- contract
- expressed contract
- implied contract
- abandonment
- consent
- Good Samaritan Act
- Americans with Disabilities Act
- standard of care
- negligence
- malpractice
- fraud
- Health Insurance Portability and Accountability Act of 1996 (HIPAA)
- electronic data interchange (EDI)
- covered entity

OUTLINE

- defamation
- breach of confidentiality
- privacy rule
- protected health information (PHI)
- individually identifiable health information
- privacy practices notice
- minimum necessary
- personal representative
- privacy officer
- mitigation
- security rule
- administrative safeguards
- technical safeguards
- physical safeguards
- code of professional conduct
- code of ethics

As a dental office administrator, you will work on behalf of the patient as well as the dentist to ensure a high level of professional excellence in delivering oral health care.

In the process of doing this, you will be faced every day with making decisions that have serious legal and ethical implications. Such decisions can affect not only the health and well-being of your patients but also the liability and reputation of your dental office and colleagues and the very future of your career. For example, if the dental office administrator received a telephone call from a patient who requested a refill of his or her pain reliever prescription, the dental office administrator would know that there are federal laws that govern prescription writing and medication administration that apply to the dentist. If the dental office administrator chose to accommodate this patient and provide him and her with a refill for the prescription by telephoning the pharmacy without first getting the permission of the dentist, the dental office administrator would be acting on behalf of the dentist and in violation of the laws in this respect. Thus, it is critical that you understand the state and federal laws that govern the dental office and to develop a strong, personal code of ethics to guide you as you work as a dental office administrator.

The purpose of this chapter is to introduce you to the legal concepts and laws that affect the dental office, especially the Health Insurance Portability and Accountability Act of 1996 (HIPAA), and to discuss how you can help ensure compliance with these laws in your role as an administrator. Additionally, this chapter presents the codes of ethics adopted by dental professional associations and covers key ethical issues you will face as a dental office administrator. Finally, this chapter equips you to establish your own ethical framework, to guide you as you make difficult decisions.

LEGAL CONCEPTS

There are many legal concepts that you will become familiar with as you progress through your academic and practical education as a dental office administrator. Some of those legal concepts are presented in this chapter and cover concepts such as contracts and consent, types of law, negligence, fraud, malpractice, litigation, and invasion of privacy, all of which affect the dental office and your practice as a dental office administrator.

Every business and profession is affected by laws. **Law** refers to a system or body of rules of conduct in society enforced through a set of institutions. Laws in the United States consist of federal laws, state laws, and common law. Box 2-1 outlines examples of these laws and how they apply to dentistry. The dental office is bound by the laws of the state and the laws set out in its state Dental Practice Act. For this reason, laws relating to the practice of dentistry may vary from state to state.

Statutory law is the law that is upheld and written by a governing authority. Each state has an agency that governs the qualifications for and the practice of dentistry within the state. This agency is known as the State Board of Dentistry and is

BOX 2-1
Examples of Laws

Federal Law

A notice available to patients is required by federal law that describes how medical information may be used and disclosed and how the patient can gain access to the information.

State Law

Licensing requirements and qualifications of dentists are mandated by the state in which licensing is sought. The unlicensed practice of dentistry is a violation of state law.

Common Law

Laws affecting the dentist-patient relationship. The legal relationship between dentist and patient can be challenged in a court of law.

also known as the "board of dental examiners." The state board of dentistry is a state government agency that governs the qualifications for dentistry and practice and outlines statutes for practice. Box 2-2 outlines areas usually governed by the state board of dentistry. The granting of a license to a professional is legal permission to practice in the profession. Both dentists and dental hygienists must be licensed to practice in the dental profession, and some states require licensure of dental assistants who perform specific duties. Both members of the dental profession and public represent the board of members.

In **civil law,** a private party, such as a patient, files the lawsuit and becomes the plaintiff. A defendant, such as a dentist, is not incarcerated in a civil law suit. Civil litigation usually is resolved by the plaintiff, or patient, being reimbursed for any losses he or she endured. The dentist-patient relationship is an area that falls under civil law. In **criminal law,** the litigation is always filed by the government, who is called the prosecution. The punishment for violating criminal law is much different from that of civil law and involves incarceration, fines paid to the government, or execution. Practicing dentistry without a license, or any dental office employee performing an illegal function on behalf of the dentist, is a violation of criminal laws. When a lawsuit is in progress, for example when a suit has been filed against the dentist, this is considered **litigation.**

Contracts

A **contract** is an agreement that is entered into between two or more parties. Because contracts are considered to be legally binding, only those who are of legal age can enter into them. Hence, minors and others requiring representatives must have their representatives enter into the contract on their behalf. For minor children, this would be their parent or guardian.

BOX 2-2
Areas Governed by the State Board of Dentistry

- Qualifications for licensure
- Issuance of licenses
- Establishment of standards of practice
- Disciplinary action against those who violate state laws

checkPOINT

1. What is a contract?

There are three elements necessary for a contract to be enforceable: (1) an offer, (2) an acceptance, and (3) consideration. In the dental office, when a patient calls to schedule an appointment, he or she is essentially offering to enter into a contract. By scheduling the appointment, the dental office representative is accepting the offer and forming the contract. The element of consideration is met once the patient has received treatment and provides the dentist with payment for the services.

Expressed Contracts

Expressed contracts consist of specific details and are expressed verbally or in writing. The responsibilities of each party involved are made explicit to alleviate misunderstandings. In the dental office, an expressed contract between the provider of dental services and the patient is not common. However, expressed contracts are commonly used in other contexts in the dental office, such as in hiring staff, leasing of office space, and vendor relationships.

Implied Contracts

checkPOINT

2. Explain the difference between expressed contract and implied contract.

An **implied contract,** on the other hand, is a type of contract in which the circumstances imply that parties have reached an agreement, even though they have not done so expressly. For example, by going to the dentist for an emergency examination of a tooth, the patient agrees to pay the costs of the service. If the patient refuses to pay after receiving the examination, the patient has breached an implied contract. The contract is implied because the actions are implied by both parties; the dentist accepted the patient and through this action it implies that an examination will be performed. The patient accepted the treatment, implying that the bill for services will be paid.

Termination of Contracts

Once the relationship has been established between the dentist and the patient, the dentist has a legal duty to provide treatment to the patient. The dentist-patient relationship can be terminated by the following:

- the patient selecting another dentist for treatment
- dentist termination of relationship

Contracts between patients and dentists can be terminated as easily as the patient choosing to see another dentist for treatment and requesting that his or her dental history or radiographs be forwarded to that dental office. If the patient states that he or she would like to continue treatment elsewhere, you, the dental office administrator, should perform the following:

- document the request in the patient's chart
- advise the patient of any incomplete treatment plans
- offer to forward patient information to a dental office of the patient's choice

Remember to treat the patient with courtesy and respect during such interactions. Patients change dentists for various reasons: moving out of the area, the need for a specialist, or switching to a spouse's dentist. It is common for patients to return to a dental office they have once left. Always ask patients why they have chosen to leave the practice; there may be a reason that could be addressed and resolved to avoid losing them. This interaction is also an opportunity to improve the practice based on the reason the patient provides. As the office administrator, it will be your job to address these requests, and letting patients know that they are welcome back anytime can make the difference between seeing them again or not.

In some cases, the dentist may have cause to end the care of a patient. Reasons for ending the dentist-patient relationship may include long-term noncompliance

checkPOINT

3. What process should be followed when a patient requests to change dentist?

what IF ?

A patient in the dental clinic has just cancelled her third consecutive appointment in a 1-month period. After explaining her last-minute cancellations as work-related commitments that she could not get out of, she informs the office administrator that she is terrified and is just working up the nerve to continue treatment. The office administrator shows concern by expressing the importance of continuing the treatment the dentist has started and follows up by explaining the office policies regarding short-notice cancellations and the inconvenience it can cause. The patient becomes irritable and insists on making another appointment. The office administrator becomes frustrated with this patient and asks her politely to "take her business elsewhere." What legal implications does this action have?

with treatment, consistent rudeness to office staff, or nonpayment of account. If the dentist decides to terminate the dentist-patient relationship, the patient must be notified in writing, and this task is often the responsibility of the dental office administrator. The letter should be sent by certified mail, in which a signature can be obtained for confirmation of receipt. The letter must contain the reason for terminating the relationship, the date the relationship will cease, name and contact information of the local dental association for the patient to contact for new provider information, an offer to provide interim or emergency care for the patient until another dentist is found, and an offer to provide the patient records to a dentist of his or her choice. The dentist should also outline the current status of dental care or future dental care the patient may require. The goal is to assist the patient in a smooth transition to a new dental provider and, as such, continuing care should be available until the patient begins visiting the new provider. All staff members should be informed when a patient relationship has been terminated. If the patient were to telephone the office to schedule an appointment at the office after the date specified in the letter, the dentist-patient relationship could be reestablished.

The importance of this process and the information contained in the letter cannot be stressed enough. If a dentist, or you, the administrator acting as the representative of the dental office, chooses to terminate a patient relationship without ensuring that the proper steps were followed, particularly if the patient required additional treatment, the dentist could be charged with patient abandonment. **Abandonment** is a unilateral discontinuation of services without reasonable notice provided to the patient after treatment has been started but before it is completed. Furthermore, a dentist cannot terminate a patient relationship on the basis of the age, sex, race, religion, or disability of a patient. The state law regarding patient abandonment should be consulted prior to action being taken because of various laws among states.

Consent

By law, patients must **consent** to treatment with the dentist. This means that the dentist must have the patient's agreement to being treated prior to treatment being performed. This consent can be given to the dentist verbally or in writing. When someone arrives as a new patient in the dental office, he or she may be given a consent form to sign, which authorizes the dentist to perform general treatment for the duration of the relationship with the patient. Figure 2-1 provides an example of this. Other types of treatment, such as surgery with a dental specialist or comprehensive periodontal treatment, may require a separate consent-for-treatment signature from the patient. Figure 2-2 is a consent-for-treatment form for this type of situation. Children who require consent for treatment will have a parent or guardian provide the consent.

A consent form must include the following information:

- Name of the dentist performing the treatment
- Name of the patient accepting the treatment
- Type of procedure
- Length of time or number of appointments to complete treatment
- Statement indicating that all patient questions have been addressed
- Statement indicating alternatives presented
- Patient, dentist, and witness signatures
- Date of signing

The form that the patient signs must be in a language that is understandable to the patient, and the patient must sign the consent form willingly. Patients who are not willing to sign a consent form for treatment must be informed of their right to alternative treatment and their right to select another dentist.

Patient Information

Name____________________ Address____________________

City____________ Province________ Postal Code________ Home Phone________

Work Phone____________ Birthdate __/__/__ (DAY MTH YR) Health Care #____________

SIN____________ Employer____________________

Insurance: Name____________ Group Policy No________ ID No.________

Physician's Name____________ Referred by____________

Consent for Treatment

I do hereby authorize the performance of diagnostic services and dental treatment for the above patient by the staff of this dental clinic, their assistants and designees. I further authorize the administration of such anesthetics and medications as are deemed necessary by the staff. I understand that all diagnostic aids, including radiographs, are the property of the clinic.

Office Policy

Office policy is that your portion of the services are paid for at each visit as they are performed. In certain circumstances special arrangements for payment may be made by consulting the doctor and\or the office manager. We will prepare necessary reports to help collect your benefits from insuance companies. However, each fee is individual with the patient and not based on the assumption that the insurance company will pay all our charges. Interest will be charged on all overdue accounts at the rate of 1.8% per month after 30 days.

Signature of patient or guardian ____________ Date____________
Relationship of responsible agent ____________ Witness____________

MEDICAL ALERTS

FIGURE 2-1 Patient consent form: general.

CONSENT FOR ORAL SURGERY

PLEASE INITIAL EACH PARAGRAPH AFTER READING. IF YOU HAVE ANY QUESTIONS, PLEASE ASK YOUR DOCTOR BEFORE INITIALING.

You have the right to be informed about your condition and the recommended treatment plan to be used so that you may make an informed decision as to whether or not to undergo the procedure after knowing the risks and benefits involved. This disclosure is not meant to alarm you but is rather an effort to properly inform you so that you may give or withhold your consent.

PATIENT NAME: ______________________________ **DATE:** ____________

_______1. I hereby authorize Dr. Henderson, and any other agents, assistants, or employees selected by him, to treat the condition(s) described as:

____

_______2. The procedure(s) necessary to treat the condition have been explained to me and I understand the nature of the procedures to be:

____

_______3. I have been informed of the following possible alternative methods of treatment (if any), including no treatment, and the associated risks:

____

_______4. My doctor, or his agent, has explained to me that there are certain inherent and potential risks and side effects in any surgical procedure and in this specific instance such risks include, but are not limited to the following:

a. Postoperative discomfort and swelling that may require several days of at-home recuperation.
b. Prolonged or heavy bleeding that may require additional treatment.
c. Injury or damage to adjacent teeth or fillings.
d. Postoperative infection that may require additional treatment.
e. Stretching of the corners of the mouth that may cause cracking and bruising and may heal slowly.
f. Restricted mouth opening for several days, which is sometimes related to swelling and muscle soreness and sometimes related to stress to the joints of the jaw (TMJ).
g. The decision to leave a small piece of the tooth in the jaw when its removal would require extensive surgery to risk other complications.
h. Fracture of the jaw (in more complicated extractions or on medically compromised patients).
i. Injury to the nerve underlying lower teeth resulting in numbness or tingling to the chin, lip, gums and/or tongue which may persist for several weeks, months, or in some cases, permanently.
j. Opening of the sinus (a normal cavity situated above the upper teeth) requiring additional surgery.

_______5. It has been explained to me that during the course of the procedure(s) unforeseen conditions may be revealed which will necessitate extension of the original procedure(s) or different procedure(s) from those set forth in Item 2 above. I authorize my doctor and his staff to perform such procedure(s) as are necessary and desirable in the exercise of professional judgment.

_______6. I understand that I have the option of being referred to a specialist in oral and maxillofacial surgery for the procedures previously described and that Harrison Family Dentistry, PLLC will make a copy of my records, including radiographs, and mail or give to the patient to hand deliver to the oral and maxillofacial surgeon.

_______7. I have been made aware that certain medications, drugs, anesthetics, and prescriptions which I may be given can cause drowsiness, loss of coordination and lack of awareness which also may be increased by the use of alcohol and other drugs. I have been advised not to operate any vehicle or hazardous machinery, and not to work while taking such medication, or until fully recovered from the effect of the same. I understand this recovery may take up to 24 hours or more after I have taken the last dose of medication. If I am to be given sedative medication during my surgery, I agree not to drive myself home and will have a responsible adult drive me home and accompany me until I am fully recovered from the effects of the sedation.

_______8. It has been explained to me, and I fully understand, that a perfect result is not, and cannot, be guaranteed or warranted. I am further advised that I can get additional explanation of risks before treatment by asking my doctor.

_______9. I certify that I have read and fully understand this consent for surgery, and that all blanks were filled in prior to my initials and signature.

PLEASE ASK IF YOU HAVE QUESTIONS CONCERNING THIS CONSENT FORM.

____
Patient's (or legal guardian's) signature — Date

____
Witness's signature — Date

____
Doctor's signature — Date

FIGURE 2-2 Patient consent-for-treatment form. Courtesy of Nathan Henderson, DDS.

LAWS THAT APPLY TO DENTAL PROFESSIONALS

In addition to the legal concepts presented above, you should also be familiar with the laws that govern the dental profession. In particular, legal changes have been implemented over the past few years in the dental profession, such as the protection of patient information with the institution of privacy legislations. With these changes comes an increased accountability of the dental professional to institute them. Also, as a result of these changes, new terminology and administrative practices have been incorporated in the dental office. The dentist and other dental team members will depend on you, the dental office administrator, to ensure that the guidelines regarding patient privacy, safety, and rights and responsibilities are adhered to as much as possible.

Dental Practice Act

In the healthcare industry, many personnel are required to be licensed, registered, or certified to work in their field. As noted in Chapter 1, a dentist, for example, must be licensed to practice dentistry. In the dental industry, such licensure, registration, and certification are governed by each state's Dental Practice Act. This legislation applies to the whole dental team: the dentist, the dental hygienist, the dental assistant, and the dental office administrator. In addition to establishing requirements that each dental professional must meet to practice, this act also determines the scope of practice of each dental profession. For example, a registered dental hygienist licensed and practicing in the state of California may perform under the direct supervision of a dentist, the administration of local anesthetic agents limited to the oral cavity. See Chapter 1 for details on the licensure, registration, and certification of dental professionals.

Good Samaritan Act

Another important piece of legislation that impacts the dental profession is the **Good Samaritan Act**, which is recognized in all states. The Good Samaritan Act, which varies from state to state, was legislated to ensure that caregivers are immune from liability in an emergency situation, as long as the care is provided in a way that a reasonable and prudent person would provide in the same situation. The Good Samaritan Act does not apply to emergency situations that occur within the dental office; it applies only to emergency acts outside of the formal practice of the dental office. This is because under the general guidelines of the Good Samaritan Act, medical professionals are not covered by the Act when performing first aid in connection with their employment. Furthermore, any first aid given must not involve any exchange of financial compensation. The dentist has insurance coverage that pertains to acts of emergency that may occur in the dental office. Should you find yourself in a situation where you make the choice to provide first aid to a person, such as cardiopulmonary resuscitation or dressing a wound, keep in mind the following guidelines:

Once first aid begins, the responder must not leave the scene until:

- It is necessary to call for medical assistance
- A person of equal or higher ability can take over providing first aid
- Continuing to give aid is unsafe (e.g., not having barriers to protect against bloodborne pathogens); a responder cannot be forced to risk his safety to provide aid to another person

Americans With Disabilities Act

The **Americans with Disabilities Act of 1990** is a civil rights law that prohibits discrimination based on a person's disability. A disability is any type of physical or mental impairment that a person has which limits a major life activity. Under this law, there are three categories of persons who are considered disabled:

1. A person who has a physical or mental impairment that substantially limits one or more major life activities
2. A person who has a record of such an impairment
3. A person who is regarded as having such an impairment but is not actually disabled

Individuals who are considered to be disabled are blind or hearing impaired, require use of a wheelchair, have a chronic illness such as diabetes, cancer, or heart disease, and are mentally retarded or learning disabled. If a person has a record of an impairment, this includes people who are currently free of a disease they once had and no longer impaired by it. An example of this would be a person who was diagnosed with cancer and received treatment, which has resulted in a state of being cancer-free.

All dental offices must adhere to the provisions outlined in the Americans with Disabilities Act. This means that dentists are required to make certain modifications to the dental office in order to facilitate access for disabled persons. Within a reasonable scope, these modifications may include rearranging the physical layout of the office, such as ramps for wheelchair access, or changing office policies to reflect inclusion, by providing auxiliary aids. Auxiliary aids may be required for patients who require interpretation, such as a deaf patient requiring sign language interpretation.

Negligence and Malpractice

Other laws are in place to protect patients from poor care or medical errors. Dentists, like other healthcare professionals, are held to a reasonable **standard of care** in their profession that members of the public who are not dentists are not held to. A standard of care refers to the degree of care and skill that would be exercised under similar circumstances by reasonable and prudent members of the same profession. **Negligence** refers to performing an act that a reasonable and prudent person (in this case, a dental professional) would not have done or omission of an act that a reasonable and prudent person would have done. Understanding whether or not an act was negligent is often decided using the following outline, which is referred to as a test of liability:

- A duty of care was owed to the person
- A duty of care was breached
- The breach caused loss or damage to the person
- The person should be compensated for his or her loss or damage

A dentist owes a duty of care to the patients in the clinic. Since the dentist has the professional training and understanding to know what risks are involved in dentistry when treating patients, there is an obligation to take necessary precautions to avoid these risks. Knowingly putting the patient at risk and making the decision to continue doing so are a breach of the duty of care the dentist owes to the patient. If this breach of duty, that is, the particular acts or omissions to act, is deemed to be the cause of the damage or loss sustained by the patient, the dentist would be considered negligent. If negligence is decided, and it is shown that the professional standards were not adhered to, and a breach of duty was made, malpractice could be the result.

Malpractice refers to an action by a professional who has brought harm to a client or patient. Malpractice suits brought against healthcare professionals have increased over the years and, as a result, the standards of the dental office and the ethical responsibilities of dentists and staff members have been given greater emphasis. It is important for the office administrator to pay attention to areas that, if overlooked, can contribute to a malpractice suit. Those areas are maintaining thorough

checkPOINT

4. Explain what negligence is.

what IF ?

A very good friend of the dentist arrives for an appointment. As it is his first time in the clinic, you present him with a health history form and a new patient form to complete. He says that it is not required, as the dentist is such a good friend. What would you do?

legal TIP

Patients who are HIV-positive are considered disabled under the Americans with Disabilities Act. Although the use of universal precautions minimizes the threat to medical workers so that the risk of transmission is almost nonexistent, a dentist or an employees in the dental office cannot refuse to treat a patient because of this disability. All employees in the dental office act on behalf of the dentist when decisions are made and treatment is provided. Therefore, the dentist will be held liable for the acts of employees and an employee may be terminated for refusing to treat the disabled.

and accurate patient records, ensuring that informed consent is obtained prior to treatment of any type, and strictly adhering to standards of providing high-quality dental care. An integral part of the role of the dental office administrator is forming, developing, and maintaining positive relationships with patients. Throughout the relationship process, dental office administrators must ensure that the patient is aware of the treatment that is planned, make sure that the patient understands and has been made aware of the results and possible complications, and finally, that he or she agrees to and follows through with his or her financial responsibility for the treatment. If the patient relationship is positive and understanding on the patient's part is clear, avoidance of malpractice is likely. Any patient who is dissatisfied with any aspect of his or her treatment should have his or her concerns dealt with quickly. The dental office administrator should inform the dentist of unhappy patients as soon as possible. It is important to remember to document their concern and do not offer any opinions or advice to the patients, since any comment you make can be used in a court of law and could be causing damage to the dentist and yourself.

Fraud

Fraud refers to an act of deception committed for personal gain. Fraud is a crime and a violation of civil law. The most common type of fraud is defrauding people or agencies of money. The most common type of fraud that occurs in the dental office involves the billing of treatment to insurance companies. The dental office administrator is responsible for ensuring that claims sent to insurance companies are correct in all respects to avoid fraud. One example involving this type of fraud is when the date on an insurance claim form is altered. That is, the patient requests that the office administrator puts a date other than the correct one (the day treatment was performed) on the claim form in order that the benefit is paid. A patient may request that this be done in situations when their coverage is not yet in effect, they are over their yearly plan maximum, or their coverage was expired on the date of treatment. As an office administrator, you have the responsibility to act ethically by adhering to the laws governing the dental practice. By complying with the patient's request in this situation, you are violating a law and risking the dentist's license and reputation as well as your own.

Another fraud situation that may occur in the dental office involves identity theft, specifically, new patients. When an individual is first eligible to begin using the benefits, often he or she may not have a benefits card issued to him or her. In situations such as this, the office administrator may contact the insurance company by calling to verify the information needed to process the dental claim, such as eligibility and type of benefits. Once confirmation is received, treatment can begin and the claim is billed to the insurance company and payment received in the dental office. The process is correct. However, when the patient who really owns the benefit plan goes to the dentist only to discover that the maximum has been reached, and no coverage is currently available, the fraud is often discovered. The insurance company may request that the dentist return the payment to it. The prudent dental office administrator should ask for picture identification, such as driver's license, and make a copy of the identification and maintain it in the patient chart.

HEALTH INSURANCE PORTABILITY AND ACCOUNTABILITY ACT OF 1996

Probably the most important law for dental office administrators to understand is the **HIPAA.** HIPAA, a federal law, provides standards regarding the security and privacy of patients' health information. The HIPAA standards cover electronic data filing of health information, known as **electronic data interchange** (EDI), as well as written and oral communications.

BOX 2-3
General Requirements for Covered Entities

- To provide information to patients about their privacy rights and use of information
- To adopt clear and appropriate policies and procedures
- To train staff members for understanding of privacy procedures
- To designate a privacy officer to ensure that privacy procedures are adopted and followed
- To adopt adequate security policies for protecting individually identifiable health information

As in the rest of the healthcare industry, the growing use of computers to maintain and transmit patient information in dental offices has increased the concern about the privacy and protection of patients' health information. The standards and regulations mandated through HIPAA include privacy and security provisions that refer to EDI.

These provisions apply to dentists who are **covered entities.** According to HIPAA regulations, in the dental profession, a covered entity is any dentist who transmits patient information electronically. The form of electronic transmission used by the dental office must be a format that is established by the HIPAA transaction standards. Even though a dental office must transmit claims electronically to be considered a covered entity, once this happens, all forms of communication regarding protected health information (PHI) of the patient are protected by HIPAA. Box 2-3 outlines the responsibilities of a covered entity, which are discussed below.

checkPOINT

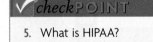

5. What is HIPAA?

HIPAA outlines regulations and standards to protect the privacy of this information. The HIPAA regulations are divided into four standards:

- Privacy
- Security
- Identifiers
- Transaction and code sets

Confidentiality and the Privacy Rule

In the dental office, all information about patients that is collected for the purpose of treatment is considered private. Each patient has a record that holds this personal information, which ranges from name and address to health and medical history. Figure 2-3 is an example of what a patient chart looks like.

The protection of collected health information from patients is of the utmost importance in the dental office. The dental office administrator plays a large role in the facilitation of patient privacy in the dental environment. The general rule is that patient information received in the dental office stays in the dental office, regardless of the medium in which the information is received. Discussing the information outside of the dental office with friends or family is strictly forbidden. Providing

PERSONAL INFORMATION PROTECTION AND ELECTRONIC DOCUMENTS ACT (PIPEDA)

In Canada, PIPEDA, or the privacy act as it applies to dental office, is very similar to the guidelines used in the United States under HIPAA. Canadian dental offices must adhere to the guidelines under PIPEDA, which can be accessed through the provincial association of which the dentist is a member.

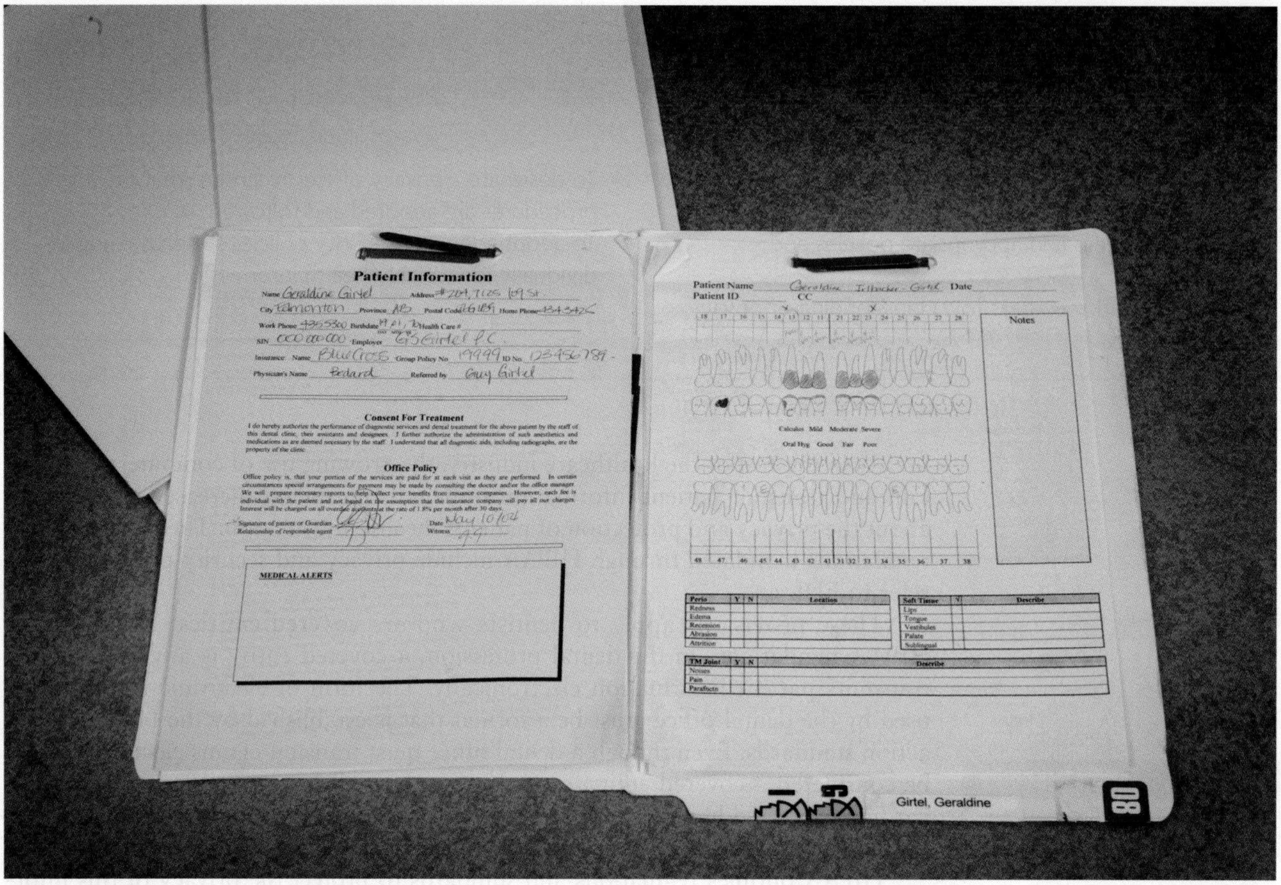

FIGURE 2-3 Patient dental chart.

> ✓ *check*POINT
>
> 6. When is it acceptable to discuss patient information?

information about patients to others, particularly if the information turns out to be false, could result in legal ramifications. **Defamation** is written or spoken injury to a person or an organization's reputation. If a dental administrator were to discuss patient information that caused harm to a person's reputation, the dental administrator could be charged with defamation of character. Disclosing information to an outside or third party, particularly to persons who do not have legal access to the patient's chart, is considered a **breach of confidentiality.**

Because of the sensitivity of this information, the HIPAA privacy regulations, collectively known as the **Privacy Rule,** have been established to mandate how patients' **PHI** is held or transmitted by a covered entity or its business associate, in any form or media, whether electronic, paper, or oral. This PHI consists of **individually identifiable health information,** which is information that pertains to a patient's health or healthcare and can be used to identify the patient. Box 2-4 outlines the information that is considered to be individually identifiable and, therefore, PHI. That is, it is believed that these items can identify who the patient is. All employees in the dental office must adhere to the privacy rule, as each member has a responsibility in collecting and protecting patient information.

So, how does this law affect you? As a dental office administrator, your position will occasionally entail facilitating patient transactions with outside business associates. An outside business associate would include such businesses that provide services in legal, accounting, data processing, management, administration, financial services, or any other service that might be contracted out by the covered entity. For example, you may have to provide information on behalf of a patient to a lawyer regarding the treatment the patient received in the dental office as a result of

BOX 2-4 Individually Identifiable Health Information

- Patient demographic data such as name, address, birth date, and social security number
- The patient's past, present, or future health condition
- The type of healthcare provided to the patient
- The past, present, or future payment of healthcare provided to the patient

a car accident. Or, the dental office you work in may use an answering service that collects information left by the patient, such as a name, phone number, or treatment information. Any contractual agreements between the covered entity and outside business associates involved in the handling of healthcare information must also adhere to the privacy rule as it pertains to them.

Besides the privacy rule, some states have other laws and regulations in place to manage health information concerns. In these situations, HIPAA is a complement to the state regulations already in place. In other words, the state rule is the prevailing law and HIPAA is an addition to those rules.

checkPOINT

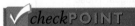

7. What is the privacy rule?

The privacy rule further addresses several issues, discussed in detail below, that are important for you to understand. These include the notice of privacy practice, the minimum necessary standard, personal representatives and minors, preemption and exception determinations, and administrative requirements.

Notice of Privacy Practice

The responsibility of the healthcare provider extends further than adhering to the correct collection and usage of patient information. The privacy rule stipulates that patients are to be provided with a **privacy practices notice** regarding their legal rights to their health information and the organization's legal duties regarding protecting this information. Usually, this is provided in the form of a brochure or a one-page document with the necessary information. Listed below are the patient rights included in the notice of privacy practices.

Under the privacy rule, patients have the right to:

- Gain access to their health records and obtain a copy if requested
- Request corrections to their patient file or provide a statement of disagreement
- Receive an accounting of how their information has been used and to whom it has been disclosed
- Request limits on access to sensitive health information
- Request confidential communications of sensitive health information
- File a complaint with the organization's privacy officer if there are problems and follow up with the complaint with the U.S. Department of Health and Human Services to achieve resolution

Upon arrival to the dental office, all new patients and any others who request it must be provided with a copy of the privacy notice. In keeping with the accountability goal of HIPAA, the dental office should obtain written acknowledgment from the patient confirming that the privacy practices notice was made available and authorizing the dentist to collect and use information (Fig. 2-4). The patient acknowledgments and authorization should be written in plain language and cover specific terms as outlined in the list of patient rights.

Figure 2-4 is an example of a patient acknowledgment of the privacy practice notice and authorization. In situations where the patient's written acknowledgment was not received, for any reason, the staff member must document the reason in the patient's chart.

HARRISON FAMILY DENTISTRY, PLLC

CONSENT FOR USE AND DISCLOSURE OF HEALTH INFORMATION

SECTION A: PATIENT GIVING CONSENT

Name: ______________________ Address: ______________________

Telephone: ______________________ ______________________

SSN: _______ - _______ - _______ ______________________

SECTION B: TO THE PATIENT—PLEASE READ THE FOLLOWING STATEMENTS CAREFULLY.

Purpose of Consent: By signing this form, you will consent to our use and disclosure of your protected health information to carry out treatment, payment activities, and healthcare operations.

Notice of Privacy Practices: You have the right to read our Notice of Privacy Practices before you decide whether to sign this consent. Our Notice provides a description of our treatment, payment activities, and healthcare operations, of the uses and disclosures we may make of your protected health information, and of other important matters about your protected health information. A copy of our notice accompanies this consent. We encourage you to read it carefully and completely before signing this consent.

*We reserve the right to change our privacy practices as described in our Notice of Privacy Practices. If we change our privacy practices, we will issue a revised Notice of Privacy Practices, which will contain the changes. Those changes may apply to any of your protected health information that we maintain.

*You may obtain a copy of our Notice of Privacy Practices, including any revisions of our Notice, at any time by contacting:

Contact Office:: HARRISON FAMILY DENTISTRY, PLLC CONTACT PERSON
Telephone: 423-344-32388479 Fax: 423-326-3552
Address: 5707 Highway 58, Harrison, TN 37341

Right to Revoke: You will have the right to revoke this consent at any time by giving us written notice of your revocation submitted to the contact person listed above. Please understand that revocation of this consent will *not* affect any action we took in reliance on this consent before we received your revocation, and that we may decline to treat you or to continue treating you if you revoke this consent.

SIGNATURE

I, ______________________, have had full opportunity to read and consider the contents of this consent form and your Notice of Privacy Practices. I understand that, by signing this consent form, I am giving my consent to your use and disclosure of my protected health information to carry out treatment, payment activities, and heathcare operations.

Signature: ______________________ Date: ______________

If this consent is signed by a personal representative on behalf of the patient, complete the following:

Personal representative's name: ______________________

Relationship to patient: ______________________

YOU ARE ENTITLED TO A COPY OF THIS CONSENT AFTER YOU SIGN IT.
Include completed consent in the patient's chart.

REVOCATION OF CONSENT

I revoke my consent for your use and disclosure of my protected health information for treatment, payment activities, and healthcare operations.

I understand that revocation of my consent will *not*affect any action you took in reliance on my consent before you received this written Notice of Revocation. I also understand that you may decline to treat or to continue to treat me after I have revoked my consent.

Signature: ______________________ Date: ______________

FIGURE 2-4 Patient acknowledgment of privacy practices. Courtesy of Nathan Henderson, DDS.

checkPOINT

8. What information is included in the notice of privacy practices?

Minimum Necessary Standard

A fundamental aspect of the privacy rule is a principle that is termed the **minimum necessary.** This term refers to the minimum necessary use and disclosure of patient information. Team members in the dental office must make every reasonable effort to obtain, disclose, and use only the PHI that is needed for the intended purpose. Policies and procedures pertaining to the uses and disclosures must be developed and followed. Furthermore, if there is a request from an outside source, the covered entity should provide only the amount of personal health information of the patient requested, that is, the minimum amount necessary. There are, however, situations in which the standard of minimum necessary does not apply. These are as follows:

- Disclosure or request to or from a healthcare provider is made for treatment purposes
- Disclosure to the individual or the individual's representative
- Disclosure authorized by the individual
- Disclosures authorized by the Department of Health and Human Services for compliance enforcement

All healthcare facilities, including dental offices, are required to integrate the minimum necessary standard into the policies and procedures carried out in their clinic or organization.

legal TIP

A patient's chart is considered a legal document. Legal representatives such as lawyers who require patient records to facilitate legal proceedings must provide a written request for copies of the chart. To provide this information, you should always ensure that signed consent to release the information was provided to the legal representative and inform the dentist of the request before releasing the information. The patient's chart is the property of the dental office, and therefore photocopies should be made and the original chart retained in the dental office.

Personal Representatives and Minors

Although there are many areas of healthcare that require the permission of the patient, such as treatment to be received, payments to be charged to the patient's account and the type of the payment, as well as the use of personal health information in the dental office, there are some situations in which the healthcare provider will not receive consent directly from the patient. These situations are when the patient has a personal representative or when the patient is a minor.

Personal Representatives In the dental office, a patient may utilize a **personal representative.** A personal representative is a person who is legally authorized to make healthcare decisions on the patient's behalf. Under the provision of the privacy rule, the healthcare members are to treat the personal representative as they would to the patient. This means that the personal representative would have the same rights regarding use and disclosure of the patient's personal health information as the patient would.

Patient as Minor When parents bring their minor children to the dental office, they are children's representatives. As a result of this, parents are afforded the same patient rights to their minor child's personal health information as if it were their own. The age at which a child is no longer considered a minor varies between states, and therefore it is wise to be aware of these laws as they pertain to the geographic area in which you are employed.

checkPOINT

9. What does "minimum necessary standard" mean?

Preemption and Exception Determinations

In some states, there are laws that are considered to be contrary to the federal rule or privacy rule. The HIPAA guidelines describe a contrary law as one that prevents the covered entity from carrying out the regulations of the privacy rule. In this situation, the privacy rule would take precedence over the state law and would preempt it. However, exemptions to this rule of preemption to contrary laws are allowed by HIPAA in situations in which the state laws protect public health, safety, or welfare need. Specifically, exemptions include cases in which the state law:

- Provides greater privacy protection to the personal health information of the patient
- Pertains to reporting child abuse, birth, or death, or for investigation or intervention
- Is used to provide reporting information such as financial or management audits

what IF ?

A patient's wife has called requesting information on the type of treatment that her husband received in the clinic today. How would you respond?

Respond politely to the patient's wife that you cannot discuss patient information without permission from the patient. Regardless of the individual making the request, patient information cannot be discussed unless written permission has been given to the dental office. Patients of the dental office may request that their information be shared with certain family members. Written permission can be obtained from the patients by using a form that names those individuals who are privy to their information.

Since there is patient health information involved in these situations, the patient or personal representative of the patient generally would be entitled to an accounting of what was reported. However, there may be some situations in which the accounting of the reporting would not be available to them.

Administrative Requirements

All covered entities in the healthcare environment must put into place policies and procedures that implement the HIPAA requirements. In the dental office, the following policies and procedures, under the privacy rule, must be a part of the policies and procedures carried out. As the dental office administrator, your role may involve the proper implementation of these policies. There are eight administrative requirements outlined in the privacy rule under HIPAA, which we will discuss here:

- privacy policies and procedures
- privacy personnel
- workforce training and management
- mitigation
- data safeguards
- complaints
- retaliation and waiver
- documentation and record retention

The size of the dental office and the nature of the environment and treatment provided will determine how these requirements are applied. For example, if the office you are employed in does not use a computer to store patient information, the method used in your office would pertain only to the physical charts or files of patient information. Although there is flexibility in these requirements, the flexibility extends only to the application of the rule in keeping with the size of the organization, the resources available, and implementation of the rule appropriate to the environment.

Privacy Policies and Procedures The dental office must include written policies and procedures that adhere to the privacy rule. Since HIPAA affects all areas of the dental office, an appropriate place to maintain these written policies is in the office procedures and policy manual. These policies and procedures would include all areas of HIPAA regulations that affect the covered entity. Chapter 12 provides discussion on the development and organization of the office policies and procedures manual.

Privacy Personnel HIPAA legislation mandates that a covered entity must assign an individual to be responsible for the implementation of the policies and procedures and ensure their compliance with HIPAA legislation. This individual carries the title of **Privacy Officer** and oversees and carries out the following:

- Develops privacy policies and procedures
- Ensures availability of privacy policies to patients through the accurate display of these policies
- Creates forms and documents needed to accurately collect and retain personal health information
- Serves as a contact for patients and third parties regarding protection and retention of health information and addresses complaints in this regard

✓ checkPOINT

10. What are four responsibilities of the privacy officer?

Because of the great level of responsibility attached to this title, in many dental offices the privacy officer is the office manager or dental office administrator. In smaller dental offices, the privacy officer may be the dentist. A sound understanding of the importance of confidentiality and protection of patient health information coupled with confidence in the practical application of these rules and regulations is crucial in this role.

Workforce Training and Management All individuals working in the dental office, paid or unpaid, must be trained on the privacy policies and procedures pertinent to the dental office and to each person's role. Everyone in the office is accountable to and must comply with these policies.

Mitigation If dental office staff or a business associate violates the privacy rule in its handling of a patient's information, mitigation is required by the dental office. **Mitigation** means that the covered entity must make every reasonable effort to alleviate any harm that resulted from the violation.

Data Safeguards Once information is collected from the patient, it is important that it is appropriately protected. The requirements for safeguarding health information under HIPAA include that a covered entity have appropriate administrative, technical, and physical protective safeguards in place. The reasonable safeguards that can be taken in the dental office depend on the size and resources available but generally include the following:

- Use of passwords on computers to enter and access patient information
- Concealing the computer monitor from the view of patients when health information is displayed
- Use of cabinets that can be locked or covered up to limit access to patient information
- Use of a private area in the dental office to discuss patient information either by telephone or in person (in some smaller dental offices, this private area may be the operatory)
- Speaking quietly when discussing patient information around others (i.e., in the waiting room)

Although technological advancements are ever present in the dental industry, the dental office is still an environment in which personal communication with patients dominates. Office administrators must be aware of their surroundings when discussing personal health information, either with patients or with staff members, and take measures to ensure confidentiality. Discussion of patients must always be done out of the hearing range of other patients. Other reasonable safeguards include keeping a neat, organized working environment in which patient charts are not left exposed for others to view and using patients' first names only, if at all, when on the telephone.

checkPOINT

11. What is important to remember regarding the safeguarding of PHI?

Complaints The privacy rule stipulates that every covered entity must provide an explanation of complaint procedures to its patients and the name of the privacy officer or other person to whom the patient can submit his or her complaint. The patient should also be informed that he or she may also file a complaint with the Department of Health and Human Services, which will investigate the complaint and settle the matter.

The privacy officer should be aware of the process to follow in addressing a complaint from a patient. First, the complaint must be held in confidence. As with any complaint, the patient must be given the time and respect to be heard, and a response to the complaint should be addressed promptly with a view to seeking an appropriate solution. A complaint of any nature should be considered carefully, and, when appropriate, changes in policies or procedures should be made to improve the dental practice.

Retaliation and Waiver Should a complaint be processed against a covered entity with the governing body, the privacy rule mandates that the covered entity may not retaliate against an individual for any of the following:

- Filing a complaint
- Assisting in an investigation of a complaint
- Being opposed to a policy or procedure that the person believes is contrary to the privacy rule

A person who files a complaint has the right to have his or her complaint protected under the privacy rule, and, therefore, the covered entity must treat this information

BOX 2-5
HIPAA Identifiers

- Name and/or initials
- Street address, city, county, precinct, ZIP code/postal code
- All elements of birth dates (except year) related to a person
- Age
- Telephone number
- Fax number
- E-mail address
- Social security number/social insurance number
- Medical record numbers/chart number
- Health insurance plan name and ID numbers
- Account numbers
- Certificate/license numbers
- Biometric identifiers, including finger and voice prints
- Full-face photographic images and any comparable images

as confidential. Furthermore, the covered entity may not expect or require an individual to waive any right the privacy rule allows him or her.

Documentation and Record Retention A covered entity, under the HIPAA regulations, is required to maintain documentation and information received from and about patients. A broad range of information is included under these guidelines (Box 2-5). All documentation regarding privacy policies and procedures must be maintained for a period of 6 years from the date they were created, updated, or last in effect (Box 2-6). If state laws require these documents to be retained for a longer period, the state laws must be adhered to.

Disposal of records and documentation in the dental office must also adhere to HIPAA regulations. All documentation ready for disposal that has individually identifiable information on it, such as a copy of the daily schedule or even a cassette tape containing a recorded telephone message with a name and phone number on it, should be shredded, not put into a trashcan. If the information being disposed of is in electronic form, it should be purged from any electronic or media device that contains it by individuals who can ensure the irreversible removal. Business associates of the covered entity must also provide to the covered entity or adequately dispose of any relevant personal health information.

Security Regulations

The security rule under HIPAA outlines the security regulations that covered entities must comply with. The **security rule** applies to all covered entities that collect, maintain, use, or transmit PHI. For example, in dental offices where claims are sent electronically to insurance companies, reasonable safeguards must be taken in compliance with HIPAA regulations to ensure integrity. Box 2-7 lists some of the standard

BOX 2-6
Documentation to Be Retained

- Policy or procedural documentation such as notice of privacy practices, consents, and acknowledgments
- Patient requests for access, amendment, or accounting of disclosures of personal health information
- Handling of patient complaints
- Procedures and policies regarding HIPAA training of office members

BOX 2-7
Common Electronic Transactions in the Dental Office

- Dental treatment claims
- Claims status inquiry
- Eligibility inquiry and response
- Coordination of benefits
- Claims attachments
- Remittance or payment advice
- Referral authorization

> **legal TIP**
>
> Patient treatment information that is transmitted to the insurance company must reflect treatment that was actually performed. Billing for dental treatment that has not yet happened is considered fraudulent activity, which has legal consequences. Each employee in the dental office is a representative of the dentist, and, as such, the dentist is responsible to a certain degree for your actions. Displaying integrity in your actions is a fundamental aspect of the position of the dental office administrator.

electronic transmissions covered by HIPAA and the ones most often seen in the dental office.

Whereas the privacy rule applies to all PHI in the dental office "in any form or medium," the security rule applies only to PHI that is electronically stored or transmitted. So, when PHI is sent electronically, the privacy rule applies generally to the collection and protection of PHI, and the security rule applies specifically to the electronic transmission of the PHI. The two rules work in conjunction with each other; one does not supersede the other.

The broader aim of the security rule is ensuring the integrity of the electronic PHI, as well as protection from unauthorized use and disclosure. The reference to integrity is twofold in this rule: (1) the trustworthiness of data, which means that the data entered are correct and reflect the circumstances and (2) the data are being transmitted by the entity it says it is from. The latter point is accomplished by each healthcare entity being given a number that identifies the entity so that each transmission of information identifies the entity. The security rule also addresses issues such as data backup, disaster recovery, and emergency operations.

There are three categories of standards identified by the security rule:

- administrative safeguards
- physical safeguards
- technical safeguards

In the dental office, computers are a regular fixture in both the administrative and clinical areas. Dental practice management software can include information such as patient accounts, demographic information, clinical data, schedules, letters, and accounting information, which, without proper safeguards, can leave a lot of very important information vulnerable to error and unauthorized use. This section provides an introduction to standards under the security rule. As you read through it, keep in mind that the size of the dental office and the availability of resources will play a role in the implementation of any of these safeguards.

Administrative Safeguards

Administrative safeguards are designed to provide accountability of covered entities in ensuring confidentiality of PHI and the integrity of the data transmitted. Under the security rule, each covered entity that transmits electronic PHI must have a contingency plan in the form of written policies and procedures. In the dental office, this means that there must be a formal process to protect the data that are stored on the computer and sent electronically in the event that the data are stolen or a disaster occurs such as a computer meltdown, a fire, or a flood. More importantly, this safeguarding process must be documented.

Developing this portion of the policy may be the responsibility of the privacy officer. As there are many staff members who may have access to electronic PHI, safeguards must be put into place. For example, in some dental offices, each person who accesses the computer files is given a unique log-in name, and that log-in name allows access to some or all data in the computer. This might mean that some

BOX 2-8
Points to Consider When Developing Administrative Safeguard Policies

- The location of copies of software being used
- The frequency of backup data, the location of the data, and which staff members have access to them
- The implementation of procedures in the event of a disaster and the recovery plan for data, software, and hardware
- What areas of data are accessible to whom?
- Are computer passwords changed regularly?
- Is the computer monitor that displays personal health information visible to patients?
- Does the staff training provided meet the HIPAA requirements?

what IF ?

A staff member approaches your work area to discuss with you the treatment that a patient has just received. There are other patients present in the area and in the process of the discussion the staff member uses the patient's full name. What would you do?

Politely inform the staff member that discussing the information at a later time may be more appropriate, or suggest continuing the conversation in a private area of the office. To avoid this type of scenario, all staff members must be familiarized to the policies and procedures of the office regarding patient privacy and information protection. This can be done at new employee orientation and reiterated at staff meetings.

employees have the capability to enter data while others do not. The HIPAA security rule requires a clear definition of which files can be accessed by each employee and which level of accessibility each employee has. Just as the privacy rule regulations under HIPAA require training be provided to staff members, so also do the security rule regulations. The development of policies in compliance with this area may also be the responsibility of the privacy officer. Box 2-8 provides points to consider when developing policies in accordance with HIPAA security rule legislation, which aims to decrease the security risks that can occur in a dental office.

Technical Safeguards

Technical safeguards under HIPAA regulations pertain to protecting the privacy and integrity of information that is transmitted electronically. Such safeguards include installing virus protection and firewall software. At a minimum, a dental office should implement passwords for system access and change them on a regular basis or use digital signatures. Furthermore, there is no guarantee that the insurance company or specialist office that sends responses to the dental office is using adequate virus protection software. In other words, making every reasonable effort to adhere to the security rule regulations in each individual office is necessary. Again, the dental office staff should be trained to implement these technological safeguards and to understand their importance.

A final point in the area of technological safeguards deals with the necessity to monitor activity on the computer system. Assigning each employee a password for access to the computer helps provide information regarding who accessed the computer and what data they created or changed. Such monitoring, via logs, is useful when investigating how errors may have occurred and is a requirement under the security rule. Most computer software programs have the capability to provide a log of when employees accessed information throughout a certain time period. The accuracy of these logs depends highly on staff members keeping their passwords confidential and not sharing them with other staff members.

Physical Safeguards

Ensuring that the PHI collected, maintained, and transmitted electronically in the dental office is not accessible to any unauthorized persons also requires physical security. Often, the dental office administrator is responsible for ensuring that office policies that apply to this area are implemented. **Physical safeguards** refer mainly to the immediate work areas where PHI may be visible to unauthorized persons, such as the cabinets or shelving units where patient files are stored, the front desk, where computer monitors may be visible and where the central processing unit may be located, and fax machines, where PHI may be received.

Taking steps to provide security safeguards, such as shredding documentation, placing computer monitors so they are not visible to others, adding a privacy screen

checkPOINT

12. What is the difference between privacy regulations and security regulations?

to the monitor or a time-out function after a few minutes of inactivity, and keeping central processing units in a secure area of the office, minimizes the risks of misuse and unauthorized disclosure of PHI. Additionally, the work area of the dental office administrator should never be left unattended. In some dental offices, the front reception area can be subject to violations of security if there are no staff members within view.

Identifiers

The National Provider Identification (NPI) is a government-issued identification number that is unique for each healthcare provider or healthcare provider organization. Each healthcare provider, such as clinics, hospitals, and group practices, must have a 10-digit NPI. Under the HIPAA legislation, this NPI must be included in the electronic transmission of PHI such as claims, claim status, eligibility inquiries, and claim attachments.

Transaction and Code Sets

In addition to the NPI, dental offices transmitting PHI electronically must use the specific procedure codes recognized under HIPAA. The American Dental Association (ADA) developed a set of uniform codes called the Code on Dental Procedures and Nomenclature (the Code), which fulfills the HIPAA requirement and which supports accurate reporting and recording of dental treatment. Dental offices submitting claims electronically, or manually on paper, must use the dental procedure codes from the most recent version of the Code.

ETHICS IN DENTAL OFFICE ADMINISTRATION

Professionals in the healthcare industry must use a high level of knowledge and skill in their role and, as such, have much responsibility. As a dental office administrator, you need to understand the reasons behind a dentist's decisions and the process required to make those decisions. If you understand the ethical dilemmas that healthcare professionals face everyday, you will be able to better protect yourself and the dental team by complying with legislation, enhance your level of professionalism, and keep ethical practice at the core of your role.

Dentists have a high ethical standard of conduct to uphold in their profession. They are ethically and morally responsible for the provision of dental care to their patients. As such, they make ethical and moral decisions each time they prepare to provide treatment. The ADA has established the principles of ethics that dentists should use to guide their behavior. The Principles of Ethics and Code of Professional Conduct (ADA Code) are essentially a public declaration of the ethical expectations that the dental profession has of its members.

Every dental assistant and dental office administrator who has certification through the Dental Assisting National Board (DANB) must adhere to the code of conduct inherent in that certification. The DANB code of professional conduct outlines the standards of professional behavior that all members of DANB must incorporate into their practice. Figure 2-5 provides the details of the code of conduct. The code of conduct provided by the state dental association should be familiar to the dental assistant practicing in that state.

Code of Professional Conduct

The **code of professional conduct** is an outline of the type of behavior, or conduct, that is required of dentists based on the principle in question. The primary responsibility

DANB's Code of Professional Conduct

To promote quality and ethical practice and to assist DANB Individuals* in understanding their ethical responsibilities to patients, employers, professional colleagues, including fellow DANB Individuals, the dental assisting profession, and the public, DANB has established the following *DANB Code of Professional Conduct*. The *DANB Code of Professional Conduct* includes a DANB Individual's responsibilities to patients, employers, colleagues, the profession, the public, and DANB.

Individual Autonomy and Respect for Human Beings

The dental assistant has a duty to respect each patient's individuality, humanity, and autonomy in decision making.

DANB Individuals shall

- Respect the autonomy of each person to decide from among treatment options, including refusing treatment.
- Respect the legal and personal rights, dignity and privacy of all patients in whose treatment they assist.
- Maintain professional boundaries in relationships with patients.

Health and Well-Being of Patients and Colleagues

The dental assistant has a duty to refrain from harming any patient. The dental assistant has a duty to promote each patient's welfare. The dental assistant has a duty to protect the health and well-being of colleagues.

DANB Individuals shall

- Always act in the best interests of each patient.
- Make patient health and safety the first and most important consideration in all actions and decisions.
- Undertake assignments only when qualified to perform them competently.
- Respect the health and safety of self, colleagues, and patients.
- Practice without impairment from substance abuse, cognitive deficiency, or mental illness.
- Diligently perform all duties designed to protect themselves and their colleagues from workplace hazards.
- Enhance professional competency through continuous learning, incorporating new knowledge into daily performance of delegated services.
- Refuse to conceal incompetent acts of others and report acts with a potentially dangerous outcome.

Justice and Fairness

The dental assistant has a duty to treat people fairly.

DANB Individuals shall

- When providing appropriately delegated oral healthcare services, behave in a manner free from bias or discrimination on any basis.
- Behave ethically, without a conflict of interest.
- Report unethical acts of others.

All DANB Individuals must abide by the *DANB Code of Professional Conduct and must maintain high standards of ethics* and excellence in all areas of professional endeavor.

Violating the *DANB Code of Professional Conduct*, including but not limited to commission of any act specifically prohibited in *DANB's Disciplinary Policy and Procedures*, may result in disciplinary action and the imposition of sanctions.

Truth

The dental assistant has a duty to communicate truthfully.

DANB Individuals shall

- Conduct themselves with honesty and integrity at all times.
- Provide patients with truthful assessment(s) of problems and potential treatments, including risks, within the DANB Individual's authorized scope of practice.

Confidentiality

The dental assistant has a duty to respect each patient's right to confidentiality.

DANB Individuals shall

- Maintain patient confidentiality.
- Safeguard all patient and practice information that is confidential in nature.

Responsibility to Profession, Community, and Society

The dental assistant has a duty to know the law, to act within the law, and to report to the proper authorities those who fail to do so.

DANB Individuals shall

- Obtain and maintain knowledge of governmental laws, rules and regulations that govern the dental assisting profession in the states where they work.
- Comply with their state's dental practice act and related rules and regulations, and any other local, state, and federal statutes that promote public health and safety.
- Refuse to accept assignment of duties that violate the state's dental practice act or administrative rules or regulations.
- Report illegal acts of others.
- Report violations of the state dental practice act, administrative rules or regulations to the proper authorities, such as the state board of dentistry, state department of environmental protection, state bureau of radiological health, etc.

Continued on next page

* *DANB Individuals* is an inclusive term that refers to all DANB examination applicants, DANB examination candidates, DANB Certificants (CDAs, COAs, CDPMAs, COMSAs), and those who hold DANB Certificates of Competency (RHS, ICE). See Definitions section for additional detail.

FIGURE 2-5 DANB code of conduct for dental assistants. Reprinted with permission from Dental Assisting National Board, Inc.

Responsibility to the Dental Assisting National Board, Inc. (DANB)

The dental assistant has a duty to know DANB policies and procedures, to act within them, and to report to DANB those who fail to do so.

DANB Individuals ***shall***

- Maintain current knowledge of DANB Certification and Recertification Requirements.
- Uphold the integrity of DANB credentials by representing credentials earned with complete accuracy.
- Report to DANB any misuse or misrepresentation concerning DANB credential designations or DANB trademarks by others.
- If certified, maintain DANB Certification in accordance with the rules and procedures established by DANB.
- Refrain from any action or behavior prohibited in DANB's Disciplinary Policy and Procedures.

DANB Individuals ***shall not***

- Engage in cheating or other dishonest behavior that violates examination security (including unauthorized reproducing, distributing, displaying, discussing, sharing or otherwise misusing test questions or any part of test questions) before, during or after a DANB examination.
- Obtain, attempt to obtain, or assist others in obtaining or maintaining eligibility, certification, or recertification through deceptive means, including submitting to DANB, the individual's employer or state regulatory body any document that contains a misstatement of fact or omits a material fact.
- Manufacture, modify, reproduce, distribute, or use a fraudulent or otherwise unauthorized DANB certificate.

DANB Definitions

The term ***DANB Certificant***efers to DANB Certified Dental Assistants (CDAs), Certified Orthodontic Assistants (COAs), Certified Dental Practice Management Administrators (CDPMAs), and Certified Oral and Maxillofacial Surgery Assistants (COMSAs). Those who have earned these credentials at one time but have not maintained them by complying with DANB Recertification Requirements are no longer DANB Certificants and may not use any DANB acronyms.

The term ***DANB examination applicant*** or ***candidate*** refers to those individuals who have applied for any DANB examination but who have not yet taken an examination, including national CDA, COA, CDPMA, RHS, ICE, GC, or OA examinations. DANB has contracts with many state regulatory bodies to develop, administer and score state-specific dental assisting examinations*DANB's Code of Professional Conduct* applies to individuals taking these examinations, as well, as long as a particular state Code of Professional Conduct, if one exists, does not supercede*DANB's Code of Professional Conduct. For a complete list* of DANB state examinations, go to www.danb.org, and click on State-Specific Requirements.

The term ***DANB certificate of competency holder*** refers to those individuals who have taken and passed DANB's RHS and/or ICE examinations.

DANB defines a ***Certified Dental Assistant (CDA)*** as a dental assistant, dental hygienist or dentist who

- Meets the education and/or experience prerequisites established by the Dental Assisting National Board (DANB) ***AND***
- Passes DANB's Certified Dental Assistant (CDA) exam, which is comprised of component exams covering Radiation Health and Safety (RHS), Infection Control (ICE), and General Chairside Assisting (GC), ***AND***
- Is currently CPR certified, ***AND***
- Continues to maintain the credential by meeting DANB Recertification Requirements (including continuing education, current CPR certification and annual fee).

DANB defines a ***Certified Orthodontic Assistant (COA)*** as a dental assistant, dental hygienist or dentist who

- Meets the education and/or experience prerequisites established by the Dental Assisting National Board (DANB) ***AND***
- Passes DANB's Certified Orthodontic Assistant (COA) examination, which is comprised of component examinations covering Infection Control (ICE), and Orthodontic Assisting (OA), ***AND***
- Is currently CPR certified, ***AND***
- Continues to maintain the credential by meeting DANB Recertification Requirements (including continuing education, current CPR certification, and annual fee).

DANB defines a ***Certified Dental Practice Management Administrator (CDPMA)***as a dental assistant, dental hygienist or dentist, or person with management experience who

- Meets the education and/or experience prerequisites established by the Dental Assisting National Board (DANB) ***AND***
- Passes DANB's Certified Dental Practice Management Administrator (CDPMA) exam, ***AND***
- Is currently CPR certified, ***AND***
- Continues to maintain the credential by meeting DANB Recertification Requirements (including continuing education, current CPR certification, and annual fee).

DANB defines a ***Certified Oral and Maxillofacial Surgery Assistant (COMSA)*** as a dental assistant, dental hygienist or dentist, or other healthcare professional who

- Meets the education and/or experience prerequisites established by the Dental Assisting National Board (DANB) ***AND***
- Passed DANB's Certified Oral and Maxillofacial Surgery Assistant (COMSA) examination, ***AND***
- Is currently CPR certified, ***AND***
- Continues to maintain the credential by meeting DANB Recertification Requirements (including continuing education, current CPR certification, and annual fee).

Effective January 1, 2000, the COMSA examination was discontinued because of low participation. However, DANB continues to recognize those who have earned the COMSA credential and maintain it annually by meeting DANB's Recertification Requirements.

The DANB *Code of Professional Conduct* represents the minimum standard of professional behavior to which all dental assistants should adhere. Dental assistants Certified by DANB, those seeking Certification through DANB, and those who have applied for or taken and passed DANB national exams, are subject to review under DANB's *Disciplinary Policy and Procedures for violation of any tenet* of the *Code of Professional Conduct . DANB has published* its *Disciplinary Policy and Procedures*which are available on DANB's website,www.danb.org. DANB's *Disciplinary Policy and Procedures addresses appropriate professional* conduct with greater detail and specificity. DANB encourages all DANB Individuals to review and uphold the tenets describe in both of these documents.

Dental Assisting National Board, Inc. (DANB) • 444 N. Michigan Ave., Suite 900, Chicago, IL 60611 • www.danb.org • 1-800-FOR-DANB

FIGURE 2-5 *(Continued)*

CANADIAN PRACTICE: CANADIAN DENTAL ASSOCIATION CODE OF ETHICS

The Canadian Dental Association Code of ethics is designed as a framework to guide the relationship between the dentist and the patient, as well as the dental profession and the community it serves. The dentist's first responsibility is to the patient he or she treats. The dentist is obligated to uphold the profession and adhere to the legislation under which it falls by conducting himself or herself in an honorable and dignified manner. For a detailed look at the code of ethics, the dental administrator can access the Canadian Dental Association Web site at: www.cda-adc.ca.

The Canadian Dental Assistants Association code of ethics reflects values upheld by the profession of dental assisting that include veracity, integrity, and respect. All dental assistants have an obligation to understand the code of ethics and incorporate the code of ethics into their practice. To develop and maintain public trust in the abilities of dental assistants to provide high-quality oral health care, the principles outlined in the code of ethics must be adhered to. The code of ethics for dental assistants can be accessed by going to www.cdaa.ca.

of a dentist is first and foremost to the patient. As the treatment options expand, adding to the dynamics of the doctor-patient relationship, the code of ethics and professional conduct is a document that changes to reflect these dynamics. The code of professional conduct is binding on the members of the dental association and, as such, any member who violates the code of professional conduct may face disciplinary action. The code of professional conduct applies strictly to the dentist. However, as the dental office administrator, you are acting on behalf of the dentist through your employment in the dental office and the actions and decisions you make, for which the dentist is responsible. For example, if you filed a claim to an insurance company for treatment that was not completed, the dentist is responsible for this false claim, even though he or she did not personally complete the claim. An understanding of the code of ethics for dentists and the responsibilities to patients will equip you with very important knowledge required for the position in being a successful dental administrator.

Principles of Ethics

The **code of ethics** is a guideline of professional conduct dentists adhere to in their practice. These principles are the goals that are aspired to in the profession.

There are five overarching themes that can be found in this code of ethics:

- patient autonomy
- nonmaleficence
- beneficence
- justice
- veracity

Box 2-9 outlines the five principles listed above.

Patient Rights and Responsibilities

Dentists and their patients have an agreement with each other whereby the rights and responsibilities of both parties must be considered and respected. A patient who makes an appointment at a dental office has made the choice to receive treatment from that dentist. The patient is under no obligation to see a specific dentist when making a selection and may choose freely from among all the available dentists. The first right in the dental patient's bill of rights (Box 2-10) refers to this selection process: the right to select one's own dentist.

checkPOINT

13. What is the difference between nonmaleficence and beneficence?

BOX 2-9 ADA's Dental Code of Ethics

Principle: Patient Autonomy ("self-governance")

The dentist has a duty to respect the patient's rights to self-determination and confidentiality.

This principle expresses the concept that professionals have a duty to treat the patient according to the patient's desires, within the bounds of accepted treatment, and to protect the patient's confidentiality. Under this principle, the dentist's primary obligations include involving patients in treatment decisions in a meaningful way, with due consideration being given to the patient's needs, desires, and abilities, and safeguarding the patient's privacy.

Principle: Nonmaleficence ("do no harm")

The dentist has a duty to refrain from harming the patient.

This principle expresses the concept that professionals have a duty to protect the patients from harm. Under this principle, the dentist's primary obligations include keeping knowledge and skills current, knowing one's own limitations and when to refer to a specialist or other professional, and knowing when and under what circumstances delegation of patient care to auxiliaries is appropriate.

Principle: Beneficence ("do good")

The dentist has a duty to promote the patient's welfare.

This principle expresses the concept that professionals have a duty to act for the benefit of others. Under this principle, the dentist's primary obligation is service to the patient and the public at large. The most important aspect of this obligation is the competent and timely delivery of dental care within the bounds of clinical circumstances presented by the patient, with due consideration being given to the needs, desires, and values of the patient. The same ethical considerations apply whether the dentist engages in fee-for-service, managed care, or some other practice arrangement. Dentists may choose to enter into contracts governing the provision of care to a group of patients; however, contract obligations do not excuse dentists from their ethical duty to put the patient's welfare first.

Principle: Justice ("fairness")

The dentist has a duty to treat people fairly.

This principle expresses the concept that professionals have a duty to be fair in their dealings with patients, colleagues, and society. Under this principle, the dentist's primary obligations include dealing with people justly and delivering dental care without prejudice. In its broadest sense, this principle expresses the concept that the dental profession should actively seek allies throughout society on specific activities that will help improve access to care for all.

Principle: Veracity ("truthfulness")

The dentist has a duty to communicate truthfully.

This principle expresses the concept that professionals have a duty to be honest and trustworthy in their dealings with people. Under this principle, the dentist's primary obligations include respecting the position of trust inherent in the dentist-patient relationship, communicating truthfully and without deception, and maintaining intellectual integrity.

Reprinted from the American Dental Association. Available at: http://www.ada.org/prof/prac/law/code/ada_code.pdf. Accessed March 4, 2009.

Patients also have the right to hold their dentists accountable to the highest standard of care. As discussed earlier in the chapter, the code of ethics outlines this principle, whereby dentists are to develop their skills and knowledge in their practice. Patients should be able to expect that the level of care they are receiving is of the highest standard and that the decisions they are making regarding the selection of treatment are based on the accurate information provided by the dentist, namely, that the benefits, risks, and prognosis of the treatment are fully explained.

Patients have the right to expect moral and ethical conduct from the dentist they select. Trustworthiness, honesty, and professionalism are all qualities that patients should expect from the dentist and the dental team. Even if the patient has not regularly visited the dentist or has not followed recommendations made by the dentist, he or she has the right to expect that the dentist will provide care (even emergency care) if and when needed.

BOX 2-10
Patient Rights and Responsibilities

Dental Patients' Bill of Rights

- To select your own dentist
- To hold your dentist accountable for the highest standard of care in the dental community
- To expect your dentist to be of the highest professional, ethical, and moral conduct
- To expect your dental health care team to maintain current continuing education
- To receive responsive urgent care and to be treated with courtesy, respect, and dignity
- To know in advance the type and anticipated cost of treatment
- To expect prompt appointment scheduling and a right to privacy
- To expect appropriate infection and sterilization protocol for all dental care
- To inquire about treatment alternatives and be advised of the risks, benefits, and cost of each option
- To know the education and training of your dental health care team

Patient Responsibilities

- To provide accurate and complete information and health history
- To ask questions until there is clear understanding on planned treatment
- To complete treatment as agreed upon and comply with all recommendations toward prevention
- To maintain appointments in a timely manner
- To treat dental team with respect and consideration
- To pay for services in a timely and agreed-upon manner

Regardless of the type or reason for the treatment, the patient has the right to be informed of the cost of the treatment before accepting it. This is a great advantage to the office administrator, who is responsible for collecting payment from the patient, as it eliminates any surprises for the patient.

As discussed above, the patient has the right to privacy of information as well as the right to proper infection and sterilization protocols. A patient should feel confident that the sterilization and infection techniques used are up to the recommended standard as a safety measure for both patient and staff.

Finally, patients have the right to know what the credentials of the dentist are, that is, what training the dentist received and the right to see the professional association membership and licensure. This document is usually displayed prominently where it is visible to patients.

Given the rights that patients have, this equates to many responsibilities for the dentist and the staff members. Since the relationship between the patient and the doctor depends on both parties participating in its survival, the patient also has responsibilities to the dentist.

In the dental office, staff members work very hard to provide care in a fair and efficient manner to all patients. In return for this right, the patient has the responsibility to be considerate of the staff members and other patients in the clinic. This means treating staff and patients with the same respect they would prefer. To receive high-quality care from the dentist and staff, patients have the responsibility of providing the dentist with up-to-date and complete information regarding their health history, which includes illnesses and medications they may be taking. If presented with treatment options, patients have the responsibility to ask questions about that which they do not understand. Additional responsibilities of patients include arriving promptly for their appointment, providing adequate notice for rescheduling, and paying for the services they received. Patients also have the responsibility to inform staff members of the dental office when they feel their rights have been violated.

checkPOINT

14. List five rights and responsibilities of patients.

Chapter Summary

Many dental offices currently implement several of the HIPAA regulations established to protect the privacy of a patient's health information. In general, the privacy rule under HIPAA requires healthcare providers to inform patients about their privacy rights and how the provider intends to use their information. Each dental office must implement privacy rules and procedures in accordance with HIPAA and follow those rules in the office by providing all staff members with proper training. A privacy officer or designated individual must be given the responsibility of ensuring that privacy rules and regulations are implemented correctly and followed.

Review Questions

Multiple Choice

1. The federal law that provides standards regarding the security and privacy of patients' health information is known as
   a. HIPAA.
   b. PHI.
   c. EDI.
   d. privacy rule.

2. Failure to take reasonable precautions to prevent harm to a patient is referred to as
   a. malpractice.
   b. negligence.
   c. mitigation.
   d. consent.

3. Written or spoken injury to a person or an organization's reputation is called
   a. breach of confidentiality.
   b. defamation of character.
   c. minimum necessary.
   d. malpractice suit.

4. The patient's agreement to being treated prior to treatment being performed is known as
   a. expression.
   b. expressed contract.
   c. implied contract.
   d. consent.

5. A dental office that transmits dental claims electronically is known as a(n)
   a. electronic data interchange.
   b. covered entity.
   c. personal representative.
   d. privacy officer.

6. A copy of the office's privacy notice provided to the patient is called the
   a. privacy rule.
   b. privacy practice notice.
   c. technical safeguards.
   d. physical safeguards.

7. The Code of Ethics is a document that
   a. provides a guide of professional conduct that dentists adhere to in their practice of dentistry.
   b. expresses the type of behavior, or conduct, that is required on the basis of the principle in question.
   c. explains the right of patients to make an independent decision about their treatment.
   d. is an agreement entered into between two or more parties.

8. An individual responsible for the implementation of policies and procedures and compliance with HIPAA legislation is known as the
   a. office administrator.
   b. HIPAA officer.
   c. privacy officer.
   d. office manager.

9. An example of a physical safeguard in the dental office would be
   a. leaving the work area unattended.
   b. placing patient charts in covered shelving units.
   c. using covered garbage cans.
   d. placing the computer monitor for patient viewing.

10. The "minimum necessary" refers to the amount of patient information that is
    a. transmitted electronically.
    b. taken from the patient.
    c. used and disclosed.
    d. given to the dentist.

Critical Thinking

1. How would you react to a patient who is calling to have his or her dental chart sent to another dentist?

2. Why is it necessary to have physical safeguards for patient information? What would you do if you were in an office where these safeguards were not used?

3. Why should the dental office administrator be familiar with the ADA's Code of Ethics and Professional Conduct if it is a guideline for dentists?

4. Why do you think is it necessary for patients to be aware of the licensure of the dentist?

5. Based on what you have read so far, what do you think is the most important aspect of HIPAA in the dental office, and how is it beneficial to patients and dental personnel?

HANDS-ON ACTIVITY

You have been hired as the office administrator for a brand new dental office in your area. The dentist has given you the title of Privacy Officer and has asked you to implement any policies and procedures necessary to bring the office up to compliance. Develop a brochure of privacy practices in the office that can be given to patients.

Web Sites

American Dental Association—Code of Ethics
http://www.ada.org/prof/prac/law/code/principles.asp

U.S. Department of Health and Human Services
www.hhs.gov

HIPAA Information
http://www.hhs.gov/ocr/hipaa/

chapter THREE

Infection *Control*

OBJECTIVES

After completing this chapter, you should be able to do the following:

- Spell and define key terms
- Describe how disease can be transmitted in the dental office
- Identify key agencies and regulations pertaining to infection control
- Explain the role of the office administrator related to infection control procedures
- Describe the use and purpose of personal protective equipment
- Properly perform and discuss the importance of hand washing
- Explain how and why equipment is sterilized
- Classify waste and discuss the importance of waste management in the dental office
- Discuss the material safety data sheet and how it relates to the role of the office administrator
- Identify the responsibilities of the dental patient in infection control

KEY TERMS

- occupational exposure
- infectious disease
- pathogens
- direct transmission
- indirect transmission
- cross-contamination
- bloodborne transmission
- parenteral
- sharps
- airborne transmission
- infection control
- standard precautions
- personal protective equipment
- biohazardous waste
- regulated waste
- nonregulated waste

OUTLINE

As an administrative member of the dental team, you need to understand not only the business aspects of the dental office but also some of the clinical facets. As the first person with whom the patient has contact in the dental office, you will be directly involved in proper infection control procedures through the collection of up-to-date and accurate health history information from the patient. Furthermore, controlling the occurrence of cross-contamination in the dental office is the responsibility of every member of the dental team. This chapter provides you with an introduction to disease transmission, agencies and regulations related to infection control, infection control techniques, waste management, and the dental patient's role in infection control, with emphasis placed on areas that directly relate to the dental office administrator.

DISEASE TRANSMISSION AND OCCUPATIONAL EXPOSURE

According to the Occupational Safety and Health Administration (OSHA), the clinical tasks and procedures that are carried out by dental office employees are classified into categories of occupational exposure. **Occupational exposure** refers to any reasonably anticipated skin, eye, or mucous membrane contact with blood or infectious materials that may result from the performance of duties. The nature of the duties that clinical staff members perform on a regular basis would put them at a higher risk of exposure to disease than computer clerks in the same office. Clinical staff, such as dentists, dental hygienists, and dental assistants, are regularly exposed to blood and saliva. Occasionally, the dental office administrator and other administrative staff members may be exposed to blood and saliva through their contact with clinical areas. This exposure may happen while sterilizing an operatory, moving instruments from one area to another, or assisting a patient who is coughing or sneezing. Table 3-1 shows the categories of occupational exposure in the dental office, as discussed above.

Methods of Disease Transmission

To become adept at avoiding the spread of infectious disease in the dental office, it is important to understand how it is transmitted. We will briefly discuss six methods of disease transmission: direct, indirect, cross-contamination, bloodborne, parenteral, and airborne.

Infectious disease is a disease that is contagious or can be spread from one person to another in some way. **Pathogens,** which are the organisms that cause disease, require a means of entering the body to infect an individual and are transferred from one host (person) to another.

One way of spreading an infectious disease is through **direct transmission.** Coming into direct contact with body fluids, such as blood and saliva, provides a mode of transfer for infection. Viruses and bacteria such as human immunodeficiency virus (HIV) and hepatitis are spread through direct contact with these body fluids. The clinical members of the dental team, such as the dentist, the hygienist, and the dental assistant, are exposed to blood and saliva each time they treat a patient.

Indirect transmission occurs when a surface or an instrument is contaminated by infectious microorganisms and then touched by a person. When a person

TABLE 3-1 OSHA Occupational Exposure Categories

Category/Class	Staff Members Included	Definition of Category
I	Dentists, dental hygienists, dental assistants, and sterilization assistants	Regular occupational exposure to blood and saliva while performing regular duties
II	Dental office administrators, office managers, and other administrative staff	Occasionally exposed to blood and saliva while performing duties involved in the clinical areas
III	Computer or insurance clerk	Never exposed to blood or saliva

legal TIP

OSHA conducts inspections of healthcare facilities from time to time to ensure compliance with OSHA standards. Citations for violations of these standards can be issued. Usually one employee in the dental office is responsible for OSHA compliance. This individual is often either a clinical staff member or the dental office administrator.

transmits microorganisms to an object, these microorganisms can easily be transmitted to another person if necessary precautions are not taken. **Cross-contamination** refers to the transmission of microorganisms from one source to another, whether the transmission is from one person to another, as in direct transmission, or through the use of an intermediary object, as in indirect transmission.

Clinical employees working in a dental office are well versed on the issue of **bloodborne transmission** of infectious diseases. Bloodborne transmission refers to the spread of an infectious disease by contamination of the blood. The bloodborne pathogens that are carried by infected individuals can be spread to others. The most common examples of bloodborne diseases are hepatitis B, hepatitis C, and HIV infection. The single most important source of these viruses is blood.

Exposure to blood in the dental operatory is common. Body fluids, particularly saliva, are frequently contaminated with blood. Blood may be present in saliva, even though it may not be visible. For this reason, standard precautions are taken in which the healthcare professional treats all human body fluids as though they were contaminated. In the dental office, bloodborne diseases can be spread through blood on instruments that are not sterilized properly, and the risk of transmission increases when standard precautions are not followed.

The risk of being infected with a bloodborne disease also increases when there has been a **parenteral** exposure to blood. The term *parenteral* refers to the piercing of the skin or the mucous membrane. Transmission via such parenteral exposure can occur when the dental employee has been cut or stuck with an infected instrument or needle. Instruments used for cutting or those that have pointed ends, such as scalpel blades and needles, are referred to as **sharps** (Fig. 3-1). Thus, proper handling, sterilization, and disposal of sharps are necessary to avoid parenteral exposure to bloodborne pathogens.

checkPOINT

1. Name and describe two methods of disease transmission in the dental office.

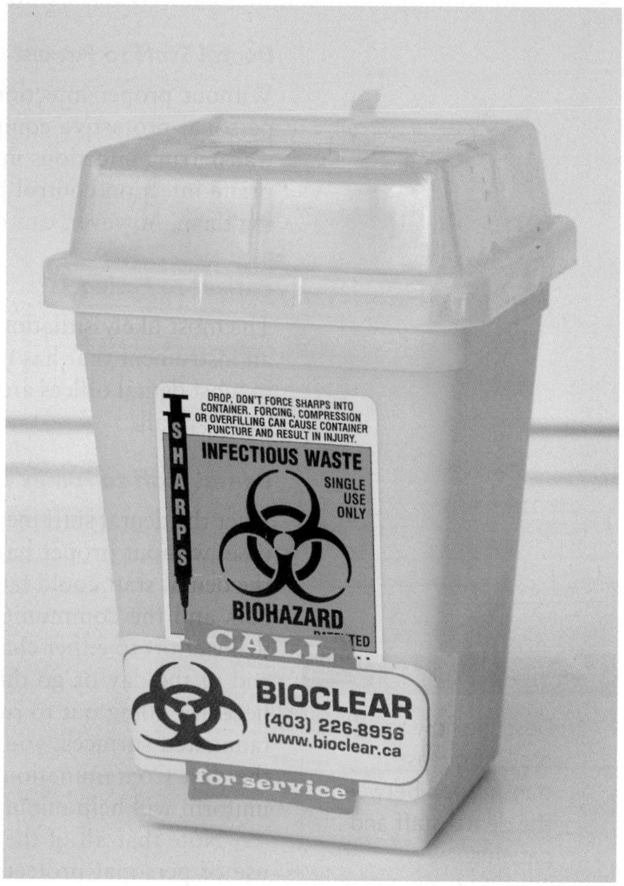

FIGURE 3-1 Sharps container.

Airborne transmission of infectious disease is present in many environments, from the movie theater to the grocery store. **Airborne transmission** refers to contact with droplets containing microorganisms that can remain in the air for long periods of time. Droplets are transmitted when an infected person coughs, sneezes, or exhales and another person nearby inhales this air. Respiratory infections are often transmitted through the air. In the dental office environment, personal protective equipment such as those listed later in the chapter prevents infection via airborne disease transmission.

Disease Transmission in and out of the Dental Office

In the dental office, all dental team members are exposed to infection and communicable disease, which can lead to illness. This exposure could also lead to patients, family members, or friends becoming ill if they are in turn exposed to the communicable disease. Specifically, transmission between people can occur in each of the following ways:

- patient to dental staff
- dental staff to patient
- patient to patient
- dental staff to family and community

Patient to Dental Staff

There are many ways in which patients can transmit infectious microorganisms in the dental office. As patients receive treatment in the operatory, their blood or saliva may contact staff members, or as they enter or leave the clinic, their exhaled breath, cough, or sneeze could transmit droplets into the air that could be inhaled by staff members. If the staff member should happen to touch any contaminated surfaces in the operatory without gloves, infection can spread.

Dental Staff to Patient

Without proper infection control procedures in place, such as hand washing and personal protective equipment standards, the possibility of a dental staff member transferring infectious microorganisms to the patient would be high. Having appropriate infection control procedures in place and staff members consciously following them, however, can minimize this risk.

Patient to Patient

The most likely situation for disease transmission to occur between patients is with an instrument that has not been sterilized. Because the infection control procedures in most dental offices are advanced and very strict, the chances of this happening are low, if at all.

Dental Staff to Family and Community

After the dental staff members have been exposed to a patient with an infectious disease, without proper hand-washing techniques and personal protective equipment, the dental staff could facilitate the spread of infectious disease to their family members and the community. If scrubs are the accepted uniform in the dental office, make effort to either change into street clothes before leaving the dental office at the end of the day or go directly home and change before spending time either in the house or going out to run errands. With the exposure to aerosols, spatter, and contaminated surfaces, your uniform traps some of these microorganisms throughout the day. Contamination can occur without visible stains. Promptly washing your uniform will help minimize the spread of these microorganisms.

Note that all of the scenarios discussed above have one thing in common: the use of personal protective equipment, combined with hand washing and correct

checkPOINT

2. Describe how to prevent disease transmission between the dental staff and patients.

sterilization techniques, minimizes the risk of infectious disease transmission in the dental office. These preventive measures are discussed in detail later in the chapter.

INFECTION CONTROL AGENCIES AND REGULATIONS

Because of the significant risks that infection poses to both healthcare workers and the general public, several key federal agencies and regulations have been established to reduce these risks. Because these agencies and regulations will impact your role in the dental office, it is important that you develop a basic understanding of them.

Centers for Disease Control and Prevention

The Centers for Disease Control and Prevention (CDC) is one of many components that make up the Department of Health and Human Services. It is a federal agency that monitors infectious diseases occurring around the world and issues reports that provide recommendations and guidelines with a view to managing disease incidence. The CDC (2003) provides guidelines for the dental offices in the United States, which impacts the management of infection control and disease transmission. This document, titled "Guidelines for Infection Control in Dental Health-Care Settings—2003," provides recommendations and procedures for assisting dental office employees in delivering safe oral healthcare. The document provides recommendations in areas such as the following:

- Personnel health elements of an infection-control program
- Preventing transmission of bloodborne pathogens
- Hand hygiene
- Personal protective equipment
- Contact dermatitis and latex sensitivities
- Sterilization and disinfection of patient-care items
- Environmental infection control
- Dental unit waterlines, biofilm, and water quality
- Special consideration topics in dentistry

Most of the items in the document are covered in this chapter. The document provides a very detailed and informative discussion about the CDC recommendations for dental office infection control. This document can be accessed through the American Dental Association (ADA) Web site and is a valuable document to have in the dental office.

Occupational Health and Safety Administration

An association within the Department of Labor, OSHA, sets standards and guidelines for employers to follow to ensure the safety and health of workers in all industries. Training, outreach, and education are provided through OSHA with a focus on continual improvement in workplace health and safety. Under the standards set forth by OSHA, employers in the dental profession must ensure that employees in the dental office are provided with correct and appropriate protective equipment from infectious disease. Box 3-1 outlines the rules governing healthcare providers, specifically dental care providers.

OSHA requires that all dental offices maintain a program whereby dental employees are given adequate training in the area of hazardous materials in the dental office, specifically regarding identification of hazardous materials, proper labeling, and maintaining an up-to-date listing of the materials in the dental

BOX 3-1
OSHA Rules Specific to the Dental Office

OSHA requires that the following standards are adhered to in a dental healthcare environment:

- A list of staff members who are exposed to blood-borne diseases on a regular basis by virtue of their occupation must be maintained.
- An exposure control plan, including postexposure procedures, must be available for employees to refer to in the event of accidental exposure.
- The employer must make available protective clothing that provides a proper fit.
- Training for all employees regarding exposure control standards.
- Hepatitis B vaccine must be provided to employees working directly with body fluids.
- Warning labels on biohazardous products and access to the material safety data sheets that accompany them.

office. Hazardous wastes commonly generated by the dental office include the following:

- photo processing water—x-ray fixer, developer, and cleaner
- suction line cleaner wastes
- amalgam wastes
- chemical sterilant wastes—chemiclave solutions for sterilizer
- universal wastes—batteries, fluorescent light bulbs

All employees in the dental office must be trained in hazardous waste management and disposal. This includes proper handling, suitable storage, disposal of materials, spill cleanup procedures, and reporting. Employees should be given a yearly refresher on hazardous waste training when changes occur in the procedures or methods; retraining should be provided. Furthermore, employees must be able to read, understand, and know the location of a material safety data sheet (MSDS). A dental office must also maintain a detailed list of all hazardous materials, how they were wasted, how the waste is managed, and how it is disposed of. The dental office administrator in conjunction with a clinical staff member often maintains these records. Examples of records to be maintained include the following:

- *Hazardous waste disposal log*: Dental offices should maintain records of all hazardous wastes generated and disposed of. Even though the waste may be disposed of off-site, it must be recorded in the log.
- *Amalgam separator maintenance log*: Regular service maintenance must occur for the amalgam separator, with a record maintained.
- *X-ray developer and fixer log*: A record of how and where used x-ray developer and fixer were disposed of must be maintained.
- *Employee training log*: A record of training activities and employees who participated should be maintained.

Labeling hazardous materials and waste appropriately is required in the dental office, and the label must provide the following information:

1. the date materials were first placed in the container
2. name and address of the generator of the waste (office name and address)
3. the type of hazard the material generates, for example, flammable, corrosive, or reactive

Laws regarding the disposal and shipment of hazardous wastes may vary from state to state. As the office administrator, it may be your responsibility to know the state laws in this regard as well as the OSHA guidelines. You can find this information by contacting your state environmental office.

Implementing Office Policies and Maintaining Records

The ADA provides all its members with written documentation regarding guidelines for practice as well as the administrative tools necessary for putting those practices into play, such as form templates and the details required on the forms. The dental office administrator and dental manager often consult the documentation and administrative tools provided by the ADA because they provide a framework for effectively running the dental office and keeping within laws and regulations. The *Regulatory Compliance Manual* includes information for the dentist and forms for use by the dental office administrator regarding compliance with federal OSHA guidelines. The guidelines provided focus on the following:

- train employees regarding infection control and hazardous waste procedures as mandated by OSHA
- create and implement an exposure control plan to protect employees from pathogens
- implement and maintain the hazard communication program
- keep records of your training and other compliance efforts
- find a facility for recycling amalgam waste in your geographical area

The dental office administrator will be privy to the forms and information provided by the ADA since part of the role of this position is to maintain office policies and procedures. Office policies relating to health protection of employees should be available for all employees to access through the office policy manual. The dental office administrative should be aware of the policies and could likely be involved in their development. The inclusion of each of the following should be found in a comprehensive office policy manual and adjusted to fit the office:

1. Immunization requirements for Class I, II, and III employees
2. Postexposure procedures
3. Exposure prevention
4. First-aid and emergency procedures
5. Exposure training and education

checkPOINT

3. How do the CDC and OSHA regulate infection control practices in the dental office?

Boxes 3-2 and 3-3 provide the information that a dental office administrator will need in the event that an employee or a patient is exposed to bloodborne pathogens in the dental office. The details regarding procedure to follow and the information required in the incident report are provided.

INFECTION CONTROL TECHNIQUES

Infection control refers to all procedures in both the clinical and administrative areas of the dental office that are to protect patients and dental team members from exposure to infectious agents. The safety measures taken in the dental office are

CANADIAN PRACTICE: INFECTION CONTROL REGULATIONS

The Public Health Agency of Canada outlines infection control guidelines for Canadian healthcare workers. In addition to recommendations made that apply to all healthcare settings and workers, such as training, management, and development regarding infection control guidelines (much the same as the guidelines used by American dental offices), the document specifically points out the higher risk of infection as a dental employee in that there is a high risk of glove puncture, increased risk of spatter, and use of instruments that transfer bloodborne pathogens. For more information regarding this document, visit http://www. phac-aspc.gc.ca.

BOX 3-2
Postexposure Report Documentation

The following information should be included in the exposure report, recorded in the patients' chart, and provided to the healthcare professional performing postexposure follow-up:

- Date and time of exposure.
- Details of the procedure being performed, including where and how the exposure occurred and whether the exposure involved a sharp device, the type and brand of device, and how and when during its handling the exposure occurred.
- Details of the exposure, including its severity and the type and amount of fluid or material. For a percutaneous injury, severity might be measured by the depth of the wound, gauge of the needle, and whether fluid was injected; for a skin or mucous membrane exposure, the estimated volume of material, duration of contact, and the condition of the skin (e.g., chapped, abraded, or intact) should be noted.
- Details regarding whether the source material was known to contain HIV or other bloodborne pathogens, and, if the source was infected with HIV, the stage of disease, history of antiretroviral therapy, and viral load, if known.
- Details regarding the exposed person (e.g., hepatitis B vaccination and vaccine-response status).
- Details regarding counseling, postexposure management, and follow-up.

From Centers for Disease Control and Prevention. (2003). Guidelines for infection control in the dental healthcare setting—2003. Available at: http://www.cdc.gov/mmwr/preview/mmwrhtml/rr5217a1.htm.

known as **standard precautions.** Standard precautions are safety procedures used before and during treatment for each patient to prevent the transmission of infectious diseases. The body fluids of all patients are treated as if they were infectious. These standard precautions are determined by the CDC and the ADA. The justification for using standard precautions is that it is difficult to identify patients who are infectious, and therefore all patients must be treated the same, that is, as if they may be infectious. Several key infection control techniques are covered below: immunization, personal protective equipment, hand washing, and sterilization.

checkPOINT

4. What are standard precautions?

Immunization

Employees in the dental office who are directly exposed to bloodborne diseases as a result of their employment duties are encouraged, for their safety, to be immunized against bloodborne diseases. The hepatitis B vaccine is an effective vaccination and is also available as a treatment for postexposure. According to the standards set down by the OSHA, every dental office must gather and maintain medical records

BOX 3-3
Guidelines for Postexposure Procedure

1. The individual who has been exposed must receive first aid immediately.
2. Report the incident to the dentist, office manager, or safety coordinator in the office.
3. Select a testing facility/practitioner for postexposure follow-up and cover all expenses involved in the follow-up.
4. Complete a postexposure report or an incident report. Also, see Box 3-2 for details of this report.
5. Ensure that consent forms have been signed by affected individual for permission to begin postexposure follow-up.
6. Maintain confidentiality of all individuals involved throughout the process.

FIGURE 3-2 Employee declination statement. From the U.S. Department of Labor, Occupational Safety and Health Administration (OSHA). Available at: http://www.osha.gov/SLTC/etools/hospital/hazards/bbp/declination.html.

Employee Declination Statement

I understand that due to my occupational exposure to blood or other potentially infectious materials I may be at risk ofacquiring hepatitis B virus (HBV) infection. I have been given the opportunity to be vaccinated with hepatitis B vaccine, at no charge to me; however, I decline hepatitis B vaccination at this time. I understand that by declining this vaccine I continue to be at risk ofacquiring hepatitis B, a serious disease. If, in the future I continue to have occupational exposure to blood or other potentially infectious materials and I want to be vaccinated with hepatitis B vaccine, I can receive the vaccination series at no charge to me.

Employee Signature:____________________ Date:_______________

for its employees who have occupational exposure to bloodborne pathogens, such as hepatitis B and hepatitis C virus and HIV. OSHA requires that employee medical records are kept for Class I and II employees. The medical record should contain the vaccination status of the employee and any information related to immunizations such as declinations and any follow-up of postexposure management. According to the CDC, dental workers may be at a greater risk for contracting or transmitting some vaccine-preventable diseases and, as such, documentation of immunity to these diseases is recommended. These diseases are hepatitis B, influenza, measles, mumps, rubella, and varicella-zoster virus infection (chickenpox). OSHA requires that documentation regarding immunization for hepatitis B include all dates of immunization. Hepatitis B vaccine is administered in three injections over a 7-month duration. Each date must be documented. In addition to the disease-preventing vaccines recommended, vaccination against tuberculosis and tetanus are two immunizations that are also recommended for healthcare professionals, since the risk of contracting or transmitting these diseases is higher, given the nature of the work and frequency of exposure.

If an employee declines to be immunized for any of the infectious diseases, for reasons known to him or her, such as religious views, previous reaction to the immunization, or simply not wanting the vaccine, an employee declination form must be provided to the employee and a copy given to the employee and one maintained in the employee medical file. Figure 3-2 is a sample of an employee declination statement for the hepatitis B virus vaccination. Promoting the prevention of vaccine-preventable diseases ensures health and safety among dental employees and within the dental professional. As a dental office administrator, promoting your own health and safety contributes to this.

The dental office administrator should be familiar with the procedure to follow in a situation where an employee or a patient is exposed to bloodborne pathogens. Box 3-3 outlines the actions that must be taken to address the concern. Even though vaccination is not available for all infectious diseases, following office protocol regarding standard precautions will lower the risk of infection significantly. The importance of understanding and adhering to safety procedures and infection control by all dental office employees is necessary to reduce the risk of transmission. Hand washing, the use of personal protective equipment, care and cleaning of instruments and surfaces, as well as the implementation of injury techniques all contribute to minimizing the risk of transmission to persons. Box 3-4 provides a list of the diseases and their mode of transmission in the dental office.

legal TIP

The code of professional conduct mandates that a dentist has an ethical obligation to immediately inform any patient whom he or she suspects may have been exposed to blood or any infectious material while in the dental office of the patient's need for postexposure follow-up and services. The dentist should refer the patient to a qualified healthcare practitioner who can provide these services. If the dentist or other employee is the source individual of the pathogen, he or she should submit to, or be encouraged to submit to, testing to assist in the examination of the patient. The incident must be documented in the patient's chart, and any follow-up actions taken should also be noted.

Personal Protective Equipment

As a member of the dental team, there may be occasion for the administrative staff to provide help in the clinical areas, such as cleaning the laboratory area, sterilizing operatories, and organizing supplies. For this reason, it is imperative that the dental administrator be aware of the necessary precautions to take to become confident in this area of the dental clinic. One of these precautions is the use of **personal**

BOX 3-4
Diseases and Modes of Transmission in the Dental Office

Airborne	Contact
Varicella-zoster virus infection (chickenpox)	Varicella-zoster virus infection (chickenpox)
Measles	Hepatitis A
Tuberculosis	Herpes
Droplet	**Bloodborne**
Mumps	Hepatitis B
Rubella	Hepatitis C
Influenza	HIV infection

protective equipment, items the healthcare worker wears to prevent from being infected by pathogens.

Examples of personal protective equipment are as follows:

- face masks and eyewear
- medical gloves
- uniforms

To carry out appropriate standard precaution procedures in the dental office, the use of personal protective equipment is recommended.

Masks and Eyewear

Masks and protective glasses, or face shields, must be worn during dental procedures to protect the eyes, nose, and mouth from contact with blood and saliva, which commonly spatter clinical personnel during treatment. Some staff members may require the use of prescription eyeglasses as a matter of necessity and will prefer to wear their own glasses. Protective eyewear often resembles safety glasses, with or without side shields and made of lightweight plastic. A dental mask should be worn by all dental staff members during procedures, while performing sterilization techniques, or when cleaning up an operatory. There are two commonly worn styles of masks, known as cone-shape or ear-loop masks (Fig. 3-3). Masks are made of lightweight breathable material, are available in various colors, and can be shaped to fit the face comfortably by a bendable strip over the nose. A new mask should be used for each patient and changed during lengthy procedures. Dental office administrators who help out in the clinical areas with wiping down operatories or laboratory areas should wear a protective mask.

Gloves

Dental personnel are most likely to contact blood with their hands. Gloves provide good protection from microorganisms that can be found in blood and are particularly needed if you have small breaks in the skin of your hands, such as paper cuts and hangnails (Fig. 3-4). Medical gloves must be worn during all dental procedures with a patient. A new pair of gloves is worn for each patient. Gloves must also be worn during cleanup of operatories and when handling any instruments. Gloves are available in latex and nonlatex types. Some patients, as well as some dental team members, may have sensitivities or allergies to latex products. For this reason, medical gloves are available in nonlatex varieties. It is important to note, however, that there are many sources of latex in the dental office that can cause an allergic reaction in some patients. These items include masks, goggles, rubber dams, orthodontic

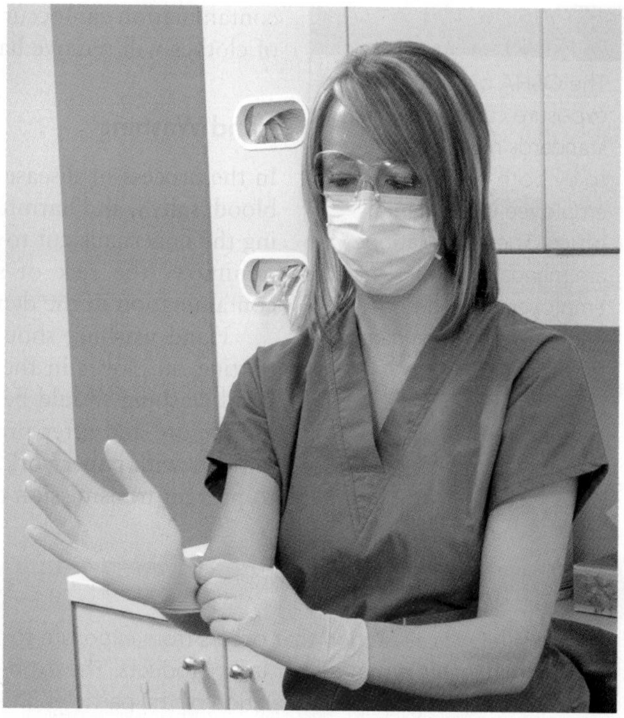

FIGURE 3-3 Personal protective equipment.

elastics, and mixing bowls. An appropriate time of day to schedule appointments for patients who have a high sensitivity to latex is the first opening in the daily schedule. Throughout the day, glove powder can infiltrate the air and collect on uniforms. An early morning appointment would avoid this risk.

Uniforms

In the dental office, many types of uniforms are worn by clinical personnel. The most commonly worn uniforms are scrubs, a lab coat over clothes, or employer-issued clothing. If you anticipate assisting the clinical staff, including working in the sterilization or laboratory areas or sterilizing the operatory, protect your clothes from contamination by wearing a lab coat or come prepared by wearing a uniform.

If your clothes do become visibly contaminated with blood, change them. It is important to wear clean work clothes each day to the dental office, whether you wear scrubs or street clothes, and launder your work clothes regularly, since

> **checkPOINT**
>
> 5. List and describe the purpose of three personal protective items.

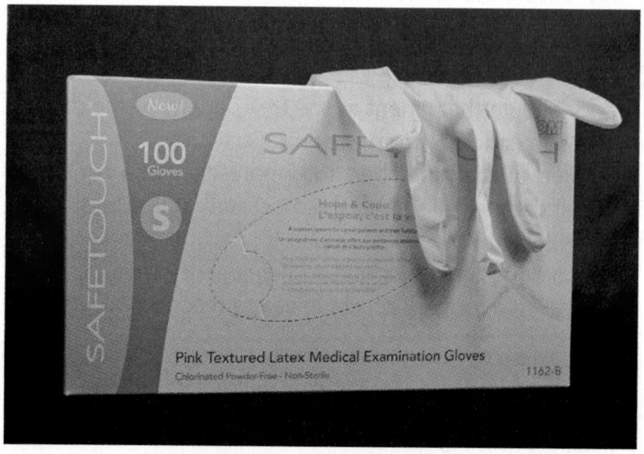

FIGURE 3-4 Gloves.

contamination can occur and not be visible to the eye. Normal washing and drying of clothes will remove harmful microorganisms.

legal TIP

The OSHA occupational exposure categories and standards must be adhered to by both employer and employee in the dental office. These regulations are mandated, and employers who do not implement the standards may be fined.

Hand Washing

In the process of disease transmission, our hands can be a vehicle for transmitting blood, saliva, and harmful microorganisms, particularly under the fingernails. Keeping the fingernails cut to a short, functional length and ensuring that they are clean minimizes the risk of spreading infection. Controlling and preventing cross-contamination in the dental office can be accomplished through hand washing.

Hand washing should be done after interacting with each patient and before putting on gloves in the clinical environment. In the administrative environment, hand washing should be done periodically throughout the day, such as before eating, before and after providing help with cleaning operatories, and after assisting patients with paperwork. See Procedure 3-1 for proper steps in washing your hands to prevent transmission of infectious diseases.

Alcohol gels and rubs are also an effective and yet convenient way to prevent the transmission of pathogens through contact. Adherence to hand hygiene is easier when an alcohol-based hand disinfectant is nearby. The CDC guidelines encourage the use of alcohol-based hand disinfectants. In the dental office, hand-sanitizing solution can be made available for patient use in the reception area and for staff use in offices and lunchrooms as well as at the administrator's desk. It normally takes 15–20 seconds to perform hand hygiene using this method from start until hands are dry. If your hands dry in less time, an insufficient amount of sanitizing solution was applied. Alcohol-based sanitizers usually contain an emollient that is nourishing to skin, thus decreasing the breakdown of skin. See Procedure 3-2 for proper steps in the application of an alcohol hand disinfectant.

Hand washing can greatly reduce the potential transmission of pathogens that can be found on hands. It is considered the most important technique a dental healthcare worker can perform to reduce the risk of transmitting infectious diseases. In addition to regular hand washing, maintaining nails and the skin on hands also minimizes the risk of transmission. Consideration must be given to nail length, jewelry, and the benefits of maintaining hands free from abrasions.

Also, in most dental offices, the clinical area sinks have a foot plate activator or hands-free sensor for turning on the water flow (Fig. 3-5). This eliminates the possibility of cross-contamination from sink taps.

Administrative TIP

A latex allergy is a reaction that occurs from exposure to the protein ingredient in rubber latex products. The exposure can be through skin or inhalation of the particles. Reactions can occur quickly or have a slower onset and usually present as a skin rash, a respiratory irritation, asthma, or, in very rare cases, shock. Dental patients who have a history of latex allergies should not be exposed to products in the dental office that contain latex, such as gloves, rubber dams, orthodontic elastics, and prophylaxis cups. It is the role of the dental office administrator to provide all patients with information forms and health history forms, or health history update forms, when they come in to the dental office. Once patients have completed these forms, they are reviewed for completeness by the dental office administrator. Any question or area of the form that is not completed must be addressed by the office administrator. Sometimes patients are unaware of the importance of informing the dentist and other employees in the office of allergies and sensitivities they may have. Patients who have a latex allergy may not be aware of the severity of their allergy until they are exposed once more to the substance. For this reason, the office administrator should consider the following helpful tips when a patient with a latex allergy comes in to the office:

- Schedule the patient as the first patient of the day to avoid exposure from airborne particles
- Alert all staff members to the presence of a patient with a latex allergy so that necessary precautions can be taken
- Have the office first-aid and emergency treatment kit available for easy access in case a reaction occurs

Being aware of how to proactively manage a situation with a patient who has a latex allergy will minimize the risk of exposure to the patient.

Fingernails

Keeping fingernails cut to a short length and smooth is advantageous for many reasons:

- Shorter nails are easier to keep clean.
- Most infectious organisms are found under the nails.

PROCEDURE 3-1 *Hand Washing*

The following steps outline a correct hand-washing procedure.

1. Remove all jewelry (rings, watches, bracelets).
2. Turn on the tap and run cool water at a medium stream. Use antimicrobial soap.
3. Lather hands, wrists, and forearms. Rub all surfaces using light pressure. Fingers should interlace. Wash each finger individually, rubbing with a back-and-forth motion with light pressure.
4. Rinse thoroughly under the running water, starting from the forearms to the fingertips.
5. Repeat the process.
6. Use a paper towel to dry your hands and forearms.
7. Use a paper towel to turn off the tap. Do not use hands to turn off the tap as the risk of recontamination to hands is greater.

- Sharp or pointy nails can make it difficult to wear gloves and may cause tears.
- Chipped nail polish can harbor added bacteria.
- Artificial nails carry a greater number of microorganisms, even after hand washing.

Overall, having shorter nails that are cared for by keeping them clean and smooth, with the cuticles trimmed, makes hand washing more effective, as there is a decreased chance of a large number of microorganisms harboring under the nails.

Jewelry

It is recommended that jewelry worn by dental staff be removed at the beginning of the day, since microorganisms can become embedded in small crevices of jewelry. The following points are not designed to discourage the habit of wearing jewelry to work but aim to provide techniques to make staff members more aware of the importance of thorough hand-washing techniques. Rings, bracelets, and watches are all elements that can harbor microorganisms. The first thing that should be done before hand washing is removal of jewelry. It is important to remember to wipe down jewelry as well, as spatter and other microorganisms can contaminate jewelry. Rings can provide an additional hazard in that they can create difficulty when wearing gloves by causing ill-fitting gloves or tears.

checkPOINT

6. What is the most important procedure you can perform in minimizing the spread of infectious disease?

Hand Abrasions

Wearing powdered gloves, frequent hand washing, and the use of harsh chemicals when cleaning, as well as severe weather, can cause dryness and cracks in the skin on the hands. Use of hand lotions can ease skin dryness most effectively. Leaving dry skin unattended can lead to abrasions and dermatitis, which can leave the areas susceptible to microorganisms, thus aiding the spread of infectious disease.

PROCEDURE 3-2 *Alcohol Hand Disinfectant Procedure*

The following steps outline a correct application of an alcohol hand disinfectant procedure.

1. Squirt a small amount of disinfectant onto the palm of your hand. This is usually the amount from one pump from the bottle. Automatic or sensor dispensers will dispense adequate amount when hand is placed under container.
2. Rub hands together vigorously ensuring that all areas are covered adequately.
3. Ensure that tips of fingers and areas between fingers and thumbs are covered.
4. Continue to rub the solution into hands until it evaporates and hands are dry, approximately 15–20 seconds.

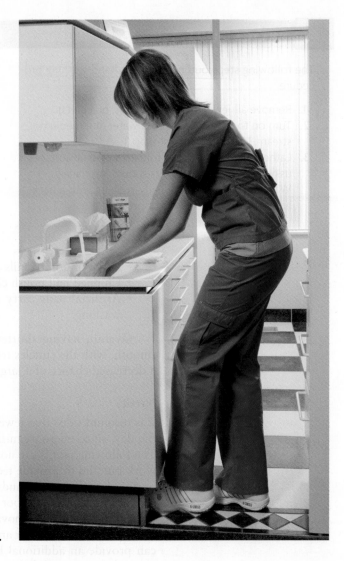

FIGURE 3-5 Foot-controlled tap in dental office.

WASTE MANAGEMENT

Maintaining a dental office that adheres to standard precautions before and after patient treatment is necessary for the prevention of spreading infectious diseases. Part of that maintenance includes the proper disposal of infectious wastes, that is, the proper removal of items used during treatment that cannot be sterilized for reuse and that may be contaminated.

There are many types of waste found in the dental office that the dental administrator will come across, for example, needles required for anesthetics, dental dams, cotton gauze, and suction instruments for blood and saliva removal. For this reason, the correct identification and proper handling and disposal of each type of waste are necessary.

Classification of Waste

There are two types of waste that the dental office administrator should be aware of and should know how to dispose of. These are biohazardous waste and regulated waste.

Biohazardous waste refers to biological hazards. These are items that are contaminated with blood and saliva during treatment and pose a risk to humans or the environment. **Regulated waste** is the term that OSHA uses to refer to biohazardous

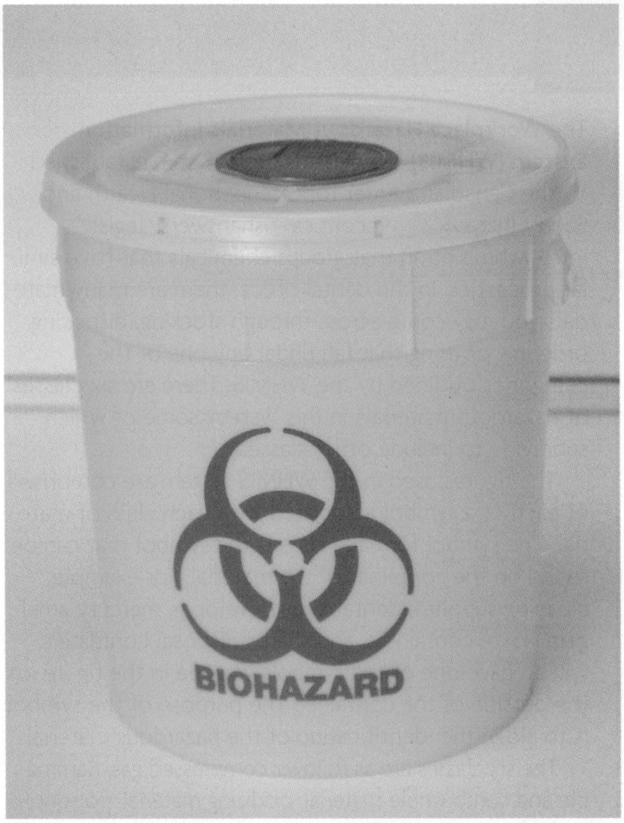

FIGURE 3-6 Biohazard symbol.

waste or medical waste. This type of waste includes blood or saliva, sharps contaminated with blood or saliva, and tissues (either hard or soft) that have been removed from the patient. Since saliva can contain blood, items that are in contact with saliva should be treated as if they were contaminated. Disposing of biohazardous (regulated) waste is usually the responsibility of the dental assistant or other member of the clinical staff, since contact with items that have been contaminated with blood, saliva, or tissues occurs during clinical procedures where the dental assistant is present. Specially marked containers and bags are used in the disposal process. Biohazard containers are generally labeled with the biohazard symbol (Fig. 3-6) so that those potentially exposed to hazardous substances will know to take precautions. Commercial regulated waste carriers are often used to collect the biohazard bags and containers from the office in order that they can be disposed of properly. It is important that the dental office administrator be familiar with what constitutes regulated waste and what is considered **nonregulated waste.** Nonregulated waste is often referred to as "garbage" or "trash." This includes paper products, disposable items, and plastic and paper wrap, all items that can be found in the dental office. If regulated waste is found in the nonregulated waste receptacle, it must be brought to the attention of the clinical staff.

checkPOINT

7. What is biohazardous waste?

Material Safety Data Sheet

The MSDS is a document that accompanies a product for the purpose of providing information regarding hazards associated with it, such as health, reactivity, fire, and environmental hazards, as well as information on how to work safely with the product. An MSDS provides the following required information:

1. Product information: name of the product and manufacturers' and suppliers' names, addresses, and emergency phone numbers
2. Hazardous ingredients

CANADIAN PRACTICE: WORKPLACE HAZARDOUS MATERIALS INFORMATION SYSTEM

The **Workplace Hazardous Materials Information System (WHMIS)** is a classification system established by the Canadian Center for Occupational Health and Safety (http://www.ccohs.ca/oshanswers/legisl/intro_whmis.html) that groups chemicals that have similar properties. In the dental office, there are many materials you may come across through stocking, disposing, ordering, or using that fall under any one of the categories outlined by the WHMIS. There are six classes of hazardous materials in this system, some of which subdivide to include other classes.

The figures used in the WHMIS system are comprised of each of a symbol associated with each class of material. The symbol for each class is the symbol that can be found on the container of the material. For example, cleaning supplies, dental x-ray developer, mercury amalgam waste containers, and sharps disposal containers will all have one of the symbols you see in the figure on the outside of the container. The purpose of the symbol is to aid in the identification of the hazardous material.

The six classes are as follows: compressed gas, flammable and combustible material, oxidizing material, poisonous and infectious material, corrosive material, and dangerously reactive material. One of the regulations concerning these materials is that they are considered dangerous goods and, as such, are not able to be transported without an MSDS, discussed later in this chapter.

Although you may not come across every one of these hazardous materials in the dental office, it is useful to study these symbols so that you will recognize any hazardous materials that are in the dental office.

Compressed Gas

The compressed gas symbol is a picture of a cylinder surrounded by a circle.

Any material that is normally a gas and contained in a cylinder is considered compressed gas. Compressed gas is considered dangerous because it is under pressure. If the cylinder is broken by misuse and handling, it can become a projectile, which could cause damage to an object or a person nearby. Also, if a cylinder of compressed gas is heated, it will explode. In the dental office, you may see a cylinder of oxygen or nitrous oxide for sedation purposes.

Flammable and Combustible Material

Flammable means that the material will burn or catch fire easily at normal temperatures. Reactive flammable materials are those that may suddenly start burning when they touch air or water or may react with air or water to make a flammable gas. The material may be a solid, liquid, or gas. Combustible materials usually have to be heated before they catch fire. In the dental office, you may see butanes or solvents with the symbol of a flame inside a circle, which indicates that the material is flammable or combustible.

Oxidizing Material

The symbol for this class of materials is an "o" with flames on top of it. Oxidizers are materials that assist in the fire process by providing oxygen. An oxidizer can be a gas, a liquid, or a solid.

Poisonous and Infectious Material

These materials can cause serious harm to a person. There are three subdivisions of materials in this class, all of which are found in the dental office, so they will receive our attention.

1. *Division 1*: Materials causing immediate toxic effects, such as poisons, cleaning supplies, or dental x-ray developer, make up this division. These materials are identified by the "skull and cross-bones" symbol.
2. *Division 2*: Materials causing other toxic effects, such as cancer, allergies, or reproductive changes, are part of this division. The symbol is a "T" with an exclamation point at the bottom. Materials such as mercury and benzene, which are found in the dental office, fall into this category.
3. *Division 3*: Biohazardous infectious waste refers to the organisms that can be produced from infectious waste and cause diseases. In the dental office, sharps are the most common form of biohazardous waste. The symbol looks like three "c's" joined together in a circle.

Corrosive Material

Corrosive material can cause severe burns if it comes in contact with skin or other human tissue and can usually burn through clothing and other material as well. The damage is permanent. The symbol for this class of materials is two test tubes pouring material, one onto a hand, the other onto a bar, and showing the items being affected. This type of material would more likely be found in a dental laboratory than in the dental office.

Dangerously Reactive Material

Most of materials classified as dangerously reactive are extremely hazardous if they are not handled properly because they can react quickly and easily. An example of this type of material would be aluminum chloride. The symbol for dangerously reactive materials is a picture of a test tube with lines coming out of the tube surrounded by a letter "R" inside a circle.

3. Physical data
4. Fire or explosion hazard data
5. Reactivity data: information on the chemical instability of a product and the substances it may react with
6. Toxicological properties: health effects
7. Preventive measures
8. First-aid measures
9. Preparation information: who is responsible for preparation and the date of preparation of the MSDS

An MSDS contains information on the use, storage, handling, and necessary emergency procedures to employ should they be required. Having one location where all MSDSs are located is one way of keeping information safe and available to all staff members in the dental office. It is important to be familiar with the hazards of the products that you are exposed to in the dental office. If there is an MSDS that accompanies the product, familiarize yourself with the safe handling and storage of the product, as well as the procedures necessary to avoid exposure or mishandling.

checkPOINT

8. What are the components of an MSDS?

INFECTION CONTROL AND THE DENTAL PATIENT

Besides the infection control procedures discussed above, it is wise to provide infection control measures for the patient and to educate the patient on his or her responsibility in infection control. First and foremost, the patient must provide a complete and accurate medical and dental history to the dentist. Second, eyewear is essential for a patient at his or her appointment. The dental assistant is responsible for making sure that each patient is provided with appropriate eyewear. If the patient is already wearing eyeglasses, he or she will be given the option to wear the protective glasses instead of his or her own or to wear the protective glasses over his or her eyeglasses. Finally, at the commencement of the appointment, a dental bib is placed on the patient. This bib protects the patient's clothing from splash and spatter that may occur during treatment. Once treatment is completed, the dental bib is removed and the protective glasses are returned.

The patient may also be given a warm towel or wiper to clean any splatter that may have occurred during the procedure. As an additional measure, antibacterial hand gel and hand wipes may be provided to patients in the reception area to use before or after appointments. When educating the patient about the importance of infection control, it is important to be able to explain the necessity of the role that both patient and dental staff members perform.

what IF?

A patient has arrived for an appointment and has expressed concern to you about the dental assistant wearing gloves during treatment. The patient feels that this is offensive since she does not have any diseases that the dental assistant should be concerned with contracting. How do you respond?

It is important to educate the patient on the meaning of "standard precautions" and what is involved with this process, particularly, how these precautions protect the dental patient and staff members. The patient needs to be aware that every patient is treated the same; that is, all members of the clinical staff wear gloves for each treatment performed on each patient.

Chapter Summary

The role of the dental office administrator is not limited to administrative duties. Often you may be required to attend to light duties in the clinical areas. Familiarizing yourself with the infection control procedures in the clinical areas provides you with an understanding of how interconnected the clinical and administrative areas are in a dental office. The confidence that comes with understanding and the excitement that results from learning new concepts and procedures in the dental office, whether it is sterilization techniques or hazardous waste symbols, will make you a much more valuable employee to the dental office and possibly expand your interests in the world of dentistry!

Review Questions

Multiple Choice

Select the best response for each question.

1. **The spread of disease through contact with contaminated surfaces such as instruments, countertops, and handles is referred to as**
   a. cross-contamination.
   b. parenteral.
   c. airborne transmission.
   d. infectious waste.

2. **A pathogen is**
   a. a disease caused by a biological agent such as a parasite or bacterium.
   b. waste capable of causing or transmitting an infectious disease.
   c. a virus or microorganism that causes disease.
   d. the contact with infectious material as a result of an employee's duties.

3. **Sharps are infectious materials to be disposed of in a**
   a. dental material garbage can.
   b. sharps container.
   c. sterilized waste container.
   d. regulated waste container.

4. **The transmission of infectious diseases from body fluids contaminated with blood is called**
   a. airborne transmission.
   b. bloodborne transmission.
   c. cross-contamination.
   d. occupational exposure.

5. **Biohazardous waste refers to waste such as**
   a. items contaminated with saliva only.
   b. items contaminated with blood only.
   c. items contaminated with blood and saliva.
   d. all items used in the dental office.

6. **The following are all examples of personal protective equipment, except**
   a. glasses.
   b. masks.
   c. shoes.
   d. lab coat.

7. **Which of the following is NOT included on an MSDS?**
   a. name of the supplier
   b. fire or explosion hazard data
   c. first-aid measures
   d. location of the product

8. **Which of the following is not an infection control technique in the dental office**
   a. immunization
   b. handwashing
   c. sterilization
   d. transmission

9. **The most likely situation for disease transmission to occur between patients is**
   a. with an instrument which has not been sterilized
   b. when patients do not wash their hands
   c. this will never occur in a dental office
   d. when employees do not wash their hands

10. **Transmission of disease in the dental office can occur in all but which one of the following:**
    a. patient to dental staff
    b. dental staff to patient
    c. patient to patient
    d. community to family

Critical Thinking

1. One of the team members in the dental office continually brings patients' charts to the front desk while still wearing gloves worn during treatment and has on occasion used pens and left them on the desk when finished. Is there anything wrong with this, and, if so, how would you deal with it?
2. As a dental office administrator, you will spend most of your time in the administrative areas of the dental office, so why do you need to understand asepsis procedures and controls?
3. How do you think a malpractice lawsuit might occur as a result of improper infection control techniques?
4. Why do you think it would be beneficial to patients if you were to educate them regarding infection control procedures in the dental office?
5. How is learning about hazardous materials useful to your role as a dental office administrator?

Hands-On Activity

Your office manager has asked you to develop a one-page patient education sheet on the necessity of standard precautions in the dental office. You have been asked to include the specifics of these precautions and how they benefit the patient. It is necessary for the information sheet to be visually appealing and easy to read, as it will be displayed in the reception area.

Create a brochure for staff use identifying the different hazardous materials used in the dental office. Include at least one example of a product found in the dental office.

Bibliography

Bloodborne pathogens. (Standards—29 CFR) 1910.1030. (h)(1). Occupational Health & Safety Administration Web site. Available at: www.osha.gov/pls/oshaweb/owadisp.show_document?p_table=STANDARDS&p_id=10051. Centers for Disease Control and Prevention. (2003). Guidelines for infection control in dental health-care settings—2003. *MMWR Recomm Rep*. 52(RR17):1–61. Available at: http://www.osap.org/associations/4930/files/rr5217.pdf.

Centers for Disease Control and Prevention. (2003). Guidelines for infection control in dental health-care settings—2003. *MMWR Recomm Rep*. 52(RR17):7.

Centers for Disease Control and Prevention. (2007). Recommendations for vaccination of health care workers. Centers for Disease Control and Prevention Web site. Available at: www.cdc.gov/flu/professionals/vaccination/hcw.htm.

Wilkins, E. (1999). Clinical practice of the dental hygienist. 8th ed. Philadelphia: Lippincott.

Web Sites

Organization for Safety and Asepsis Procedures
http://www.osap.org

Occupational Safety and Health Administration
www.osha.gov

Centers for Disease Control and Prevention
www.cdc.gov

part TWO

Communication

chapter FOUR

Dental *Terminology*

OBJECTIVES

After completing this chapter, you should be able to do the following:

- Spell and define key terms
- Discuss the purposes of teeth
- Identify and describe the parts and tissues of a tooth
- Explain the differences between primary dentition and permanent dentition
- Describe the dental arches and the dental quadrants
- List the four types of teeth and their surfaces
- Name and describe the three tooth numbering systems
- Discuss the dental chart and how it relates to the dental office administrator

KEY TERMS

- edentulous
- crown
- clinical crown
- root
- enamel
- dentin
- dentinoenamel junction
- dentinal tubules
- dentinal fibril
- cementum
- cementoenamel junction
- periodontal disease
- pulp
- apical foramen
- primary dentition
- deciduous dentition
- resorbed
- exfoliated
- wisdom teeth
- mixed dentition
- permanent teeth
- secondary teeth
- succedaneous
- maxillary arch
- mandibular arch
- midsagittal plane
- midline
- posterior
- anterior
- diastema
- Universal Numbering System
- Palmer Notation System
- International Numbering System

OUTLINE

A familiarity with dental terminology related to the function, form, and purposes of teeth is a necessity for dental administrative personnel to answer general questions posed by patients regarding teeth and they require. Dental administrative assistants are often responsible for addressing patient concerns over the telephone and need to be able to answer general clinical questions confidently and correctly. Additionally, they must be able to read the patient's clinical chart and understand the treatment completed for billing purposes. Errors made in billing as a result of an inaccurate reading of the treatment performed can lead to problems with insurance companies and patients and a loss in revenue for the dental practice.

Thus, the study of teeth and their make-up, as well as the terminology used by dental professionals in relation to teeth, is discussed in this chapter. This chapter focuses on fundamental terms common to all general and specialty dental practices. Specifically, terms related to the purposes of teeth, the parts and tissues of teeth, dentition, arches and quadrants, types of teeth, tooth numbering systems, tooth surfaces, and dental charting are presented here. Studying the terms presented in this chapter is much like learning a new language. For some of you, the dental profession is a new world and understanding the language of the profession may seem daunting. However, correctly using dental terminology is crucial in effectively carrying out your duties.

PURPOSES OF TEETH

Educating patients on the value of healthy, functioning teeth is partly the responsibility of the administrative assistant. Although the clinical staff are well trained in this regard, administrative assistants too should understand how a healthy smile contributes to one's quality of life. Teeth serve many purposes throughout a person's life, three of which we will discuss here: speech, mastication, and esthetics.

Speech

The role teeth play in the formation and development of speech can be easily identified in the person who is without front teeth and, as a result, has a lisp. Other oral structures, such as the tongue and lips, also contribute to speech progress, but the teeth contribute directly to the formation of words in conjunction with these structures.

Speech is produced by the force of air from the lungs, through the voice box (larynx), and together the palate, tounge, lips, and teeth shape the air into sounds or speech. When making the "b" sound, for example, the lips come together to make this sound. Some letters in the English language require that contact between the tongue and teeth are made to pronounce the sound correctly. A lack of teeth in the mouth creates difficulties in this area. The pronunciation of sounds, specifically consonants, such as s, z, x, d, n, l and th, requires tongue-to-tooth contact. An edentulous individual would be unable to make these sounds. **Edentulous** means to be without teeth. An individual can be partially edentulous, some teeth are missing, or in complete edentulism, all teeth are missing.

Difficulties pronouncing speech sounds correctly can also result from malpositioned teeth in the mouth, a widening tongue caused by edentulism, and problems with the position of the upper jaw and lower jaw.

Mastication

Without teeth, the process of chewing, or mastication, of food would be impossible. Mastication breaks down food and is the first step in the process of digestion. The four different types of teeth found in the mouth assist in the act of mastication, through tearing, grinding, gnashing, and cutting. Later in this chapter, we will discuss the different types of teeth and their role in the process of mastication.

Esthetics

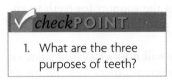

One of the first things we notice about other people is their smile. A smile, whether bright and healthy-looking or not, can affect a person's sense of well-being and self-confidence. The condition of teeth and the lack of teeth that one has can affect self-esteem. Ideally, teeth should be healthy, fully functioning, clean in appearance, with minimal space between them, and of an appropriate size for one's facial features.

> **checkPOINT**
>
> 1. What are the three purposes of teeth?

PARTS OF A TOOTH

A tooth is made up of many parts and tissues. The two main parts of a tooth are the crown and the root. The **crown** is the part of the tooth that is above the gumline unless the tooth is impacted or unerupted. The crown of each tooth varies in size, depending on the location of the tooth in the mouth and its purpose. The surface of the crown, the part that is visible and accessible during routine dental examination, is referred to more specifically as the **clinical crown.** The anatomical crown is the part of the tooth that is covered by enamel. The **root** of the tooth is the portion that is not normally visible and that lies below the gumline in the mouth. Teeth generally have one to three roots, depending on the type of tooth. For example, a molar has two or three roots, whereas an incisor will have only one. Figure 4-1 shows the parts of two types of teeth found in the human mouth.

Tissues of the tooth include enamel, dentin, cementum, and pulp. Pulp is found in the center of the tooth and contains its blood supply and nerves. The enamel, dentin, and cementum are layers that surround the pulp of the tooth. These tissues, which make up all teeth, are illustrated in Figure 4-1. Use this diagram as a reference as you read the description of each tissue below.

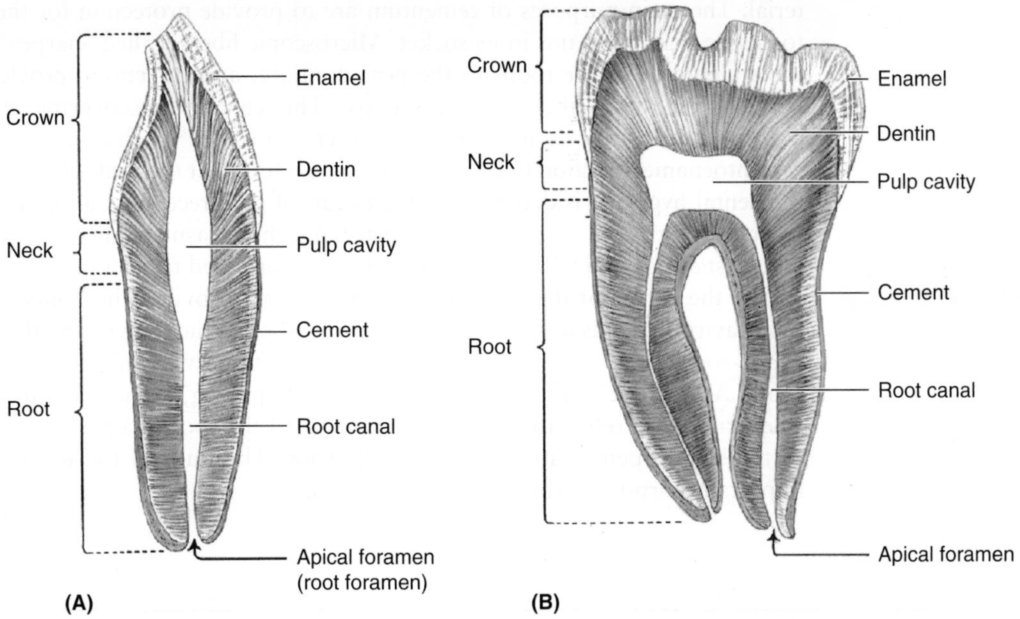

FIGURE 4-1 Anatomy and tissues of the tooth. Reprinted with permission from Moore KL, Dalley AF. Clinical oriented anatomy. 4th ed. Baltimore, MD: Lippincott Williams & Wilkins, 1999.

Enamel is the hard, outer tissue that covers the crown of the tooth. Enamel is made up of mostly calcified inorganic matter, such as calcium hydroxyapatite, and a small amount of organic matter, such as enamel matrix, as well as water. Enamel is the hardest material in the body. Given the amount of chewing, crushing, and grinding of food that that is required of teeth, enamel must withstand great force. The combination of the strength of enamel and softness of the dentin underneath it, as well as the cushioning support of the gums, provides the support for teeth to endure such force. However, as strong as it is, enamel is also brittle and can still chip or break and theoretically is incapable of self-repair.

If you look at your teeth and those of others, you will notice that the color or shade varies. That is, some people have whiter teeth, whereas others have yellow or gray shades to their teeth. The variations in shades are actually a result of the degree of translucency of the enamel. Underneath the enamel in teeth is a layer of a material called dentin. The translucent properties of enamel allow light to pass through which actually reveals the color of the dentin beneath the enamel. The combination of enamel and dentin affect the overall color of teeth. There are, however, other contributing factors to tooth coloring, such as disease, antibiotic use, drug use, and external staining caused by certain foods and liquids such as tea, coffee, red wine, or blueberries and tomato sauce. Other factors include cigarette smoking, decay, restoration on the teeth, and color variations in dentin. Furthermore, as a person gets older, teeth tend to reveal changes in color, which is a result of an increase in the translucency of the enamel.

Dentin comprises a large part of the tooth and is the main tissue surrounding the pulp. Most commonly it is yellow material that lies below the enamel and cementum and gives teeth their bulk. Dentin is covered by enamel in the crown and by cementum in the root. The dentin in teeth is not an exposed tissue, unless the tooth has been cut open or the enamel has been worn through but is visible on a radiograph. The surface of the enamel that joins to the dentin is termed the **dentinoenamel junction.** Dentin contains microscopic S-shaped tubes, called **dentinal tubules,** that extend from the pulp canal to the enamel of the crown and the cementum of the root. Within the dentinal tubules lie fibers, termed **dentinal fibril,** that assist the dentin in providing nourishment to the tooth and transmitting pain stimuli. Dentin consists of about 70% inorganic material and 30% water and organic substances.

Cementum covers the root of the tooth and consists of about 55% inorganic material. The main purposes of cementum are to provide protection for the tooth and to ensure that it remains in its socket. Microscopic fibers, called Sharpey's fibers, aid the attachment of the tooth to the periodontium, and cementum provides a rough surface for these fibers to adhere to. The cementum covering the root of the tooth meets the enamel covering the crown of the tooth at a point called the **cementoenamel junction (CEJ).** The CEJ can be found at the neck of the tooth. When the dental hygienist is determining the extent of gum recession, an indication of **periodontal disease** or aggressive toothbrushing, the measurement between where the gum tissue ends and where the CEJ begins is determined using a probing instrument.

At the center of the tooth is the **pulp.** Dentin provides the boundaries for the pulp cavity, which is made up of the pulp chamber, in the crown, and the pulp canal, in the root. Pulp is a soft tissue that contains the nerves and blood supply of the tooth. At the base of the tooth's root is a small opening, termed the **apical foramen.** The term *apical* refers to the apex, or tip end, of the root of a tooth; *foramen* refers to the small opening in the apex of the root. The pulp of the tooth serves very important purposes, which Box 4-1 outlines.

checkPOINT

2. What are the four tissues found in the tooth?
3. What is the apical foramen?

DENTITION

Dentition is the arrangement of teeth in the jaw. Throughout the human life, two dentitions, or sets of teeth, are present at different times.

BOX 4-1
Purposes of the Dental Pulp

Protection: responds to injury or decay of a tooth by forming reparative dentin.
Sensation: nerve endings in the pulp chamber provide the necessary sensory messages.
Nutrition: provides a method of transportation of nutrients from the bloodstream to the dentin in the tooth.
Formation: cells in the pulp termed dentin-producing cells continuously produce dentin throughout the life of the tooth.

Primary Dentition

Primary dentition, also referred to as "baby teeth," is the first set of teeth that a human possesses. The primary teeth can also be termed the **deciduous dentition,** which refers to the fact that primary teeth are shed, or fall out, and replaced by permanent teeth. The primary dentition consists of 20 teeth, when they are all fully erupted. Beginning at the age of approximately 6 months, the primary dentition starts to erupt, and this process continues over a 2-year period, until all primary teeth have erupted. There is no exact age at which a child's teeth will erupt, as developmental stages for children are different. For this reason, an approximate time is often given to parents who inquire about when they can expect their child's teeth to erupt or fall out. As the permanent teeth begin to erupt, the roots of the primary teeth are **resorbed,** this term referring to the wearing away or absorption of the root of the primary teeth caused by pressure from the permanent teeth erupting. The crown of the tooth is **exfoliated** or shed and replaced by the permanent tooth.

Mixed Dentition

The process of shedding the primary teeth begins when a child is about 6 or 7 years old and continues over about a 6-year period. At age 12 years, all or most of the permanent teeth have replaced their primary teeth, with the exception of the third molars, or wisdom teeth, which may never fully erupt or erupt later, in the teen to early adult years. **Wisdom teeth** are so called because they erupt when the person is entering early adulthood. Because both primary and permanent teeth are present in the oral cavity at the same time during this 6-year period, this stage of dentition is referred to as **mixed dentition.**

Permanent Dentition

Permanent teeth and **secondary teeth** are terms used to refer to adult dentition. Once all primary teeth have exfoliated, they are replaced by permanent, or **succedaneous,** teeth. "Succedaneous" refers to the fact that these teeth succeed or follow the primary teeth, occupying the space they previously had. There are 32 teeth in the permanent dentition. The first, second, and third molars in the permanent dentition are the only teeth that are not succedaneous. The primary molars are replaced by the premolars or bicuspids in the permanent dentition. Figures 4-2 and 4-3 show the permanent and primary dentitions, respectively.

*check*POINT

4. What is a mixed dentition?

ARCHES

There are two dental arches in the mouth: the upper arch and the lower arch. The upper dental arch is referred to as the **maxillary arch,** and the lower arch is referred

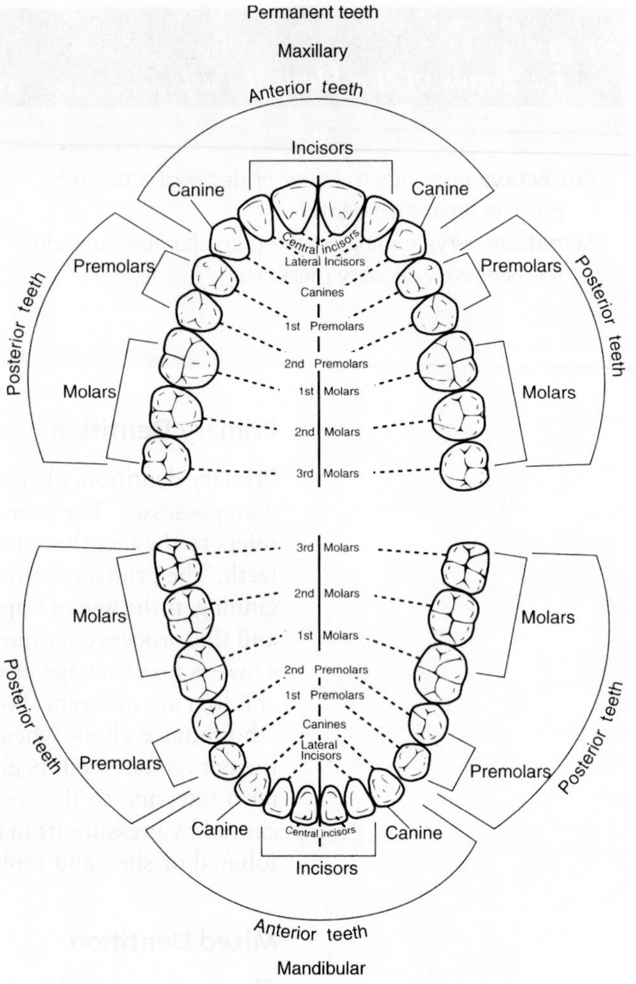

FIGURE 4-2 Permanent dentition. Reprinted with permission from Woelfel JB, Scheid RC. Dental anatomy: its relevance to dentistry. 6th ed. Baltimore, MD: Lippincott Williams & Wilkins, 2002: p. 4, Fig. 1-2.

checkPOINT

5. What are the two dental arches?

to as the **mandibular arch.** The maxillary arch is so named because the bone in which the upper teeth are set is the maxilla or maxillary bone. The maxilla is attached to the frontal bones and the skull and, as a result, is fixed in place and cannot move. Contrary to this, the mandibular arch, or the mandible, in which the lower teeth are set, does move.

QUADRANTS

In anatomy, body reference planes are used to indicate the locations of structures of the human body. Reference planes are imaginary lines that are used to divide the body into sections. The reference plane that runs longitudinally (up and down) and separates the right and left sides of the body is referred to as the **midsagittal plane.** This reference plane, also known as the **midline,** is the most commonly used one in the dental environment in reference to teeth. The upper and lower arches are divided by the midline into right and left sides, creating four sections, or quadrants, of the dentition. Each quadrant in the adult dentition contains eight teeth, and each quadrant in the primary dentition contains five teeth. The importance of the quadrants will become evident later in this chapter, when we review the numbering systems used for teeth. Each quadrant is abbreviated as follows: quadrant 1 (Q1), quadrant 2 (Q2), quadrant 3 (Q3), or quadrant 4 (Q4). Below are the names of the four quadrants:

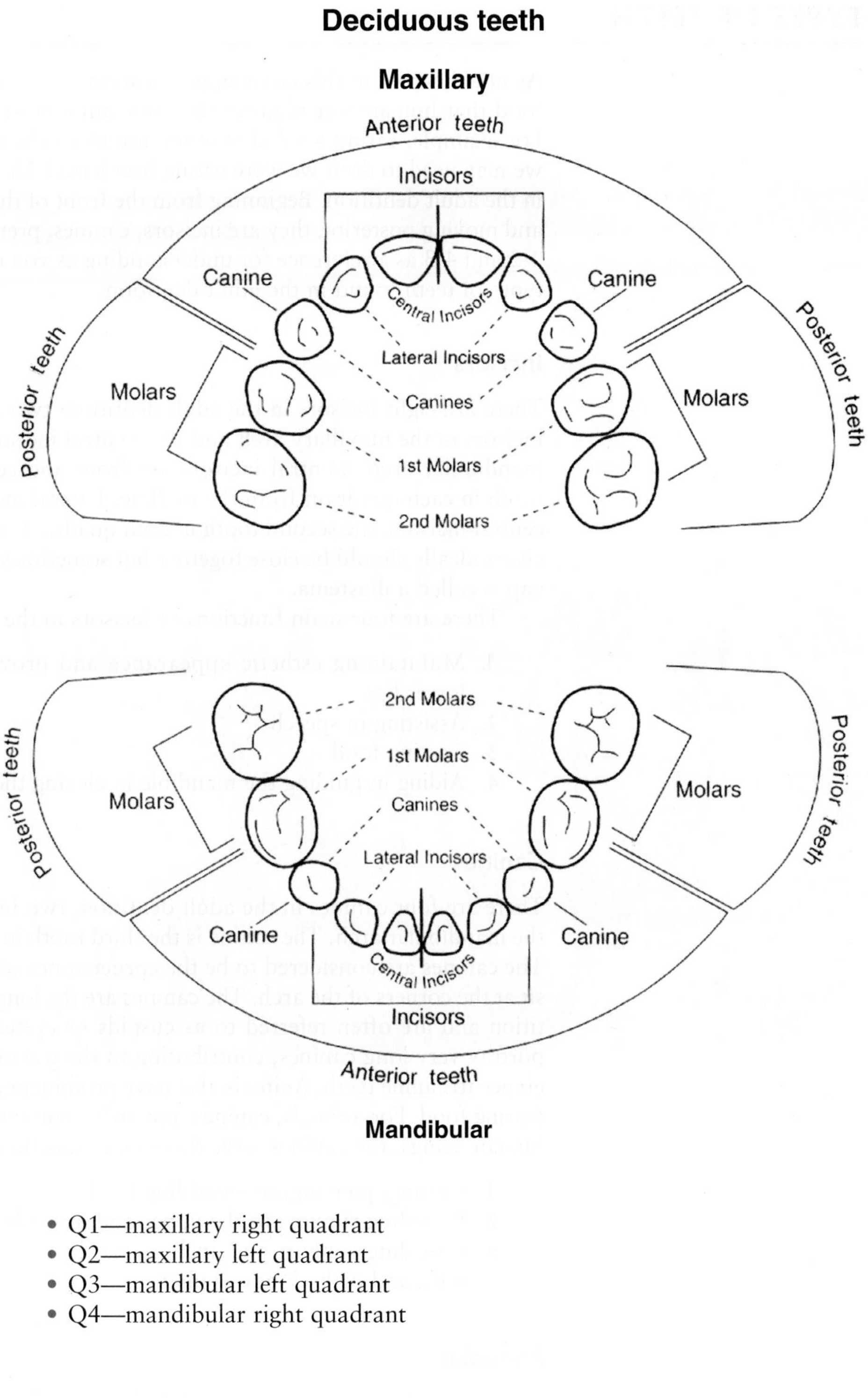

FIGURE 4-3 Primary dentition. Reprinted with permission from Woelfel JB, Scheid RC. Dental anatomy: its relevance to dentistry. 6th ed. Baltimore, MD: Lippincott Williams & Wilkins, 2002: p. 2, Fig. 1-1.

- Q1—maxillary right quadrant
- Q2—maxillary left quadrant
- Q3—mandibular left quadrant
- Q4—mandibular right quadrant

ANTERIOR AND POSTERIOR TEETH

Anterior and posterior are terms used to refer to the location of teeth in the oral cavity. Teeth are **posterior** if they are toward the back of the mouth and **anterior** if they are toward the front of the mouth. Anterior teeth are the teeth visible from the front of the mouth. These teeth include the first three teeth from the midline in each quadrant, which are the central incisors, lateral incisors, and canines. Posterior teeth include the premolars and molars. Figures 4-2 and 4-3 show anterior and posterior teeth.

TYPES OF TEETH

As noted earlier in this chapter, mastication is one of the purposes of teeth. Not all food that humans eat requires the same amount of force or effort from our teeth. For example, eating a salad may require us to chew, but not to tear the food, like we may need to do if we were eating beef jerky! There are four types of teeth found in the adult dentition. Beginning from the front of the anterior portion of the mouth and moving posterior, they are incisors, canines, premolars, and molars. Use Figures 4-2 and 4-3 as a reference for understanding as you read through this section on the types of teeth found in the adult dentition.

Incisors

There are eight incisors in the adult dentition: two central incisors and two lateral incisors in the maxillary arch and two central incisors and two later incisors in the mandibular arch. Central incisors are front and center in the dentition, the first tooth in each quadrant from the midline. Lateral incisors are beside (lateral to) the central incisors, the second tooth in each quadrant from the midline. The central incisors ideally should be close together but sometimes have a gap between them. This gap is called a **diastema.**

There are four main functions of incisors in the adult dentition:

1. Maintaining esthetic appearance and provide support to the upper and lower lips
2. Assisting in speech
3. Cutting food
4. Aiding in guiding the mandible in closing the teeth together

Canines

There are four canines in the adult dentition, two in the maxillary arch and two in the mandibular arch. The canine is the third tooth in the quadrant from the midline. The canines are considered to be the cornerstones of the dental arches because they sit at the corners of the arch. The canines are the longest teeth in the permanent dentition and are often referred to as cuspids or eyeteeth. Pictures of vampires often portray very long canines, contributing to the use of the slang term "fangs" in reference to canine teeth. Animals also have prominent canine teeth, which they use for tearing food. For animals, canine teeth are essential to their survival in the wild. For human beings, the canines serve three main functions:

1. Cutting, piercing, or shredding food
2. Providing support to the upper and lower lips
3. Providing support and anchors for dental appliances, such as bridges, partials, and orthodontic appliances

Premolars

There are eight premolars in the adult dentition, two in each quadrant. They are the fourth and fifth teeth in the quadrant from the midline. The premolars are so named because they replace the primary molars found in the primary dentition. They are also referred to as bicuspids. There are four main functions of premolars in the adult dentition:

1. Chewing food
2. Assisting canines in cutting food
3. Supporting the corners of the mouth and cheeks to keep them from sagging
4. Assisting in maintaining the vertical proportions of the face

Molars

There are 12 molars in the permanent dentition. In each quadrant, there are three molars: the sixth, seventh, and eighth teeth from the midline. Molars are the largest and strongest teeth in each dental arch. The last molar in the dental arch is named the wisdom tooth. Unfortunately, the wisdom tooth has garnered a negative reputation among dental patients for creating crowding and being difficult to keep clean, particularly to floss. Dentists commonly surgically remove wisdom teeth. Often, because little space is available for the tooth to erupt, much discomfort results as the tooth attempts eruption. All of the molars provide a large part of the chewing surfaces used in mastication, and not having all or some permanent molars can create problems for patients. The molars have four main functions:

1. Chewing and grinding food in mastication
2. Assisting in maintaining the vertical proportions of the face
3. Maintaining alignment among all other teeth in the dental arch
4. Maintaining support for cheeks and keeping the chin at a proper distance from the nose

checkPOINT

6. Name the types of teeth.

TOOTH NUMBERING SYSTEMS

All dental team members must help maintain accurate patient records. To identify a tooth in a patient's chart that has just been treated and to maintain accurate and consistent records, dental team members must use a common numbering or coding system. For example, if a patient receives root canal therapy on a tooth, that information must be recorded in the patient's chart. Instead of writing "maxillary left first molar root canal therapy," it would be more efficient to use a tooth numbering system and abbreviation guide. In this section, we will introduce three tooth numbering systems used throughout the world in dental offices. As not all dental offices use the same system, it is best to be familiar with all three. The tooth numbering systems are the Universal Numbering System, the Palmer Notation System, and the International Numbering System. Each system is different in how the teeth in the adult and primary dentitions are numbered.

Universal Numbering System

The **Universal Numbering System** is the tooth numbering system most often used in the United States and was adopted for use in 1975. All dental insurance providers accept and recognize the Universal Numbering System. This numbering system uses the format of numbering each tooth in the adult dentition with the numbers 1 to 32. It begins with the maxillary right third molar as number 1 and follows the maxillary arch to the left third molar as number 16, and then drops down to the mandibular arch on the same side, with the left mandibular third molar as 17, and follows the mandibular arch around to the right third molar, which is number 32. Figure 4-4 A and B provides an example of this numbering system, using the permanent and primary dentitions. The Universal Numbering System for the primary dentition uses the alphabet, letters A through T, for identification of the 20 primary teeth, beginning with the maxillary right second molar as letter A and following the maxillary arch to the left second molar as letter J, then dropping down to the mandibular arch on the same side, with the left mandibular second molar as the letter K, and following the mandibular arch around to the right second molar, which is T.

Palmer Notation System

The **Palmer Notation System** is a tooth numbering system that uses brackets to represent the quadrant of the tooth, with the tooth number appearing inside the bracket. Each tooth in the adult dentition is numbered from 1 to 8 in each quadrant, starting

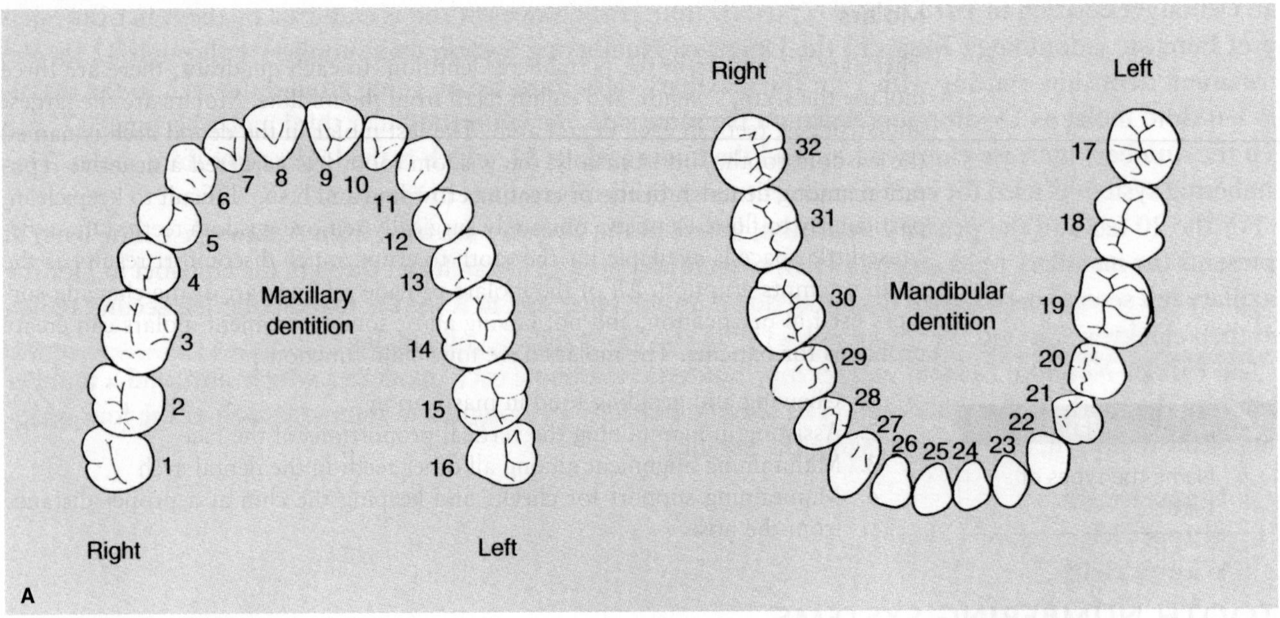

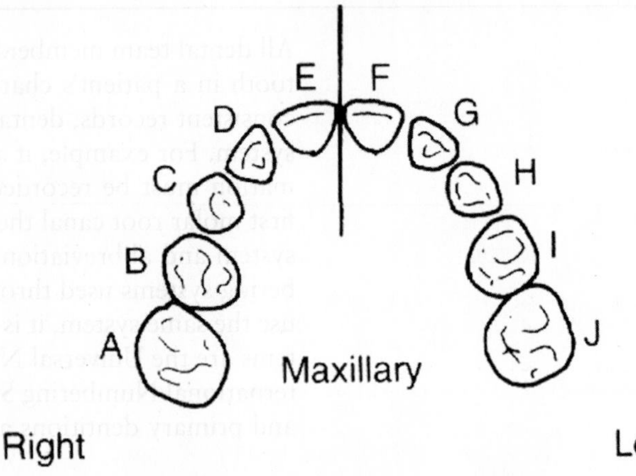

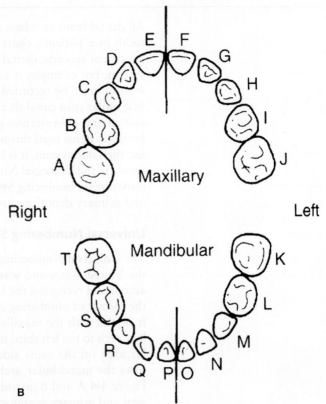

FIGURE 4-4 Universal numbering system. **A)** Permanent dentition. **B)** Primary dentition. Reprinted with permission from Woelfel JB, Scheid RC. Dental anatomy: its relevance to dentistry. 6th ed. Baltimore, MD: Lippincott Williams & Wilkins, 2002: pp. 80, 262; Figs. 3-1, 9-1.

with the central incisor as tooth 1 and moving away from the midline to the third molar, which is number 8. Each quadrant is assigned a bracket to represent it, as follows:

- _| represents the maxillary right quadrant
- |_ represents the maxillary left quadrant
- ‾| represents the mandibular right quadrant
- |‾ represents the mandibular left quadrant

For example, the maxillary right canine would be identified as 3|. For the primary dentition, the same bracketing system is used to denote in which quadrant the tooth is located, but letters A through E are used to represent the five teeth found in each quadrant. For example, starting with the tooth closest to the midline and moving posterior, the central incisor is labeled A, the lateral incisor B, and so on, with the second being labeled E.

International Numbering System

The **International Numbering System** (Federation Dentaire Internationale) assigns each primary and permanent tooth a two-digit number. The first digit signifies the quadrant of the tooth and the second signifies which tooth in the quadrant. In the permanent dentition, each tooth in a quadrant is numbered 1 through 8, starting with the tooth closest to the midline. For example, tooth 13 is the maxillary right canine, and tooth 33 is the mandibular left canine. In the primary dentition, each tooth in a quadrant is numbered 1 through 5, starting with the tooth closest to the midline (the central incisor) as number 1 and ending with the second molar as tooth number 5. The quadrants in the International Numbering System are labeled as follows:

1 = Permanent dentition, maxillary right
2 = Permanent dentition, maxillary left
3 = Permanent dentition, mandibular left
4 = Permanent dentition, mandibular right
5 = Primary dentition, maxillary right
6 = Primary dentition, maxillary left
7 = Primary dentition, mandibular left
8 = Primary dentition, mandibular right

Note that the quadrants in the permanent dentition are assigned numbers 1 through 4 and the quadrants in the primary dentition are assigned numbers 5 through 8. The numbers in the range 11–48 are permanent teeth, and numbers in the range 51–85 represent primary teeth. For example, a tooth with the number 51 represents a primary tooth in the maxillary right quadrant (5) and a central incisor (1). If this system seems confusing, consult Table 4-1, which shows all three numbering systems.

It is important to note how the international system requires that teeth numbers be spoken. In the Universal System, tooth 17 is said as "tooth seventeen." The International System requires that tooth 17 is said as "tooth one-seven." That is, each digit is pronounced individually and not as part of a double-digit number. This is important to remember because tooth one-seven (maxillary right second molar) is a different tooth from tooth seventeen (maxillary left second molar).

The remainder of this chapter and this textbook will use the Universal Numbering System.

checkPOINT

7. What are the three different tooth numbering systems used?

TOOTH SURFACES

Not only are individual teeth uniquely identified, but the surfaces of each tooth are also uniquely identified. When a patient receives treatment for a tooth, such as a restoration (filling), there are particular surfaces of the tooth that the dentist restores. To accurately and proficiently record the treatment, knowledge of both the tooth numbers and surfaces is necessary for the dental administrative assistant.

Each tooth in both the adult dentition and primary dentition has five surfaces. The surfaces each have a name, which are as follows:

1. Facial or labial (vestibular or buccal)
2. Lingual
3. Incisal (occlusal)
4. Mesial
5. Distal

TABLE 4-1 Tooth Numbering Systems

Tooth Name	Universal System Right	Universal System Left	FDI System Right	FDI System Left	Palmer System Right	Palmer System Left
Permanent dentition						
Maxillary						
Central incisor	8	9	11	21	1┘	└1
Lateral incisor	7	10	12	22	2┘	└2
Canine	6	11	13	23	3┘	└3
First premolar	5	12	14	24	4┘	└4
Second premolar	4	13	15	25	5┘	└5
First molar	3	14	16	26	6┘	└6
Second molar	2	15	17	27	7┘	└7
Third molar (wisdom tooth)	1	16	18	28	8┘	└8
Mandibular						
Central incisor	25	24	41	31	1┐	┌1
Lateral incisor	26	23	42	32	2┐	┌2
Canine	27	22	43	33	3┐	┌3
First premolar	28	21	44	34	4┐	┌4
Second premolar	29	10	45	35	5┐	┌5
First molar	30	19	46	36	6┐	┌6
Second molar	31	18	47	37	7┐	┌7
Third molar (wisdom tooth)	32	18	48	38	8┐	┌8
Primary dentition						
Maxillary						
Central Incisor	E	F	51	61	A┘	└A
Lateral Incisor	D	G	52	62	B┘	└B
Canine	C	H	53	63	C┘	└C
First molar	B	I	54	64	D┘	└D
Second molar	A	J	55	65	E┘	└E
Mandibular						
Central Incisor	P	O	81	71	A┐	┌A
Lateral Incisor	Q	N	82	72	B┐	┌B
Canine	R	M	83	73	C┐	┌C
First molar	S	L	84	74	D┐	┌D
Second molar	T	K	85	75	E┐	┌E

FDI, Federation Dentaire Internationale.

The names in parentheses in this list are the ones used specifically for posterior teeth. Some of the surfaces are so named as a result of their relation to other structures in the oral cavity and the direction that the surface faces. As we review each surface, this explanation will become clear. Each of the surfaces is given an abbreviation to represent the surface. The reason for this is for conciseness in charting and in correspondence with external agencies, such as insurance companies and other dental offices. For example, if a patient requires a restoration on the maxillary right first molar on the mesial, occlusal, and lingual surfaces of the tooth, this would be recorded in the chart as 3 MOL. As a dental administrative assistant, you must be able to recognize and properly interpret this abbreviation. When a restoration such as the one in our example is charted, the letters of each surface are pronounced separately; for example, 3 MOL is pronounced "three, M – O – L." The following are definitions of each surface name to assist you in understanding where the surfaces exist on each tooth:

- *Facial (labial or buccal)*: On anterior teeth, the names facial and labial are used. The facial surface is that surface of the tooth closest to the face; the labial surface is named in reference to the surface that is closest to the lip. It is referred to as the front of the tooth on an anterior tooth. On a posterior tooth, the name buccal is used to refer to the surface that is closest to the cheek.
- *Lingual*: The lingual surface of the tooth is the surface closest to the tongue.
- *Incisal (occlusal)*: On an anterior tooth, the main biting or chewing surface is referred to as the incisal edge. On a posterior tooth, the main chewing surface is referred to as the occlusal surface.
- *Mesial*: The mesial surface is the surface of the tooth that is toward the midline.
- *Distal*: The distal surface of the tooth is the surface furthest away from the midline.

checkPOINT

8. Name the tooth surfaces found on anterior teeth.

If you imagine a box with a closed top, you can count the four sides of the box and include the top as a fifth side, the bottom of the box would represent the roots. Now imagine a molar in place of the box, and you can see how there are five sides to a tooth. Figure 4-5 provides examples of the surfaces found on a molar. Anterior teeth, although thin and shaped differently from posterior teeth, also have five sides,

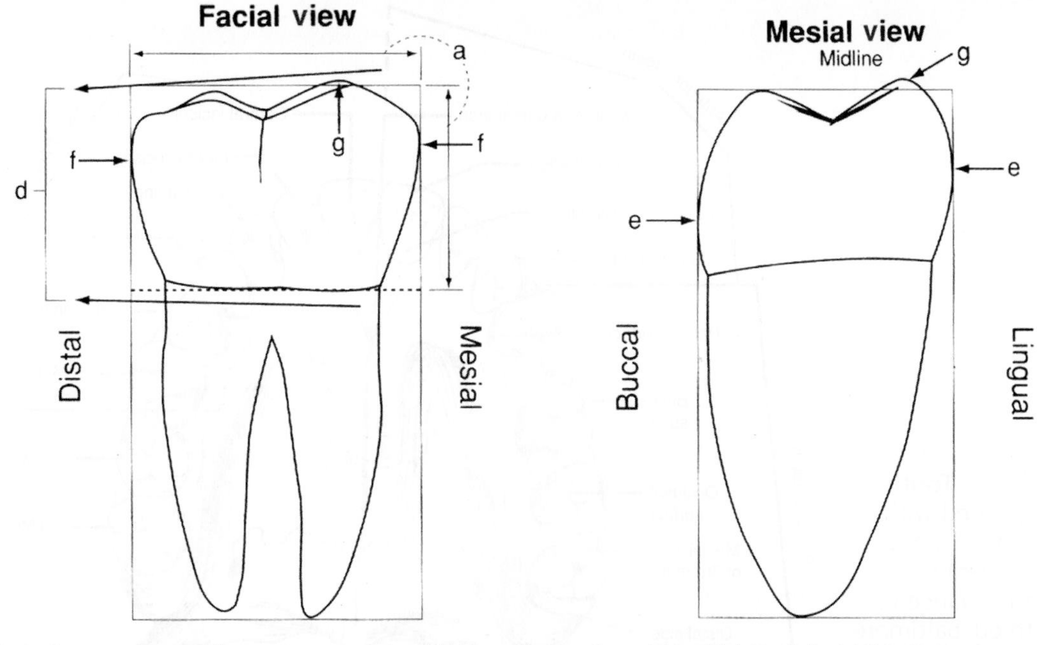

FIGURE 4-5 Molar surfaces. Reprinted with permission from Woelfel JB, Scheid RC. Dental anatomy: its relevance to dentistry. 6th ed. Baltimore, MD: Lippincott Williams & Wilkins, 2002: Appendix, p. 7. (*continued*)

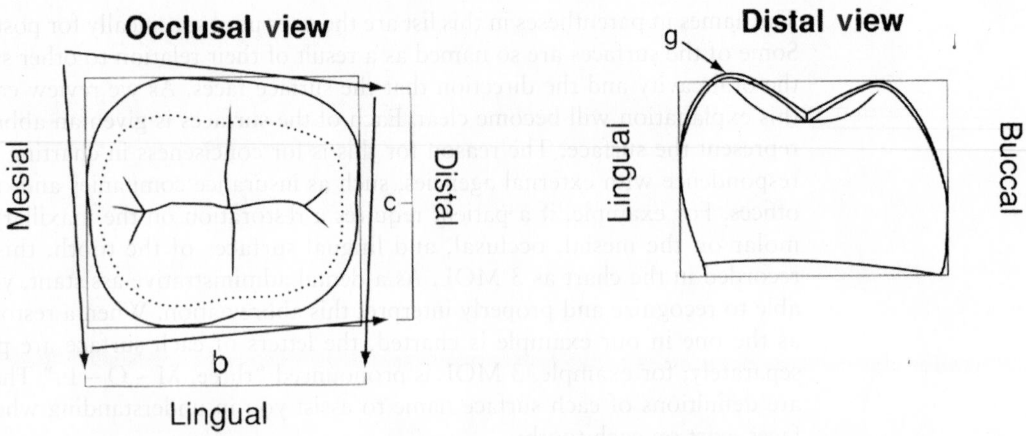

FIGURE 4-5 *(Continued)*

with the sides being much thinner. If you picture a rectangular box standing on end and replace this image with an incisor or a canine, you can see how these teeth also have five sides. Figure 4-6 shows the surfaces of teeth in reference to the above definitions. As you review the diagram, go over the surface definitions again to reinforce your understanding.

DENTAL CHARTING

As a dental administrative assistant, you should be able to read and interpret the dental chart and the charting notations that the dental assistant, hygienist, or dentist records in the patient's chart. To accurately charge for services rendered and maintain a correct dental report of the patient's treatment, it is critical to pay particular attention to the methods of treatment recording in the dental office. Each dental office may be different in the methods chosen for recording. That is, one dental office

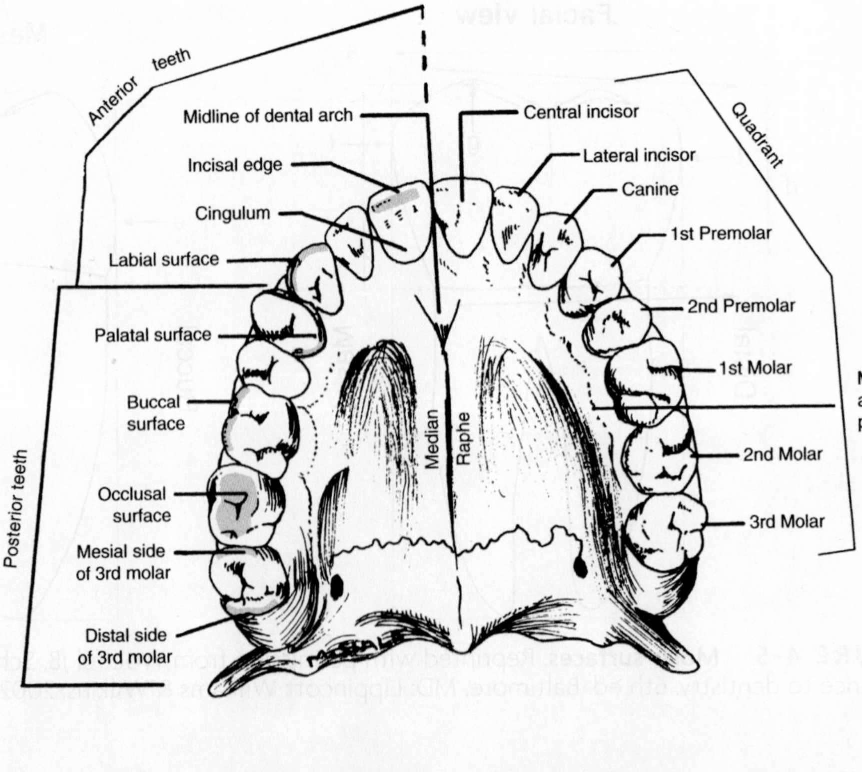

FIGURE 4-6 Tooth surfaces. Reprinted with permission from Woelfel JB, Scheid RC. Dental anatomy: its relevance to dentistry. 6th ed. Baltimore, MD: Lippincott Williams & Wilkins, 2002: p. 84, Fig. 3-3.

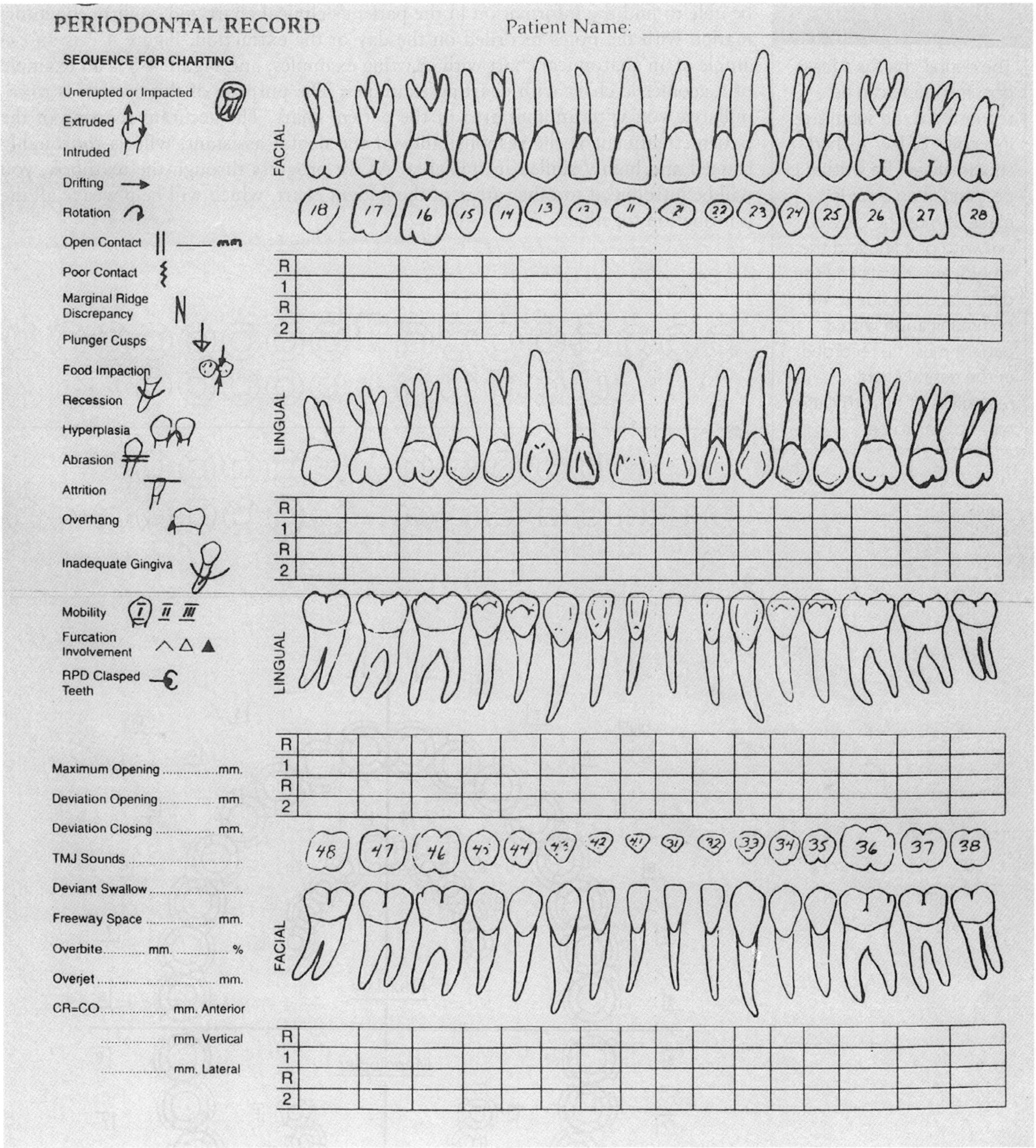

FIGURE 4-7 Anatomical chart.

may use the Universal Numbering System for tooth identification, another may use the International Numbering System, and still another may use the Palmer Notation System. Unfortunately, tooth numbering systems are not something that can be learned over night, and, as such, efforts must be made to differentiate among them.

It is important for the dental administrative assistant to know that a patient's tooth has been extracted or that a fixed bridge has been placed in a patient's dentition. For example, if a representative from a patient's insurance company were to contact the dental office and ask when the patient had a tooth extracted, you must

> **legal TIP**
>
> The dental chart is a legal document and can be requested to be submitted in a court of law. A chart should always be written in pen, and, if an error is made, it must be crossed out with one line and the employee's initials and the date placed beside it. All communication with a patient must be recorded in the dental chart, regardless of how trivial it may appear to be.

be able to find the information in the patient's clinical chart and confirm the information with the notes recorded on the day of the extraction. Figure 4-7 is an example of an anatomical chart with charting examples, and Figure 4-8 is an example of a geometric chart with charting examples. The purpose of this section is to familiarize you with another area of the patient chart. The accurate charting of the patient treatment is the responsibility of the dental assistant, who is thoroughly trained and highly skilled in this area. As we progress through the textbook, you will be introduced to other areas of the patient chart, which will help weave all the information together.

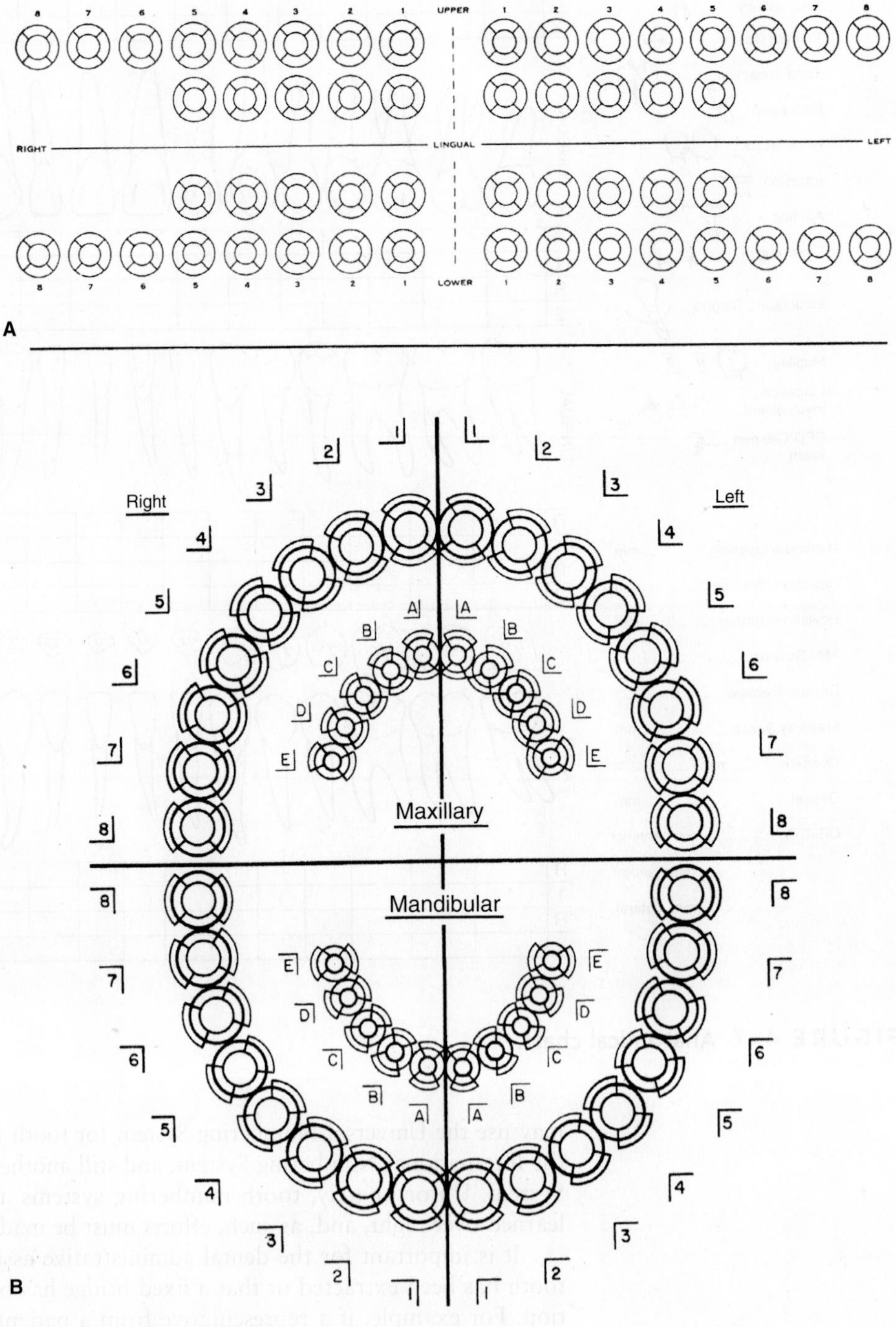

FIGURE 4-8 Geometric chart. Reprinted with permission from Wilkins EM. Clinical practice of the dental hygienist. 9th ed. Baltimore, MD: Lippincott Williams & Wilkins, 2005: p. 101, Fig. 6-4.

The anatomical chart is named in reference to the way the teeth are represented on the chart. They are shown in a very lifelike representation, from the groves in the occlusal and incisal surfaces to the number and shape of the roots of the teeth. The geometric chart is named in reference to the shape of the geometric shape used to represent each tooth and the five surfaces. Note the detail provided by the anatomical chart.

Chapter Summary

This chapter focuses on dental terminology that you must be most familiar with as you embark on your career in the dental profession. Specifically, this chapter provides an introduction to the morphology of the tooth, the numbering systems of teeth that may be encountered in the dental office, as well as a brief introduction to the patient's clinical chart. Without a basic clinical introduction to the practice of dentistry through terminology, reading and interpreting treatment rendered and completing billing procedures would be a frustrating task.

Review Questions

Multiple Choice

1. **The root of the tooth is**
   a. the portion of tooth that lies above the gumline.
   b. the anchor of the tooth.
   c. the portion of the tooth that lies below the gumline.
   d. the most important part of the tooth.

2. **Tooth number 15 in the Universal Numbering System is the**
   a. maxillary right second premolar.
   b. maxillary right second molar.
   c. maxillary left first molar.
   d. maxillary left second molar.

3. **Tooth number 28 in the International Numbering System is the**
   a. mandibular left third molar.
   b. maxillary left third molar.
   c. mandibular right third molar.
   d. maxillary right third molar.

4. **The mesial surface on a posterior tooth is the surface of the tooth that is**
   a. furthest from the midline.
   b. closest to the midline.
   c. on the chewing surface.
   d. toward the cheek.

5. **The following are functions of premolars except**
   a. chewing food.
   b. assisting the molars in cutting food.
   c. supporting the corners of the mouth.
   d. keeping the cheeks from sagging.

6. **The imaginary line used to separate the right and left sides of the dental arches is called the**
   a. quadrant.
   b. midline.
   c. dental arch.
   d. maxillary.

7. **The lower arch is termed the**
   a. maxillary.
   b. mandibular.
   c. dentition.
   d. quadrant.

8. **The dentinal tubules transmit pain stimuli and provide nourishment to the tooth.**
   a. true
   b. false

9. **The main biting or chewing surface on a posterior tooth is termed the**
   a. incisal edge
   b. occlusal surface
   c. labial surface
   d. mesial surface

10. **The hard, outer tissue that covers the crown of the tooth is termed the**
    a. crown
    b. enamel
    c. dentin
    d. pulp

Critical Thinking

1. What is the difference between the anatomical crown and the clinical crown of a tooth?
2. How are the different shades of teeth explained?
3. How would you relieve the anxiety of a patient who is concerned with her son's permanent dentition not erupting when the guidelines say it should?
4. What is the purpose of understanding and interpreting clinical charts in the administrative area of the dental office?

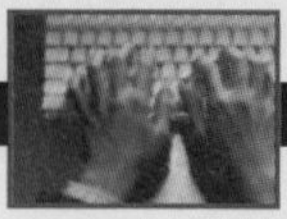

Hands-On Activity

1. For the following teeth: 8, 16, 20, 27, describe (1) where the tooth is located; (2) name the surfaces of the tooth; and (3) provide the name of the tooth.
2. Develop a patient handout that describes the types of teeth found in the permanent dentition and the purpose of each one.

References

Woelfel J, Scheid R. Dental anatomy: its relevance to dentistry. 6th ed. Baltimore, MD: Lippincott, 2002.

Wilkins E. Clinical practice of the dental hygienist. 9th ed. Philadelphia, PA: Lippincott, 2004.

chapter FIVE

Communication *in the Dental Office*

OBJECTIVES

After completing this chapter, you should be able to do the following:

- Spell and define key terms
- Explain the differences between verbal communication and nonverbal communication
- List and demonstrate the techniques used for successful communication
- Name and explain common barriers to communication
- Describe the role of culture, stereotypes, and language in communication
- Explain how to communicate effectively with dental team members

KEY TERMS

- communication
- sender
- receiver
- message
- channel of communication
- interpersonal variables
- environment
- feedback
- verbal communication
- vocabulary
- conciseness
- inflection
- timing
- meaning
- nonverbal communication
- facial expression
- eye contact
- posture
- gestures
- proximity
- active listening
- attitude
- empathy
- reflecting
- paraphrasing
- open-ended questions
- summarizing
- clarification
- bias
- discrimination
- stereotype

OUTLINE

During your employment as a dental administrator, you will find that 90% of your daily activities are centered on communicating. Answering phones, greeting patients as they arrive at the clinic, discussing treatment with the dentist or dental assistant, and phoning patients on behalf of the dental hygienist are just some of the ways the dental administrator communicates on the job. **Communication** is the act of sending and receiving information through verbal and nonverbal forms. Effective communication with patients, doctors, and other team members is crucial to the role of the dental administrator.

Your communication skills create the first impression of the dental practice for patients when they phone or arrive at the dental clinic. Receiving and interpreting the messages that patients communicate to you enable you to respond to patients in an accurate manner. Developing and maintaining positive, long-lasting relationships with patients can be achieved through effective communication skills.

The relationship between the dental office administrator and the patient is a dynamic one. Successful oral health care requires efforts from both the patient and the dental health care professional. The dental office administrator plays an integral role in the development of the relationship the patient has with the dental health care team. Understanding the patient perspective that influences the dynamics of the relationship will assist in the development of successful oral health care for the patient. The first relationship the patient develops is with the dental administrator. Often the patient will provide information to the dental administrator about how he or she feels about dental treatment and its outcome and may disclose difficulties he or she might have regarding compliance with treatment, such as lack of time commitment or financial concerns. The dental administrator has a unique perspective of the patient and his or her attitude toward dental health and can assist in enabling the patient to follow through with treatment. Proficiency and skill in communication are required by the dental administrator to successfully manage the patient relationship.

MASLOW'S HIERARCHY OF NEEDS

A psychologist by the name of Abraham Maslow (1970) developed a theory on the basis of the premise that all people have needs and that it is in the desire to fulfill these needs that people are motivated. There are many needs that people desire to fill, but Maslow has categorized these needs into five classifications. A pyramid shape is used as a visual to illustrate the hierarchy in which these needs are met as they are arranged from a person's most basic needs such as food, water, and oxygen up to higher needs such as self-actualization (Fig. 5-1). To fulfill higher needs, a person must fulfill basic needs. Once a need is satisfied, it no longer motivates a person. For example, a person who is starving is greatly motivated by the need to obtain food and is unable to achieve any of the higher needs until this need is met. Once the person meets the need to obtain food, he or she is no longer motivated by the need. The five needs of the hierarchy are physiological, safety and security, love and belonging, esteem, and self-actualization.

Physiological needs are needs for oxygen, food, water, and homeostatic body conditions. These needs are fundamental to achieving higher-order needs effectively. These needs are considered the strongest needs a person has because the deprivation of one of these needs would create a high level of motivation for the person to meet the need.

Safety and security needs can become active when all physiological needs are no longer motivating the person's behaviors. Children are sensitive to situations of insecurity and express the need to be safe. Adults, however, have the ability to create a secure situation for themselves such as finding adequate

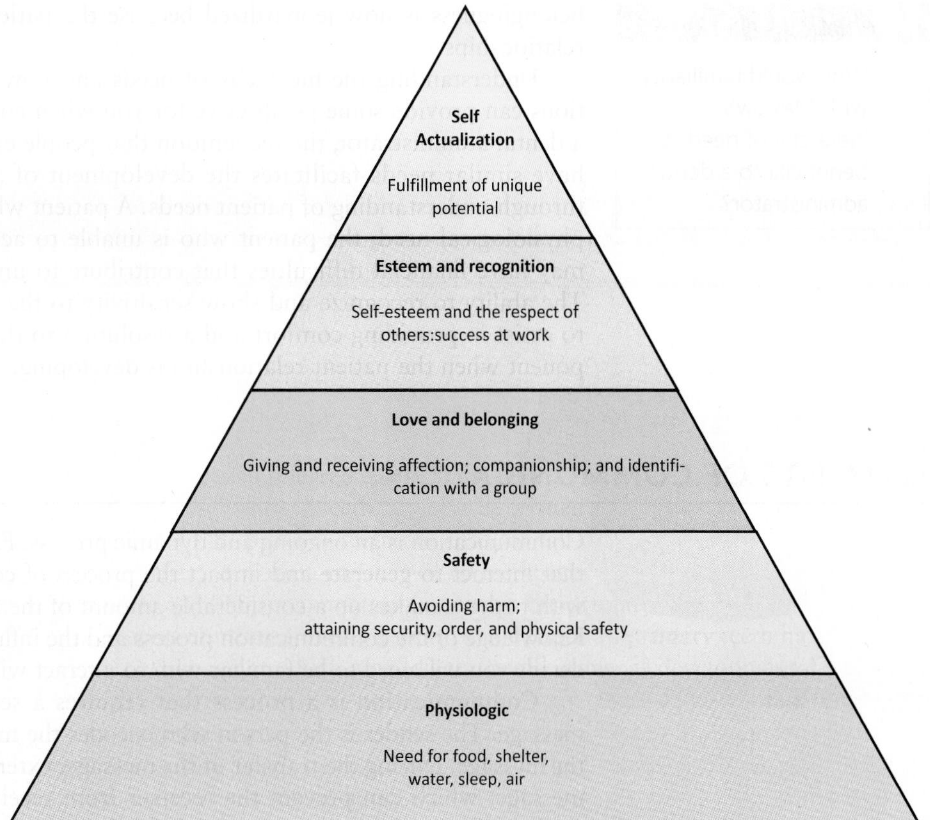

FIGURE 5-1 Maslow's hierarchy of needs.

shelter, obtaining employment for income, and living in an environment conducive to remaining safe.

Love and belonging needs are sought by people to overcome feelings of loneliness and alienation. An inherent quality of human beings is to communicate with others. Through the development of friendships and social acquaintances, people develop a sense of belonging with both formal and informal groups. Through the development of relationships with others, the need for love and belonging is satisfied.

Esteem needs involve both self-esteem and the esteem people receive from relationships formed with others. Human beings have a need to achieve self-respect from other people and when this need is met the person feels confident and as a valued member of society. When the need for esteem is not met, the person may feel inferior and worthless to themselves and those around them.

Need for self-actualization refers to a person's need to be and do that which the person was born to do. When all of the prior needs on the hierarchy are met, the need for self-actualization is desired. Individuals who are motivated to becoming self-actualized desire to achieve a greater goal and recognizing that there are no unmet needs on the hierarchy.

People do not always meet all needs of one level of the need hierarchy and move continually upward. That is, a person can have all needs met on one level and become motivated by needs at the next level yet have a setback that places them on a lower level of the hierarchy. For example, a patient of the dental practice calls to cancel her appointment because she has developed pneumonia and has been hospitalized. The patient, who normally has a very active social calendar, is now in the hospital with a respiratory condition and is not up to seeing visitors. The physiological need of being healthy is now desired and the previous need of a sense of

> ✓ checkPOINT
>
> 1. Why would familiarity with Maslow's hierarchy of needs be beneficial to a dental administrator?

belongingness is now jeopardized because the patient is not able to maintain her relationships.

Understanding the hierarchy of needs and how they affect a person's motivations can provide some perspective for you when communicating with patients. As a dental administrator, the recognition that people experience similar emotions and have similar needs facilitates the development of a positive patient relationship through understanding of patient needs. A patient who arrives in pain has an unmet physiological need; the patient who is unable to accept treatment due to the cost may have financial difficulties that contribute to unmet safety and security needs. The ability to recognize and show sensitivity to the patient by making every effort to assist in providing comfort and a resolution to the unmet need is a critical component when the patient relationship is developing.

ELEMENTS OF COMMUNICATION

Communication is an ongoing and dynamic process. Figure 5-2 illustrates the elements that interact to generate and impact the process of communication. Communicating with patients makes up a considerable amount of the role of the dental administrator. Knowledge of the communication process and the influence of its components provide details you will need to be familiar with to interact with patients effectively.

Communication is a process that requires a sender, receiver, and intentional message. The **sender** is the person who encodes the message and the **receiver** decodes the message. During the transfer of the message, external components can distort the message, which can prevent the receiver from receiving the message as it was intended. The way a message is encoded affects the intended meaning. For example, stating the message in a certain way by using a particular tone will affect the

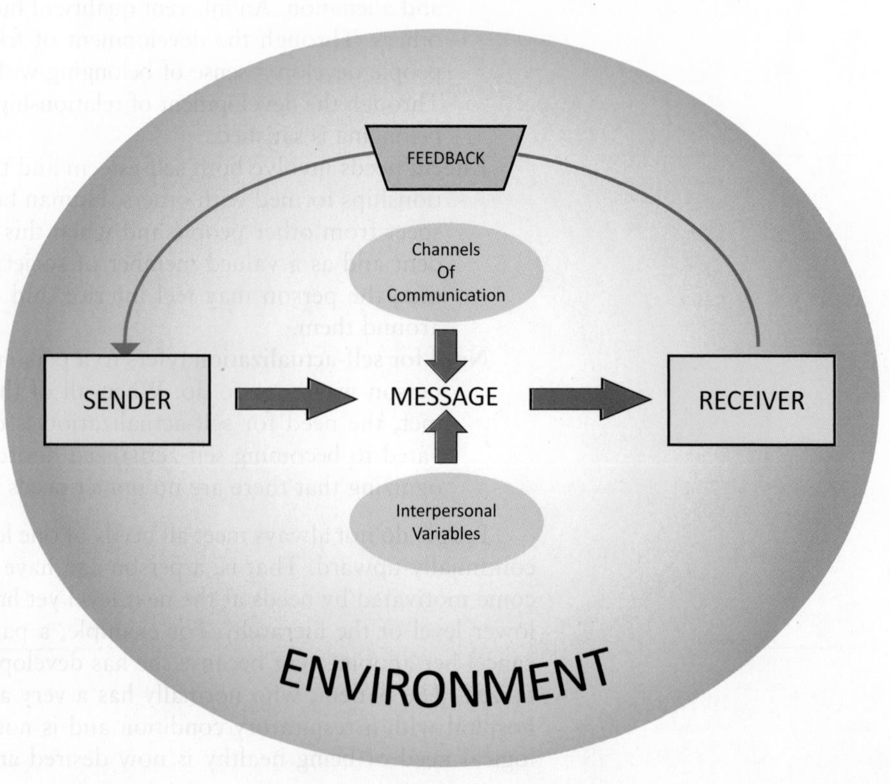

FIGURE 5-2 Process of communication.

meaning. The receiver of the message must then decode the message that is sent. Decoding involves the receiver deciphering of the words, tones, and gestures used by the sender and can result in the message being distorted. There are many components involved in both the encoding and decoding activities of the communication process. The more methods used by the sender to communicate, the more effective the communication of the intended message becomes. Using nonverbal communication techniques can increase the likelihood of the intended message being decoded accurately or greatly distorted. Later in this chapter we will focus on nonverbal communication techniques.

The **message** being sent and received involves both verbal and nonverbal aspects of communication and is the main subject of the communication. Consideration must be given to the receiver and the understanding of the message being sent. The understanding of one message by two different people can vary on the basis of their separate interpretations of the message. Communication with patients can also be influenced by the level of education of the subject the receiver holds. For example, "You require a crown on tooth 7 of the fourth quadrant" means the same as "You require a crown on the lower right molar"; however, patients often better understand the latter explanation. How the message is sent is referred to as the **channel of communication.** Verbal, written, and technological methods to communicate are used by the dental administrator on a regular basis. For example, telephone conversations, fax, and e-mail messages, as well as speaking with patients in person, are the more common forms used.

Interpersonal variables greatly influence the communication process. For example, you may say to a patient, "How has your day been going so far?" Your intent is to make the patient more comfortable by striking up a conversation that involves the added benefit of getting to know the patient better. One patient may perceive that you are friendly and caring, another patient may perceive this as being invasive and unwelcome. The perceptions that a patient holds are created by experiences and expectations and each person's perception is unique. Therefore, a person's interpretation and understanding of things around them influence how a message is interpreted. There are many variables that influence a person's interpretations, these include education, culture, values and beliefs, gender, and physical health status. In the dental office, patients may present with a high level of pain or anxiety, which also alters the communication process.

In addition to the perceptions people hold, the environment in which communication occurs also affects how a message is encoded or decoded. The **environment** is the surroundings in which the communication occurs. Imagine you answer the telephone in a very noisy dental office and the patient calling asks to book an appointment to see the dentist on the 5th of January and because of the noisy environment you misheard the patient and mistakenly scheduled the appointment for the 6th of January. In the dental office, the noise level, lighting, temperature, and lack of privacy are all elements of the environment that impact communication.

The receiver returns a message to the sender on the basis of what is decoded and therefore interpreted to be the intended message. This **feedback** provides the sender with a confirmation that the intended message was received or that the message was distorted somehow. Imagine a group of people in a lineup, where each person must whisper a phrase to the person beside them. While this is happening, various activities such as other people talking, telephones ringing, and people arriving and leaving the room are occurring. All of these events have the potential for distorting the message when a person can hear only parts of the phrase, or a person becomes annoyed by the distractions and the phrase becomes altered, or words are misheard. Clarifying the message you send and confirming the message received help clear up misunderstandings and maintain positive relationships. The remainder of this chapter focuses on aspects of verbal and nonverbal communications used to develop effective communication strategies.

checkPOINT

2. Explain how communication is a process.

VERBAL AND NONVERBAL COMMUNICATIONS

Communication can be divided into two main categories: verbal and nonverbal. When one person attempts to communicate with another person, the communication can be distorted by nonverbal cues, misunderstanding of meanings within verbal communication, and incongruent messages perceived in the communication. Verbal and nonverbal communications are discussed below, along with how each of these communication components may be used effectively in the dental office. In addition, two related communication skills, listening and empathy, are presented.

Verbal Communication

Verbal communication is the act of conveying messages through the use of words or language. Verbal communication is the most common form of communication in the dental office and the one form of communication we rely on most. Your initial contact with patients will most likely be over the telephone when they make an appointment or in person when they come into the clinic. It is important that the verbal communication used by the dental administrative assistant is clear and direct when dealing with patients, staff members, and the dentist. Aspects of verbal communication that the dental administrator will utilize most frequently are discussed below. Specific techniques used for effective verbal communication via the telephone are covered in detail in Chapter 6.

There are five elements of verbal communication essential for effectively encoding and decoding messages in the process of communication. These elements are vocabulary, conciseness, inflection, timing, and meaning.

Vocabulary is the means by which verbal communication is expressed. You may encounter patients who speak a foreign language and are unable to fluently converse in the primary language spoken in the dental office. Establishing communication may be done through an interpreter. The communication process will not be effective if both sender and receiver are unable to connect through language. People who communicate in the same language may encounter words that have different meanings for each person, for example, when referring to dinner, some people may use the term *supper* and the time of day for this meal may be different again. One other aspect to consider is your professional vocabulary. As you develop a comprehensive dental vocabulary, it is appropriate to use it when communicating with a patient. However, all patients will not be familiar with many of these terms; therefore, it is necessary that you be prepared to explain what they mean in more familiar language. For example, if a patient has a molar that is badly decayed and the dentist suggests that a crown be placed on the tooth to restore it, the patient may be more familiar with the term *cap* instead of *crown*. It may be necessary for you to explain not only what is involved in the preparation of the tooth for the crown but also the more common names used for crowns. For example, you may have a conversation with a patient such as "Ms. Johnson, the appointment for your crown preparation will be next Friday at 3:30 PM." You notice that Ms. Johnson appears confused, and you clarify, "Dr. Milton will be placing a crown or cap on your tooth. Do you have any questions or concerns about the procedure?" If she does, you should briefly explain what is involved in the procedure or ask the dental assistant to explain it to the patient. The term *caps* for teeth is a colloquialism for the correct dental term *crown*; however, it may be more familiar to the patient. Although you should always use the correct term, clarifying by using lay terms may reinforce the patient's understanding of the procedure.

Conciseness of communication refers to the use of words that may be familiar to both the sender and the receiver in definition but may have different associations or implications. For example, the word *mother* is understood by many to be a parental figure, and in addition to the definition, there are also characteristics associated with the term, such as protection and caring. When you are required to explain treatment and finances to patients, it is important to use not only the appropriate terminology but also the terminology in such a way that it cannot be misinterpreted. Telling a patient "The dental assistant is preparing the operatory for you, please have a seat for a few minutes" can be both unfamiliar and frightening to a patient. Use of terminology such as "treatment room" in place of "operatory" will be more effective and creates concise communication.

Inflection in your voice is often conveyed through a change in tone or pitch, which is common when asking a question. Emotions are often disclosed through inflection in verbal communication. Patients who are anxious, nervous, and in pain often express a pleading or shaky tone in their voice. Angry patients may emit a louder tone in their voice. Keeping an even, calm tone in your voice as you carry on discussions with patients is necessary to avoid sending unintended messages to the patient.

The use of appropriate **timing** in communication is achieved by first assessing the patient and the situation in which he or she is presenting to you in the dental office. A patient who is wanting to pay the bill and leave because he or she is now in a hurry should be accommodated. Informing the patient of what you need to accomplish in order to exit them from the office quickly allows you to verbalize what needs to be done to help the patient. In contrast to this, a patient who arrives to the dental office experiencing pain will not likely want to engage in friendly conversation. In addition to the timing of messages, appropriate pacing in communication also contributes to its effectiveness. Speaking too quickly can create confusion in understanding for patients and lead to frustration. Leaving long pauses in between words and phrases can lead a patient to think that you are unsure of what you are saying and create feelings of distrust by the patient. Being aware of what you are saying to patients, that is, thinking about what you are going to say before saying it, will convey thoughtful and appropriate timing and pacing in communication.

Using appropriate terminology, incorporating examples, and reviewing important points of the message you are conveying will clarify the **meaning** of the message. Meaning is developed by speaking slowly and providing patients with explanations as well as using shorter explanations instead of long, in-depth explanations that can often lead to confusion. Being simple and direct in your communication is much more effective. For example, asking a patient "Which tooth is hurting?" is more effective than asking "Is the tooth which is causing you pain on the upper or lower part of your mouth and is it on the right or left side?"

As a member of the healthcare profession, you should always speak to all patients and staff members in a polite and pleasant tone, which demonstrates care and consideration and fosters a positive environment. You should also speak clearly and with proper grammar so that you can be easily understood. Of utmost importance, never use foul language or slang and racial terms, which are highly unprofessional and will likely offend patients and colleagues.

checkPOINT

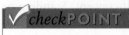

3. Describe two techniques used in verbal communication in the dental office.

Nonverbal Communication

Nonverbal communication involves communication without spoken words and includes the use of body language to encode messages. Nonverbal communication can be used in conjunction with verbal communication to enhance the verbal message and ensure effective communication. As an unconscious part of communication, nonverbal communication is often decoded by the receiver before the verbal message is received. When the verbal and nonverbal messages are incongruent, confusion can result and often the receiver determines that the nonverbal message is the intended message. The decoding of nonverbal communication can become more difficult when body language is interpreted differently by people of various backgrounds and ethnicities. For example, eye contact or touching is used in some cultures for specific purposes or avoided entirely. Understanding the impact body language has in communication will assist you in its appropriate use in communication with patients and coworkers. Body language involves several different behaviors, such as facial expression, eye contact, posture, proximity, and gestures. As the dental administrator, you should become adept at not only using your body language to effectively encode messages but also decoding the nonverbal messages that patients are sending you. Body language can reveal a lot about what others are thinking and feeling when carefully observed and interpreted.

The most expressive part of the body is the face and our **facial expression** communicates emotion; for example, happiness is shown when you smile, sadness is revealed through a frown, and anger and stress can be expressed by a furrowed brow or widened eyes. We unknowingly communicate with others, using facial expression. If you are in the midst of writing a letter that requires concentration and you are interrupted by a coworker or patient, you may have an expression of annoyance or concentration on your face and this can be interpreted by the person as disapproval. The dental office is an environment where you will encounter situations that are surprising or shocking to you, such as a person who arrives with an abscessed tooth and has a very swollen face, or a traumatic dental injury such as a broken mandible or subluxated tooth. Your facial expression must remain neutral or show signs of concern in this situation. Showing expressions of shock, fear, or disgust will leave the patient feeling distressed and anxious. On a regular basis, utilizing smiling as a facial expression will communicate to staff and patients that you are approachable and friendly.

Eye contact is an important facet of nonverbal communication. Engaging a person in communication begins with eye contact. Maintaining eye contact with patients and colleagues encourages communication and conveys interest in what the speaker is saying (Fig. 5-3A). Conversely, looking at the floor, ceiling, or wall while communicating sends a message other than one of genuine interest. As stated earlier, eye contact can have different and profound meanings in some cultures, and as such the use of eye contact may be avoided. Eye contact is effective in situations in which you must assert your autonomy; for example, when a patient is angry and argumentative about the treatment or cost of treatment he or she received, it is helpful to keep eye contact at the same level as the patient. If the patient is standing over you at your desk, stand up to face him or her; likewise, if the patient is in a seated position, take a seat across from him or her to have the discussion.

As you communicate with people, you should remain conscious of your **posture.** The way you sit or stand reveals your attitude and self-concept. Standing or sitting straight shows that you are confident and have a sense of well-being and conveys interest in what someone is saying while he or she communicating with you, whereas slouching implies that you could be tired or depressed. Leaning slightly forward toward the person is helpful in communicating that you are interested. Turning your back toward the person who is speaking or to whom you are speaking communicates disinterest.

The use of **gestures**, or actions, can also facilitate communication. During communication, using gestures assists in emphasizing and punctuating words. On its own a gesture can be effective and can convey meaning to a person, but used in conjunction with verbal communication, the message is more likely to be decoded accurately. For example, putting your hand on a coworker's shoulder as you say "You give 100% when you are here, no wonder you go home tired at the end of the day!" is effective in sending the unspoken message that you care and appreciate the person. The gesture alone can be effective but can have several meanings. While you are communicating with patients, using gestures such as nodding your head while using phrases such as "Okay" and "Uh huh" and lightly touching their arm facilitates the conversation (Fig. 5-3B). Nodding your head can be used to show understanding or agreement that encourages the speaker to continue and provides positive reinforcement as well as affirmation that you are listening to. The key to using gestures effectively is to ensure that the verbal message you are sending is congruent with the gesture you are using. Informing a patient that you are pleased to see

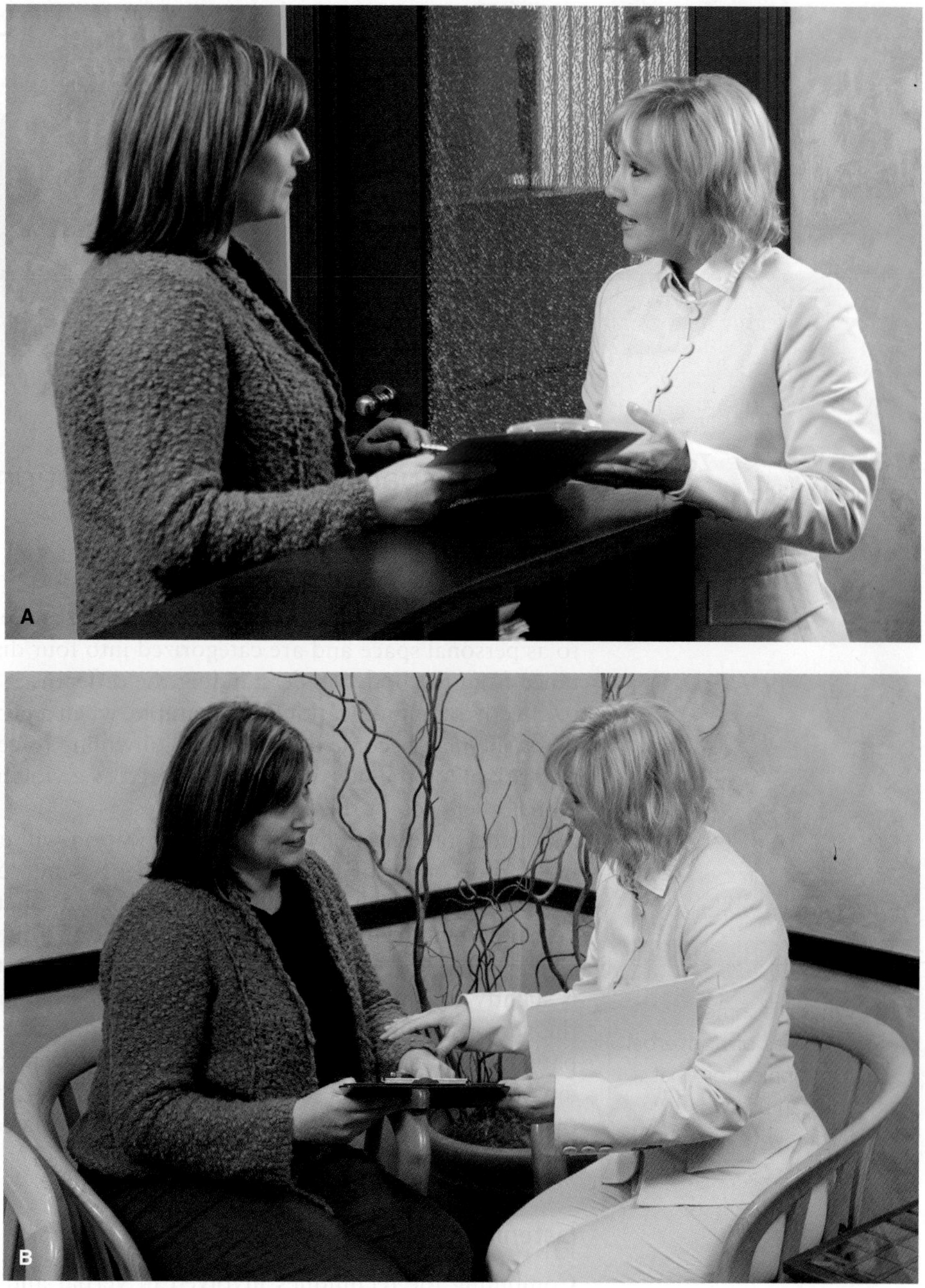

FIGURE 5-3 Dental administrator using effective nonverbal communication with a patient. **A)** Maintaining eye contact. **B)** Lightly touching patient's arm.

him or her while typing up a letter on the computer does not send a message that is genuine and congruent.

Maintaining a comfortable distance between yourself and the patient during communication enables the communication process by eliminating the frustration caused by violating one's personal space. **Proximity**, standing too close or too far away from the receiver, may have negative implications for the communication process. While interacting, people maintain a certain distance between them, depending on the relationship they have with the person, their cultural beliefs, and the environment in which they are communicating. For example, you may stand closer and speak more quietly to a close friend or spouse while talking than you would when speaking with a patient in the dental clinic. The amount of space you choose to keep around yourself is referred to as personal space. There are four zones of

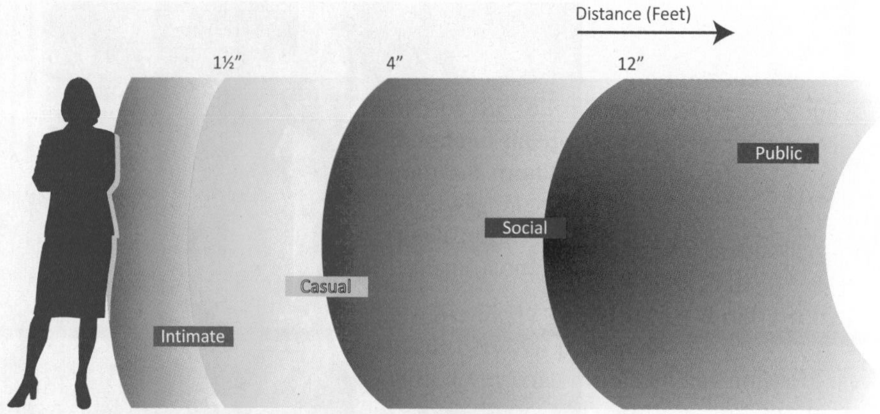

FIGURE 5-4 Zones of personal space.

Personal spaces for social interaction

personal space, which are described in Figure 5-4. The physical space around us is considered part of our personal territory. The spaces around a person are referred to as personal space and are categorized into four distinct zones on the basis of distance from the body. Understanding the differences among these zones contributes to effective communication. For example, when a person's intimate space is invaded, he or she may become defensive and unwilling to communicate. Sitting too closely to a person on the bus may be considered as a violation of personal space for some, while others accept this level of closeness.

Understanding nonverbal communication will enable you in your understanding and decoding of messages that patients send you, whether intentional or not. Sometimes, nonverbal cues reveal more about what a person is feeling than their verbal communication, especially when the two messages are incongruent. If you ask a patient how she is and she says, "I'm doing just fine," but you can see that she is slightly pale and shaking her leg, the nonverbal messages are not consistent with the verbal response. As a dental administrator, you will become skilled at reading patients and knowing when they are masking feelings such as nervousness and anxiety. Review Table 5-1, which provides examples of communication cues that are open and facilitate communication and those that are closed and that discourage communication.

checkPOINT

4. What are some examples of nonverbal communication that you can use when talking with a patient?

Listening

Combining the techniques involved in verbal and nonverbal communications is known as **active listening.** Active listening in the dental office means giving your full attention to patients to facilitate a positive dental experience. When you actively listen to another person, you are listening to the content of what he or she is saying. That is, attention is paid to the message that is being conveyed. For example, if you are listening to a patient who is concerned with the cost of dental treatment and the patient is pointing out treatment costs on the invoice, you should allow the patient to finish explaining all aspects of his or her concern and then, after getting the whole message, you can provide the best response. If you are actively listening to the patient, you will not select the content of his or her concerns that you agree or disagree with, you will respond on the basis of all of the information the patient provides. To be a successful active listener, you must allow all information to be presented by the other party before you form your opinion or provide a response.

Part of getting the complete message in communication involves nonverbal communication. In the active listening process, understanding the whole message involves the assessment of the speaker's nonverbal cues. For example, a patient who

TABLE 5-1 Communication Cues

Open Communication Cues	Closed Communication Cues
Relaxed demeanor	Rigid demeanor
Direct eye contact	Avoidance of eye contact
Open hands or arms	Arms folded across chest
Smiling	Frowning or scowling
Leaning into conversation	Leaning away from conversation
Standing or sitting up straight	Moving away from person
Hands away from face	Hands covering mouth
Affirmative head nodding	No response to sender
Sitting with feet apart, relaxed	Legs crossed, foot tapping
Paying attention to speaker	Looking around the room

is nervous about receiving dental treatment is sitting in a chair in the reception area, arms crossed and nervously tapping one foot on the ground. When you ask the patient whether he or she is feeling nervous about the dental treatment, he or she responds by saying, "I'm not nervous. I've never liked dental offices, I'm always this way." This is conflicting information. The patient's physical cues are not congruent with what he or she is saying. In this situation, the active listener uses the speaker's nonverbal communication to understand the complete message from the patient. Responding to this patient requires careful control by the dental administrator. If it seems that the patient is nervous on the basis of his or her nonverbal cues, yet he or she responds in the negative, you would not respond to the patient by saying, "You seem nervous!" Using empathy and being nonjudgmental to the patient are important in this communication process. In active listening, the goal is to try and understand the speaker's position and the message he or she is sending. Appropriate responses to this patient may include asking questions such as "Do you have any questions about the treatment?" or "Can I get you a glass of water?" Subtle attempts to comfort the patient are often successful and can include talking to the patient about current news or sports events as a distraction. There are five components that make up the active listening process. Box 5-1 outlines these components and provides explanations for each.

Attitude

Your outlook and how you choose to portray it represent your **attitude.** Patients arriving at the dental clinic will be exposed to your attitude before anything else in the office, and the representation of the type of service and treatment delivered in the dental office is often predetermined through the attitude of the office administrator. Consider the following scenario: upon arrival to the dental office for an appointment, the patient is not greeted by the dental administrator immediately, and furthermore, his or her presence is not acknowledged for the first 5 minutes after arrival. After 5 minutes, the dental administrator addresses the patient with "The assistant should be out in a few minutes to get you" and then returns to completing paperwork. In this situation the patient is left feeling unimportant and sensing the uncaring and poor attitude of the dental administrator, which has set the tone for the appointment. The patient is likely apprehensive that for the remainder of the appointment poor attitudes from staff will be encountered. A more appropriate

BOX 5-1
Active Listening Components

Face the person you are speaking with. Facing the person you are speaking with provides a physical demonstration to the person that you are interested in what he or she is saying.

Maintain eye contact. Eye contact is critical for maintaining interest, developing trust, and creating relationships with patients. Maintaining eye contact lets patients know that you are interested in what they are saying and sends the message that you are listening to what they are saying. Avoiding eye contact sends the message that what the person is saying is not important enough to listen to or that the person should not trust you.

Lean toward the person while conversing. Leaning toward the patient while communicating illustrates a genuine interest in what the patient is communicating and that you wish to be involved in the interaction.

Demonstrate open posture. Refraining from keeping your arms and legs crossed sends the message that you are approachable and willing to listen. Crossing your arms while talking with someone in person might imply an uptight or defensive position. This can also evoke a defensive attitude from the person you are communicating with.

Stay relaxed. Remaining in a relaxed state while communicating with patients contributes to the positive, relaxed office environment. Feelings of anxiousness or restlessness can be sensed by the patient and can lead to concerns or doubt about the responses you are providing. Showing that you are relaxed while communicating with the patient sends the message that you are confident and capable in your position.

scenario would be, when the patient arrives at the clinic he or she is greeted and his or her presence is acknowledged immediately. By acknowledging patients, you are sending the message that they are important and that you care that they have arrived for their appointment.

It is common for a personal event or a situation at the workplace to create negative emotions that affect our attitude. If the negative emotions are evident to patients, it creates an unfavorable environment. In the dental office where communication with people makes up a large part of the daily activities, keeping a positive attitude is essential. Remaining consciously aware of your attitude in the dental office is important for generating a positive environment.

Assess your mood. A person's mood can influence his or her attitude. For example, arriving late to work because the car would not start can put a person in a bad mood. Arriving at the office in a bad mood and allowing that mood to be demonstrated to coworkers and patients through actions such as slamming doors, being short with responses, or having a scowl on your face can be perceived as a negative attitude. Allow yourself a few minutes at the start of each day to take an inventory of your mood. Being aware of your emotions will create the control you need to set your negative mood aside when dealing with coworkers and patients in a positive, friendly way.

Conceptualize your attitude. If you are aware that you are in a bad mood or your negative emotions are showing, it is preferable that your attitude does not portray this. Being aware of negative emotions allows for the conceptualization of the attitude we would like to have. Visualize yourself being in a positive mood, or visualize leaving your negative emotions outside of the office.

Be flexible. Communicating with people on a regular basis requires great flexibility in adapting your attitude to suit the situation. A patient who is in pain may express anxiousness and urgency, and your attitude should create a sense of calmness and demonstrate empathy for the patient. A patient who is angry because he or she cannot get an appointment with the dentist for a week and feels it is your fault will require that your attitude become one of empathy for him or her yet assurance that you are being as accommodating as possible.

Avoid negative talk. Being in an environment of negativity can breed negativity. If you bring your bad mood and negative attitude to the dental office, you will impact others. Prepare yourself for a positive attitude by telling yourself that you will be positive and accounting for all the things about your position or yourself that are positive. For example, if you work with colleagues you respect and you feel part of the team, remind yourself that you are respected and needed by them. Avoid bringing negativity into the office by speaking about the situation that upset you to any person you come across. Unsolicited negative talk of any type creates a negative climate.

Be enthusiastic. A positive attitude allows for enthusiasm to be displayed. Showing that you are excited and interested in being in your position as a dental administrator contributes to a positive attitude and pleasant office atmosphere and contributes to the confidence patients and colleagues have in your abilities. Choosing to be enthusiastic each day will lead to increased effectiveness in your communication abilities.

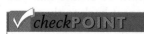

> ✓ *check*POINT
>
> 5. How does your mood influence your attitude?

In Chapter 11, the effect that attitude can have on the necessity of working as a team member in the dental office is discussed.

Empathy

Empathy is the accurate recognition of emotions of others and the ability to communicate your understanding to them. Empathy is often referred to as the ability to "put yourself in someone else's shoes." As a dental office administrator, you will have the opportunity to express empathy for patients when communicating with them. Expressing empathy entails providing comfort and support to patients, such as offering a glass of water or cool cloth to an elderly person who has arrived at the office and appears overheated. You may not always be personally familiar with the experiences patients discuss with you. In these situations, you may need to put your active listening skills to use in order to develop an understanding and exemplify your concern. Another illustration of expressing empathy is by encouraging dialogue and exercising compassion with patients who arrive at the dental clinic feeling anxious, nervous, or embarrassed about the state of their dentition. Your role as a dental office administrator is to make such patients feel safe, welcome, and not judged. Using statements that show empathy are very important because they convey that you listened and understand the emotions the patient is feeling. Empathic statements generate trust in patient relationships through their nonjudgmental tone and sensitivity. For example, you may respond to a patient who is anxious about his or her upcoming dental treatment with "It must be very upsetting for you to feel this anxiety about being here today." You can also express empathy for patients who are experiencing financial difficulties yet choose to accept a particular treatment; for example, you could say: "It must be frustrating for you to have to take care of your oral health concerns on a limited budget." When patients entrust personal information to you regarding their feelings or financial situation, it is imperative that you uphold that level of trust through empathy and sensitivity in the communication process.

TECHNIQUES FOR SUCCESSFUL COMMUNICATION

As a dental administrative assistant, you will sometimes need to answer patients' questions about a dental procedure. It may even be a part of your duties to review the financial obligations of the patient or review a treatment plan outlined by the

> **what IF ?**
>
> Mrs. Jones has just arrived at the dental office with her 8-year-old daughter Janey. Janey's maxillary right central incisor was knocked out when she fell from her bike. A patient in the reception area saw Janey as she entered the dental office and a look of horror came across her face in reaction to seeing the child's injury. Mrs. Jones and Janey saw the look on the patient's face. Janey began to cry and told her mother she felt scared. What would you do?
>
> Many people not in the healthcare professions are shocked when they see injuries they are not used to seeing and as a result their facial expressions reflect this emotion. Nonverbal communication sends messages that the sender is unaware of and are being communicated. In this situation, and with any situation in the dental office in which patients are ashamed and embarrassed about the state of their dentition, the appropriate response is to assure the patient that his or her concerns will be attended to and that the dentist will provide the necessary treatment for the patient. Most importantly, let the patient know that this condition is common and that the dental team has effectively managed patients with similar concerns many times. Use a soothing tone of voice and proper nonverbal communication, such as sitting beside the patient, if required. If a treatment room is available, escort the patient there to provide a private area for waiting.

clinical staff. In these situations, it is beneficial for you to be familiar with the following communication techniques:

- Reflecting
- Paraphrasing
- Open-ended questions
- Summarizing
- Clarification

Reflecting

When you communicate with patients, they will provide information that must be recorded correctly. Asking questions or making statements that reflect your understanding of the information received while communicating with the patient will assist in clarification and accurate recording for clinical staff. To ensure that you understand what patients are saying, one technique is to repeat back to them part of what they have already said, which is known as **reflecting.** Besides confirming what they have said, this technique can also encourage them to provide additional information. For example, you may say to the patient, "You were saying that when you drink cold or hot liquids your tooth begins to hurt. . . ." The patient will then provide further information such as the type of pain (sharp, stabbing) and exactly when the pain occurs (while drinking, after drinking). Reflecting is a technique that is often used in healthcare settings to draw further information from the patient.

Paraphrasing

Rephrasing in your own words what you have just heard the patient say is called **paraphrasing.** Paraphrasing is a good way to ensure that you understand what the patient is saying and to demonstrate that you are listening. Begin by simply saying to the patient, "What I hear you saying, Mrs. Jones, is . . . ." After you have paraphrased the information, end with a question for clarification, such as "Is this correct?" This, again, reinforces understanding and implies that you are not assuming to be correct, but making an effort to understand correctly. Use this technique in moderation, however, as paraphrasing too many times in one conversation could become tiresome for the patient.

Open-Ended Questions

Gaining information from patients is much easier when you use open-ended questions. An **open-ended question** is one that cannot be answered with a "yes" or "no" response; thus, the person must provide substantive information to answer the question. Such questions often begin with *what, when,* or *where* and elicit answers that require patients to elaborate on their response. For example, asking patients, "What medications are you currently taking," provides an opportunity for patients to provide you with detailed information regarding their medication. Such a question is more effective than asking, "Are you taking any medication?", which elicits a "yes" or "no" answer, meaning that you will need to ask more detailed questions to get more information. Other examples of open-ended questions include the following:

- What tooth is causing you pain?
- How did you chip your tooth?
- When did the pain start?

Also, use sensitivity and tact when asking open-ended questions. Ask questions in a professional manner by using a calm voice with little inflection to avoid sounding accusatory or judgmental to the patient.

Summarizing

Summarizing is a technique in which you verbally review information with the patient that he or she has provided, after condensing it and putting it in a proper order. Again, this technique gives the patient the opportunity to affirm that the information you have is correct. When a patient calls and requests to see the dentist because he is experiencing intense pain, you may repeat back to him the information he has provided you with. For example, "You have been taking pain relievers for the past two days, and yesterday you noticed that the pain increased and the area began to swell." Summarizing the facts in the order they occurred is important, particularly when the same information is going to be relayed to the dentist or other member of the dental team. The dentist usually will review the facts with the patient before prescribing treatment.

Clarification

Asking for **clarification** of information that the patient has given to you is another very useful technique. For example, if a patient calls to make an appointment regarding pain she is experiencing from a particular area in her mouth, you may ask such clarifying questions as "What type of pain are you experiencing?" or "Please describe what the pain feels like." Asking for specific responses and examples will provide you with much-needed information necessary for the clinical team.

checkPOINT

6. What are the five techniques used in communication?

BARRIERS TO COMMUNICATION

We often assume that our communication has been understood by the receiver simply because we know what we are trying to express. Miscommunications are frequently the result of barriers or factors that confuse the intent of the communications. The three main areas of miscommunication are sender barriers, environmental barriers, and receiver barriers.

Sender Barriers

Sender barriers are factors that prevent the sender from adequately communicating the message to the receiver. Lack of clarity and conciseness is one example of a sender barrier. Mumbling or rambling can make it difficult for the patient to understand what you are saying. Proper delivery is key in avoiding this miscommunication factor.

A negative attitude on the behalf of the dental office administrator, as was discussed earlier, is also an example of a sender barrier. Attitude can be communicated verbally in your tone of voice or nonverbally through your body language. If patients sense that you do not care about them or are in a bad mood, they likely will not be receptive to the information you are trying to communicate to them.

Another sender barrier is the volume and rate of your speech. A loud voice can be disturbing and irritating to the patient. Using a loud voice can be particularly distressing for the patient when you are discussing the patient's personal information in an area where other patients may be able to overhear you. Using a low sounding voice and speaking in a pleasant tone keeps the patient at ease. Flexibility in your judgment regarding the volume, quality, and tone of your speech to use while communicating with patients is a skill utilized by the dental administrator. For example, if Mrs. Jones has arrived at the front desk to settle her account and schedule her next appointment, and you are currently assisting Mr. Green, you should ask Mrs. Jones to have a seat for a few minutes and continue to assist Mr. Green and use a lowered voice while discussing any of his personal information. You should also consider speaking at a pace slowly enough to ensure that you will be understood by the

TABLE 5-2 Terminology for Effective Communication

Old Terminology	Preferred Terminology
Waiting area	Reception area
Cancellation	Interruption in schedule
Baby teeth	Primary teeth
Adult teeth	Permanent dentition
Recall appointment	Recare appointment
Cost	Fee
Operatory	Treatment room
Checkup	Examination
Day sheet	Appointment schedule
Cleaning	Oral prophylaxis and scaling
Freezing	Anesthetic
Gum disease	Gingivitis or periodontitis
Filling	Restoration
Caps	Crown
White filling	Composite restoration
Silver filling	Amalgam restoration
Root canal	Root canal therapy

patient. The volume, quality, and rate of your speech are referred to as paralanguage, and these variables can contribute to a different meaning being decoded by the receiver than the one intended.

The language chosen to convey a message to patients can also detract from what you are trying to say. Often in the dental office, our choice of words or phrases can have negative connotations attached to them. For example, the reception area of the dental office is often referred to as the "waiting room." However, this phrase has a negative connotation, as it implies that patients are kept waiting. Table 5-2 outlines phrases that are often used in the dental office and offers alternate terminology to avoid the negative implications often associated with them.

Your appearance and personal hygiene is another potential barrier to communication and can contribute to a positive or negative image of the practice. It is important that you dress to suit the image and the message you are trying to convey. If you are wearing a stained or ripped uniform, the message you will send to patients is that you are not concerned with your personal appearance and that your supervisor is not concerned either. Maintaining a clean and neat appearance includes practicing good personal hygiene also. Brushing your teeth and flossing after you eat, as well as making sure that your breath is fresh, is expected while working in a dental office. Showering on a daily basis and using deodorant will ensure that body odor is not hindering effective communication with staff members and patients.

Lack of knowledge can be a sender barrier. Effective communication in the dental office requires being knowledgeable in your area of expertise. If you demonstrate a lack of knowledge of basic dental or office procedures, patients will likely not have much confidence in the information you convey to them. The previous chapters have provided you with some fundamental dental information.

> **checkPOINT**
> 7. How does your appearance influence the message you send?

Combining this knowledge with the communication skills presented in this chapter will facilitate your goal of being the best dental administrator you can be.

Environmental Barriers

The office environment you work in can also present barriers to communication. Creating a calm space for patients is essential, particularly for anxious patients. Factors such as noise level, caused by talking, music, or even the telephone ringing, can create an environment that leaves patients feeling stressed and unimportant. The dental office administrator facilitates the development of a positive atmosphere for patients by managing the level of noise occurring in the office, specifically in the reception area, and maintaining an organized desk.

Noise

Imagine going into a dental office where children in the waiting area are running around and yelling, the telephone at the front desk is ringing loudly, and heavy metal music is playing over the sound system. How can anyone communicate effectively amid all this chaos? What would a patient think, or feel, arriving at the clinic to this scene? As the dental administrator, you will be responsible for establishing and maintaining a positive and welcoming atmosphere in the administrative area of the dental office.

Communication with patients while children are running around can be very difficult, and such an environment contributes to messages being misinterpreted or not heard correctly. Prevent children from becoming restless while either waiting their turn to see the dentist or waiting for their parent to finish treatment by providing them with coloring or reading materials as soon as they arrive at the clinic. Although some dental offices have policies that children must be supervised by a parent for the time they are in the office, having such materials on hand can help keep children occupied and is greatly appreciated by parents. Some dental offices may even supply video games or a child's play area to keep young patients occupied. These steps will go a long way toward maintaining a calm environment.

Other noise in the dental office, such as music played over the sound system and the ringing of the telephone, can also disrupt communication. If music selection is part of your responsibility in the office, select music that is calming and is not offensive. Keep the ringer volume and pitch on the phone low so that it is less jarring for patients and staff members.

Desk Organization

Lack of organization of the front desk of a dental office is another environmental barrier to communication. On a busy day in the dental office, patient charts, mail, deliveries from laboratories, and packages from dental supply companies can pile up at the front desk and create a very unorganized work environment. Not only can this disorganized appearance form a negative association in patients' minds regarding the organization of the whole office, but such disorganization can make it difficult to find patient charts or other information needed for effective patient communication. The reception desk in the dental office makes up part of the appearance of the reception area and contributes to the calm and welcoming climate. A disorganized desk interrupts the flow of calmness aspired to in the office by transmitting a sense of confusion to the patient.

An effective method used to keep the front desk organized is to immediately address each item that is placed on the desk. Have an "in" and "out" tray on the front desk for items that cannot be dealt with as soon as you receive them. If a chart is received by a clinical staff member, the information must be recorded in the computer or on the insurance form or the chart may be placed in an area of the desk for review at a quieter time or filed away. If the mail arrives and you do not have time to sort it immediately, place it in the "in" tray and manage it during a quieter period of time. If you can, sort and distribute the mail right away. Packages that arrive at the front desk for the clinical staff should be taken to the clinical area right away and opened where patients are not present. This task is normally the responsibility of a clinical staff member.

Thus, communicating with patients either on the telephone or in person will be more effective for administrative staff when a sense of control and confidence can be conveyed. A front desk that has patient charts, documents, or mails scattered across it can convey a sense of disorder and project the message that the staff member who works at the desk is overwhelmed. A neat, clean, and organized front desk communicates to patients that the dental administrative assistant is in control of the situation, is effective, and is giving the patient his or her undivided attention.

Interruptions

Interruptions in the dental office are commonplace and are another environmental barrier to communication. The telephone rings often and patients are always arriving or leaving the clinic. While you are communicating with a patient, the telephone may ring, and you will have to stop what you are doing and answer the phone. Continual stopping and starting interrupts the flow of communication with the patient. Unfortunately, there may not be a private place where patients' accounts or treatment can be discussed while they are in the dental office. Most offices do have a private area for patient conversations to avoid the discomfort of patients having to discuss their personal information in the presence of others.

Receiver Barriers

Barriers in communication also can be related to a problem with the receiver. It is important to stay aware of these barriers as you receive messages from patients and as you send messages to them in the communication process.

Fatigue or poor health in the receiver can interfere with communication. Patients who are tired and lacking sleep or not feeling well may have difficulty concentrating on your message. Be especially patient when communicating with patients who exhibit signs of illness and fatigue.

A receiver's experiences with dental offices can create barriers to communication. A bad experience in a dental office may cause a patient to associate bad feelings with all dental offices. Such a patient may have a difficult time being in the dental office and keeping his or her scheduled appointments and regular care appointments. This can be a very big barrier to attempt to overcome. Recognizing this fact and having the dentist address it with the patient will go a long way toward developing positive communication with this type of patient. Chapter 10 introduces the various kinds of patients you will encounter in the dental office and techniques that will facilitate a comfortable and pleasant experience in the dental office.

Another barrier to communication often held by the message decoder is preconceived notions related to the message that is being sent. For example, a patient arriving at the front desk after treatment may be expecting to be informed about the fee for the treatment he or she received and may hold the assumption that the cost is going to be a high dollar amount. Prior to the dental administrator presenting the patient's account statement, the patient may be feeling defensive and sending nonverbal messages through facial expressions that say that he is not pleased with the amount he has to pay. This leads to an attitude that creates a barrier for the patient in receiving the whole message being sent by the dental administrator.

Being aware of the barriers to communication that patients may present while in the dental office calls for flexibility of the dental administrator in applying appropriate communication techniques. Recognizing the possible barriers early in the communication process allows for the opportunity to identify and correct misunderstandings.

checkPOINT

8. What are three barriers to communication?

ROLE OF CULTURE, STEREOTYPES, AND LANGUAGE IN COMMUNICATION

A person's cultural and religious beliefs influence his or her perceptions of situations and style of communication. In the dental office, you will communicate regularly with people from various cultural and religious backgrounds who will have beliefs and values that are different from your own. As a healthcare professional, you must treat each person with dignity and respect and give highest priority to his or her dental care. Any preconceived notions that you may have regarding persons of cultural and religious backgrounds different from yours must be put aside to communicate effectively with patients.

Culture

The role of culture in the communication process must be given thoughtful consideration. Earlier, we discussed the role of eye contact in the communication process. In the mainstream culture of Western countries, such as the United States and Canada, casting your eyes downward may mean that you are not telling the truth or are embarrassed, whereas looking someone directly in the eyes is a sign of respect, interest, or attention. In other countries as well as in other cultures within Western countries, looking a person directly in the eyes can be perceived as disrespectful and casting the eyes downward is seen as a sign of respect. Although it is impossible to learn the nuances of every culture in the world in order to avoid using nonverbal language erroneously, you should be aware that nonverbal language may be misinterpreted by those from cultures other than your own. Sensitivity and understanding that cultural beliefs may play a role in the communication process for some patients are important for effective communication.

checkPOINT

9. What role can culture play in the communication process?

checkPOINT

10. What is discrimination?

legal TIP

Discussing patient information where other patients can overhear can sometimes happen unintentionally in the dental office. Use the following points to minimize this from happening:

- Use a private area out of the range of hearing of others to discuss patient information.
- Use a low voice when speaking with patients in public areas.
- Never address a patient by his or her full first and last name.
- Never discuss patients outside of the dental office with other people.

Stereotypes

All patients who come to the dental clinic must be treated with dignity and respect. The race, creed, color, or sexual orientation of the patient should hold no bearing whatsoever in the communication with and treatment of the patient. Your personal **bias** should not enter into your communication with any patient. **Discrimination** is the act of making a distinction between people on the basis of some aspect such as class, race, color, sexual orientation, or disability. When you hold an opinion about a whole group of people based on an oversimplified characterization, you are **stereotyping.** Stereotyping and discrimination usually result in a lack of quality care for some patients. The possibility of establishing a positive and successful communication process between the dental administrator and the patient is limited at best. As a healthcare professional, you must treat all patients equally.

Language

Language barriers can also hamper effective communication in the dental office. Often, patients who speak a language different from English will have family members or interpreters to decipher what is being said to facilitate their dental treatment. If such is not the case, another staff member who is familiar with the language the patient speaks can provide the interpretation. The following points are useful when communicating with patients who do not speak English:

- Use gestures to try to explain to patients if an interpreter is not available.
- Speak in a slower, not louder, voice and use short, simple phrases.
- Do not use slang terminology.
- Communicate in a quiet area with few distractions.
- If an interpreter is available, speak to the patient with the interpreter in view.

COMMUNICATION WITH THE DISSATISFIED PATIENT

There will be occasions when you will have to communicate with a patient who is upset with some aspect of the service received at the dental office. All dental offices strive to achieve a 100% patient satisfaction rate, but the reality is that there will likely be some patients who will not be satisfied. Some of the most common reasons for dissatisfaction among patients in the dental office include the following:

- Waiting times
- Financial concerns
- Treatment options
- Failed treatment

Communicating effectively with these patients is a responsibility, and a fact of life, for the dental office administrator. Whether on the telephone or in the reception area, angry patients must be dealt with quickly and effectively. Following are some recommendations for dealing effectively with angry patients.

Be open and honest. Honesty and openness are two qualities that should be put into practice during daily communications with patients. This is a proactive measure put into place to avoid future misunderstandings. For example, if a patient is informed of the cost of treatment prior to the treatment appointment, collecting payment from the patient will be straightforward and surprises are avoided. Informing patients of financial obligations upfront is a responsible open and honest approach to maintaining the patient relationship.

Use a quiet space. Providing the patient with an opportunity to openly discuss concerns can facilitate a resolution. Keep in mind that every patient is unique and the treatment each patient receives is specific to his or her condition. An upset patient voicing concerns about failed treatment in the presence of other patients creates the impression that the failure was the result of practitioner error. A private environment allows you to review all the details of the situation with the patient and eliminates the possibility of other patients overhearing private information.

Do not argue. Arguing with the patient could result in the termination of the patient relationship with the dental practice. If a patient is upset enough to voice his or her concerns, he or she is likely open to negotiating an amicable outcome. Preservation of the patient–dental team relationship is given priority. If the patient is insistent and unwilling to accept a compromise, arguing will only exacerbate the situation. Depending on the policies in your office relating to patient concerns, you may have to inform the patient that he or she must discuss the issue with the manager. If you are responsible for managing concerns, you might inform the patient that you will review all the particulars of his or her situation and provide a response within a certain time period. Allowing time for yourself and the patient to reflect on the circumstances often provides clarity and a well-reasoned understanding of the concern.

Do not belittle the issue. Patients are important to the successful functioning of the dental practice. If a patient is concerned, upset, or confused about anything experienced in your office, you have the responsibility to provide clarification on the issue and set their mind at ease. Patients are not experts in the dental field and questions or concerns they have may reflect this. Being open and approachable to all patients will eliminate the risk of making them feel as if their concerns are not worthy of your time. For example, a patient in the reception area has been waiting for the hygienist who is running behind schedule. The patient approaches the administrator and says "It's now 2:15 PM and I have to leave here by 3:00 PM, will the hygienist be much longer or should I reschedule?" The response to the patient is "The hygienist won't be too much longer." In this scenario, the patient is concerned with returning to work by a certain time, the administrator did not address this concern, and the patient likely perceived this to mean that her concern was not important.

If the patient becomes threatening, solicit a manager or the dentist to escort the patient out. Attempting to reason with a patient who is belligerent or showing physical signs of aggression puts you at risk for verbal or physical abuse. Often when a person is in an aggravated state that escalates to the point of verbal or physical threats, making an effort to calm the person may only intensify the situation.

what **IF** ?

A patient arrives at the dental office and is upset about the statement she received in the mail because her insurance company did not pay for the treatment she received at her appointment. After you greet the patient in a friendly, upbeat manner, she snaps at you, asks for an explanation of the high prices you are charging in the office, and slams the statement down on the counter in front of you. There are two other patients in the reception area looking on. What would you do?

The most appropriate immediate action for you to take in this situation is to communicate to the patient that you can see she is upset by this statement and that you would like to resolve the concern. A response such as "I can see you are upset Mrs. Jones, please let me review the statement and have a look at your account information in order that I can resolve this." If a private area is available for discussion, escort the patient there. If a private area is not available, use a lowered, calm tone of voice when providing your explanation. Allow the patient to express her concerns first without interruption. Ask questions once the patient has finished talking. In this scenario, the patient was not informed of her financial obligations to the dental office and has been surprised by an unexpected invoice. A thorough explanation must be given to the patient regarding her financial responsibility outside of the payment made by the insurance company on her behalf.

One of the responsibilities of the dental administrator for maintaining the patient relationship is to be proactive in preventing misunderstandings and the resultant anger from occurring in the first place. Think about this patient who is now standing in the reception area demanding an explanation from you. This patient was likely surprised by the statement she received in the mail because she was not informed of the possibility of having to pay for treatment personally. Sometimes, a phone call before mailing the statement will keep this scenario from occurring. Most office policies prescribe that patients must be informed about financial policies, waiting times, and appointment policies before establishing a relationship with the dental team. This proactive technique can avoid future angry-patient scenarios.

COMMUNICATION WITH TEAM MEMBERS

Good communication between team members in the dental office benefits both the patients and the staff. As a general rule, be courteous in your communication with other team members. When a clinical staff member brings the chart to the front desk and provides you with the information necessary for upcoming treatment or treatment completed, remember to say "Thank you." This is a fundamental aspect of maintaining an environment conducive to communication in the office. Politeness among staff members contributes to a positive environment by showing respect for each other and the patient. Team members who show respect for each other can communicate more confidently and competently.

Throughout your career, you will have both positive and challenging communication experiences with staff members. Effectively dealing with staff members is a necessary and important part of your career process. You will depend on your colleagues and supervisors for positive references as you build your career, and your reputation will depend in part on your ability to communicate well with them. Below, we will talk more in depth about communication with team members and other professional colleagues.

Colleagues

To maintain a professional work environment, remember not to discuss your personal life with colleagues while working, especially in front of patients. As you will be spending so much time together with your colleagues, it is easy and natural to develop relationships with them and to discuss personal issues. Finding out how their weekend was, whether their child won the ball game, how the dinner at their parents' house was, and whether their son's or daughter's school play was a success are all topics that employees discuss over lunch, at coffee break, and sometimes while working. Although such camaraderie is encouraged in most dental offices, discussing topics, such as

checkPOINT

11. Why is it advantageous to maintain a positive working relationship with colleagues?

those mentioned previously, while in the presence of patients is highly discouraged. The goal is to portray a professional atmosphere overall. Talking and laughing while patients are waiting in the reception area portrays an unprofessional environment because these actions send a message to the patients that talking about personal information is more of a priority than ensuring that the patients in the clinic are seen as soon as possible. All employees must be conscious to carry on personal conversations in private, staff areas.

Keeping your relationships with your colleagues amicable and professional is important for the longevity of the working relationships and positive atmosphere in the office. Although you may be friends with your colleagues, you must also maintain the professional environment of the dental office.

what IF ?

Your supervisor has called you into his office and asked for your opinion regarding the actions of another colleague in the office. What do you do?

If you ever have to report information to a supervisor regarding another colleague, it is important that you remain professional throughout the process. You can do this by only reporting the facts about the situation. If you do not have the facts, it is best to advise your supervisor of this. Embellishing or withholding information may be discovered at a later date and could result in your termination from the position.

Dentists

The dentist in the office must always be addressed as doctor while in the presence of patients and when you are referring to the dentist when talking with patients. It is important to show respect to the dentist and never question a diagnosis or treatment in front of the patient or other staff members. Always speak to the dentist in a professional manner, as you would speak to any supervisor or manager in any position. Developing a professional rapport with the dentist is important in maintaining a professional communicative atmosphere.

Other Dental and Healthcare Facilities

If you are a dental administrator in a general dentist's office, you will from time to time call specialist offices to refer patients for treatment or you will be required to forward patient chart information to other healthcare facilities, such as when patients change dentists. Use the following key points when providing information to other dental offices or healthcare facilities:

Ensure that a written request has been received by the patient to transfer information to the requesting dental office. Submitting information of any type to another healthcare facility must be authorized by the patient. A written request from the patient should be obtained prior to the release of information regardless of the mode of transmission. The dental office you work in may have a form that the patient will complete for this purpose. Alternatively, the requesting institution or office may receive consent from the patient and submit a copy to you for the chart. There are some exceptions to this rule, which will be outlined in the office policy manual. These exceptions can often include court-mandated requests or police investigation requests for information.

Provide only the information that has been requested. If a request for patient information specifically asks for written documentation, do not include items such as radiographs and dental impressions. Most agencies requesting information are asking for particulars to obtain answers to specific questions. Furthermore, if the patient is agreeing to have specific information sent on his or her behalf, any extraneous information sent is a violation of his or her privacy.

Remain nonjudgmental of the patient. Patients are entitled to choose whatever dental or healthcare facility they wish to receive treatment from. The maintenance of a positive patient relationship includes following through with their wishes to have chart contents forwarded to another practitioner. Never assume that the patient will not return to the practice. If the patient has informed you of the upcoming transfer, inquiring about the reason is perfectly acceptable and can be viewed as an opportunity to improve the clinic if the reason alludes to that.

If the information is being mailed, confirm receipt of the information. Mailing chart information specific to a patient requires documented receipt of the information by the receiving office. It is a responsible practice by the dental administrator to ensure that the request for information was followed through correctly. Personal information that becomes lost or delivered in error to the wrong address is the responsibility of the dental office, unless a record of the information is created by the delivery service.

Chapter Summary

Effective communication is an ongoing process in the dental office and, with time, skills in this area become finely tuned. Sending and receiving messages is an involved process that includes verbal and nonverbal communications. The barriers that affect communication with patients range from barriers presented by the sender, the receiver, and the environment. Furthermore, consideration must be given to the cultural and language barriers that can impair communication. Effective communication is a primary responsibility of the dental office administrator.

Review Questions

Multiple Choice

1. **Communication is a process that**
   a. includes components such as barriers and empathy.
   b. requires a sender, receiver, and an intended message.
   c. involves mostly nonverbal communication.
   d. facilitates discussion among colleagues.

2. **Communication can be distorted by all of the following except**
   a. body language.
   b. incongruent messages.
   c. inappropriate language.
   d. misunderstanding of meaning.

3. **Nonverbal communication is**
   a. the act of conveying messages through words.
   b. referred to as body language.
   c. the most common form of communication.
   d. all of the above.

4. **Which of the following is not a technique for successful communication?**
   a. clarifying
   b. rephrasing
   c. reflecting
   d. barriers

5. **Stereotyping is**
   a. holding an opinion about a group of people based on an oversimplification.
   b. your opinion about the treatment of a patient.
   c. making a distinction between people based on race.
   d. making a distinction between people based on color.

6. **Inflection is conveyed through**
   a. changes in your emotions.
   b. change in tone of voice.
   c. change in pitch of voice.
   d. both b and c.

7. **Which of the following actions communicates interest in what the speaker is saying?**
   a. eyes drawn downward attempting to avoid gaze
   b. arms crossed and audible sighs heard
   c. leaning away from persons as they speak
   d. Nodding your head as the person speaks

8. **Which of the following is an example of conceptualizing your attitude?**
   a. Letting the patient know you are not in the mood for chit-chat
   b. Discussing your personal issues with colleagues
   c. Visualizing yourself being in a positive mood
   d. Keeping your feelings to yourself

9. **An example of an open-ended question is:**
   a. Can I get you a glass of water?
   b. Are you OK?
   c. What day would you like to come in?
   d. Did you enjoy your service today?

10. **Recognizing possible barriers to communication early in the communication process**
    a. enables you to refrain from communicating with the patient.
    b. allows for identification and correction of misunderstandings.
    c. avoids creating a negative environment in the dental office.
    d. makes the communication process flow smoother.

Critical Thinking

1. An employee in the office refuses to assist a patient at the front desk because, as she explains, she does "not like that kind of people." What should you do?
2. How would you address the patient who arrives for his appointment 20 minutes late, through no fault of his own, and insists on seeing the dentist for his appointment?
3. A parent brings her 5-year-old with her during a lengthy procedure appointment. The child becomes restless 15 minutes after the parent is taken in for treatment. How do you deal with the child and what do you say to the parent before she leaves?
4. A patient calls you and is very angry about the statement received in the mail today. He does not want to pay it and would like an explanation. What could you say to this patient to (a) calm him down and (b) convince him to pay?

Bibliography

Maslow AH. Motivation and personality. Upper Saddle River, NJ: Prentice Hall, 1970.

Molle E, Durham L. Administrative medical assisting. Baltimore, MD: Lippincott Williams & Wilkins, 2004.

Web Site

U.S. Department of Human Rights
http://www.state.gov/g/drl/hr/

chapter SIX

Telephone *Skills*

OBJECTIVES

After completing this chapter, you should be able to do the following:

- Spell and define key terms
- Identify and describe the most common features of the modern office phone
- Name and explain the basic rules of speaking on the telephone
- Demonstrate how to properly manage multiple patient interactions at the same time
- Identify key information needed when taking a message
- Explain when it is appropriate to make personal calls in the dental office and how such calls should be made
- Name and discuss some barriers to effective telephone communication
- Name and describe the types of incoming calls in the dental office
- Name and describe the types of outgoing calls in the dental office

KEY TERMS

- telecommunications relay service
- telecommunications device for the deaf (TDD)

A significant responsibility of the dental office administrator is answering the telephone. An incoming telephone call that is promptly and correctly answered speaks volumes about the dental office staff and the importance placed on their patients. The telephone is the lifeline for the dental office and, when properly managed by the dental office administrator, allows easy access to dental care. Without the telephone, new patients cannot easily contact the dental office, existing patients cannot schedule appointments without walking into the clinic, and external agencies cannot be easily contacted or contact the dental office. Even with the frequent use of e-mails and the Internet in businesses of all types today, the telephone remains an important and primary method of communication. In previous chapters, concepts regarding communication techniques were introduced. When the intended message is successfully transmitted by

OUTLINE

Office Telephone
- Placing a Call
- Transferring
- Conference
- Call Forward
- Message Waiting Indicator
- Last Number Redial
- Hold Button
- Speed Dial
- Call Display
- Cordless Telephones
- Voice Mail
  - Create a Detailed Message for Callers
  - Keep the Voice Mailbox Empty
  - Refer to the Manual
  - Multiple Recorded Greetings

Speaking on the Telephone
- Showing Respect for Patients
- Speaking Clearly
- Pronunciation and Word Choice
- Confidence and Voice Tone
- Undivided Attention

Managing Multiple Patient Interactions

Taking Messages

Personal Phone Calls

Barriers to Phone Communication

Types of Incoming Calls
- Appointment Scheduling
- Account Inquiries
- Dental Emergencies
- Treatment Inquiries
- Challenging Calls
  - Upset Patients
  - Telemarketers, Solicitors, and Unidentified Callers

Types of Outgoing Calls
- Referrals
- Prescriptions Called in/Renewed
- Patient Confirmation

Chapter Summary

the sender and correctly understood by the receiver, communication is effective. Also, when communicating with a patient in person, a combination of verbal and nonverbal communication techniques is utilized to facilitate the communication process. One of the challenges presented when communicating via the telephone with patients is that the influence nonverbal communication has on the process of sending the message is inhibited.

Thus, the goal of this chapter is to equip you with the knowledge and skills you need to effectively communicate via the telephone in the dental office (Fig. 6-1). Presented are the common features of the office phone, guidelines for speaking on the phone, various skills and barriers to phone communication, as well as the most common types of incoming and outgoing calls.

checkPOINT

1. Why is telephone answering considered a significant responsibility of the dental office administrator?

OFFICE TELEPHONE

An important part of the dental office as a business is the telephone (Fig. 6-2). Using the telephone effectively is the responsibility of the office administrator and this involves the understanding of the features of the telephone.

The following telephone calling features are commonly used in many businesses today. Depending on the type of phone used in the dental office you work in, some or all of these features will be available.

Placing a Call

Pick up the handset and dial the number you desire. Once you pick up the handset, you may have to select the line that you wish to dial out on. Often the phone will automatically select the line once the handset is lifted. Alternatively, some telephone sets may have a "handsfree" key. Pressing the handsfree key allows you to dial the

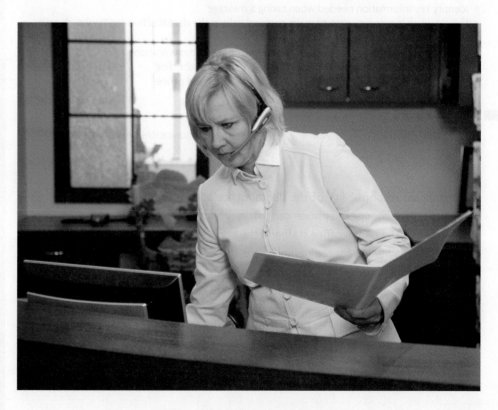

FIGURE 6-1 Attitude, skill, and confidence are necessary for effective telephone communication.

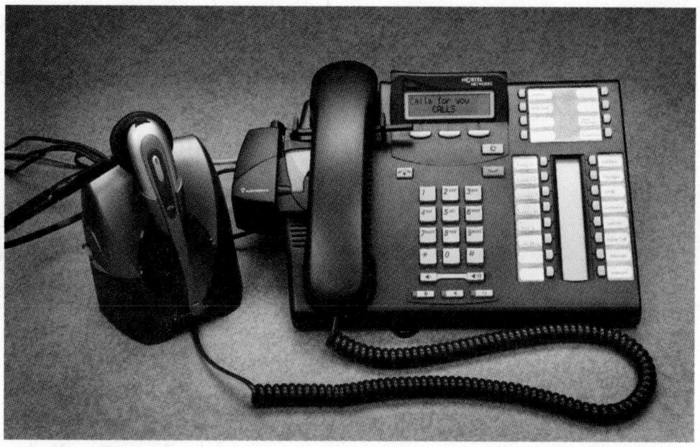

FIGURE 6-2
Telephone equipment.

number without picking up the handset in order to obtain a dial tone. This key is useful if you are gathering paperwork or accessing information on the computer to discuss with the person you are calling. The handsfree feature is also referred to as speakerphone, which is useful for having a telephone conversation without using the handset. The speakerphone feature is useful when more than one person in the room is involved in the phone call. Try to avoid using speakerphone during a phone call with a patient. If it is necessary to use the speakerphone feature, always get the permission of the patient before using this feature.

Transferring

Although most telephone calls coming into the dental office can be addressed by the office administrator, there are times when the call will be for a specific person in the office. In these instances, the call may be answered by the office administrator and then transferred to the correct person. Most telephone systems allow the call to be transferred by simply pressing the "transfer" key and dialing the extension number followed by pressing the transfer key again. Keeping an up-to-date list of the extension numbers of employees in the office will assist you in correctly transferring callers. Transferring callers to the wrong person can create frustration for the individual calling.

Conference

A conference call is a telephone call where many people can be a part of a meeting or conversation at the same time. Conference calls are an effective way of holding a meeting with individuals who are not within reasonable traveling distance from each other, and allow a meeting to occur without leaving the office. Most office telephones have a conference call feature. This is easily done by pressing the "conference" key, dialing the phone number of the desired party, and pressing the conference key again. This process is repeated until all parties are connected to the call.

Call Forward

The call forward feature is used when the person answering the phone will be away from the desk or unable to answer the phone. In the dental office the office administrator may forward all calls to the office managers' desk while she is out running an errand. If the call forward feature is used, it is often for a very short period of time. There will be a key on the phone labeled "forward," which is pressed, followed by the extension of the person who the calls will be forwarded to, the forward key is pressed again to activate the feature.

Message Waiting Indicator

Business telephones often have an indicator that tells you if a voice mail message is waiting to be heard. The indicator may be in the form of a light that flashes on the phone, a message is displayed on the telephone screen, or a beeping sound is heard when you pick up the handset. Depending on the type of indicator on the phone, you will need to listen to the voice mail message and either save or erase the message to stop the indicator. This can be done simply by entering a pass code or series of keys on the telephone to access the voice mail message. The dental office you work in will have a specific process for accessing voice mail messages.

Last Number Redial

This feature allows you to call the last telephone number that was dialed without dialing the entire number again. Generally, a key on the telephone labeled "redial" will enable you to redial the last number.

Hold Button

Pressing the "Hold" button on the telephone places the caller on hold. The telephone set may also have a feature that will prompt you if the caller is left on hold for a certain length of time. A beeping sound may be heard after 30 seconds of a caller being on hold, which is designed to remind you that the caller is waiting. To retrieve the call, pressing the line button will release the hold status.

Speed Dial

This feature allows you to place calls to frequently called numbers by entering a 1- or 2-digit code. Frequently called numbers in the dental office include the dental laboratory, insurance companies, or a specialist's office. Pressing the "Speed Dial" key on the telephone and entering a numerical code associated with the person you are calling will transmit the call.

Call Display

A telephone with a display screen that shows the name and phone number of the person calling the office has call display features. The advantage of the caller being identified before answering the telephone is that the office administrator can begin accessing the caller's information in the computer, or the chart, if the caller is a patient.

Cordless Telephones

Cordless telephones and headsets (Fig. 6-3) are commonly used in the dental office. Although the cordless telephone may not possess all the features that the desktop telephone possesses, it provides other advantages in the dental office. The use of cordless telephones allows staff members to use the telephone in any area of the dental office to schedule appointments for patients, telephone patients, or make other business-related calls. When all staff members have access to assisting with incoming telephone calls, such as using the cordless handset available, more calls will be addressed immediately. However, there will be situations in which the caller will leave a message on the voice mail system, such as when the office is closed, or during times when all telephone lines are in use.

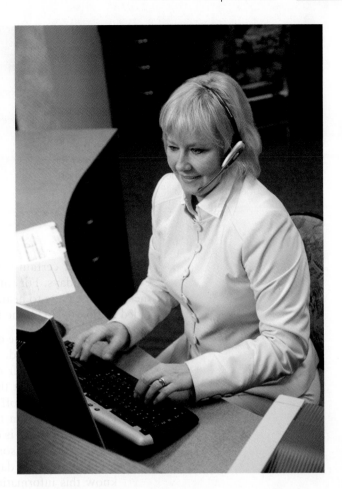

FIGURE 6-3
Telephone headset.

Voice Mail

Voice mail is a feature of telephone systems that allows the caller to leave a recorded message. When a message is left by the caller, an indicator on the telephone will inform you that a message is waiting. The indicator can be a light, an interrupted dial tone, or a displayed message on the display screen of the phone. When a caller is redirected to the voice mailbox, he or she will hear a personalized or automated greeting. An automated greeting is a greeting that is generated by a prerecorded voice telling callers that you are unavailable to answer the phone. A personalized greeting is one where a personal voice recording is made by a member of the dental team that provides information to callers about why they are redirected to the voice mailbox and when a response to the call can be expected. Usually there is an allotted amount of time for messages to be left and a maximum number of messages. This ensures that lengthy messages are not left on the voice mailbox occupying most of the space available. Accessing the voice mailbox messages is done by entering a numerical code. Once the messages are listened to and written down, they can then be deleted to create space in the mailbox.

Voice mail can be a very effective form of communication with callers. The following recommendations outline ways in which effective communication can result.

Create a Detailed Message for Callers

When callers must listen to a voice mail message, it is important to provide as much information as possible in order to gain necessary information from the caller and ultimately provide the caller with the information desired. The dental office administrator will be responsible for setting the voice mail message for the

BOX 6-1
Sample Voice Mail Message

"Thank you for calling Dr. Smith's Dental Office. Our office is open from 8:00 AM until 4:00 PM on Monday to Thursday. We are closed for lunch between 12:00 and 12:30 PM. Our office will be closed on Monday June 3 for a staff education conference. We will reopen on Tuesday June 4 at 8:00 AM. If you wish to leave a message or would like to have your call returned, please leave your phone number and the reason for your call after the tone and your call will be returned on the next business day. If you have a dental emergency, Dr. Smith can be reached by paging at 250-555-2222. Thank you for calling and have a nice day."

dental office at certain times, such as when the office will be closed for special events or holidays. For this reason you must be prepared to leave an appropriate message for callers to hear. A sample voice mail message for a dental office is provided in Box 6-1. Use the following list when creating a voice mail message:

- Always identify the office name so the caller is assured that the correct number has been dialed.
- Provide the regular operating hours of the office. This allows the callers to easily identify that they are hearing the voice mail message because they are calling outside of office hours.
- Provide the reason for the office closure and when the office will be open again. If the office is closed for a continuing education seminar, statutory holiday, or other reason, provide this information in the message and let the caller know what day and time the office will be open again. Callers like to know this information, particularly if the person is calling to make an appointment or have an emergency.
- Explain what information should be left by the caller, for example, a phone number, a reason for the call, and the best day and time the caller can be reached.
- Let the caller know of any alternatives to emergency services if the call is of an urgent nature. If there is another phone number the caller can dial, or another facility that can be accessed to help in case of a dental emergency, provide this information.
- Let the caller know when you will be returning the call. If you are returning calls on the next business day, provide this information.
- Leave a written reminder to change the voice mail message immediately on your return to the office. Leaving a message that is no longer valid is confusing to callers and also sends a nonverbal message that you are not paying attention.

Keep the Voice Mailbox Empty

Be mindful of the voice mail message indicator on the phone. If the phone does not have a visual or audible indicator, check for messages at regular intervals such as prior to beginning the day, on return from lunch, or frequently throughout the day. This is particularly important if the messages callers hear indicate that their call will be returned by a specific day or within a certain time. In other words, if the messages callers hear during the day indicate that the call will be returned within 30 minutes, make sure that this promise is kept. When obtaining messages from the voice mailbox, keep the following points in mind:

- Write down the message as completely as you can when listening to it. Voice mail includes features that will allow you to rewind messages to listen again, or fast-forward messages to gain all the information.

- Pass on messages for other staff members immediately. Make sure that the date and time of the call are written on the message. Do not save voice mail messages and ask staff members to listen to the voice mail in order to get the message.
- Return the calls in order of importance. If a patient has left a message indicating that an appointment needs to be made because of pain, attempt to call that patient first. Prioritize all calls and return them within the required time frame.
- After you have written down all the message information from each call, erase the voice mail message. Keeping the mailbox available for other callers to leave messages when necessary is much more effective for communication than a full mailbox that does not allow callers to leave a message.

Refer to the Manual

The voice mail system used in the office you work in will have a manual that outlines the features of the system. Accessing this manual will allow you to more easily familiarize yourself with the voice mail system. Familiarity with the voice mail system is a responsibility of the dental office administrator as a result of the telephone responsibilities inherent in the position. Keep the manual in a place where it is easily accessible to you and other staff members.

Being prepared by having access to and understanding how to use the voice mail features manual, keeping the mailbox available for callers to leave messages, and maintaining an up-to-date message enable the voice mailbox system to be an effective tool in communication with callers.

Multiple Recorded Greetings

During office hours, voice mail should not be the main point of contact for callers to the dental office. Most dental offices have a voice mailbox message that callers are redirected to if they call the office during office hours and all lines are busy. The prerecorded message tells callers that all lines are busy and the call will be returned within a specified time period. This voice mailbox message is different from the message callers hear when telephoning the office outside of office hours. Special attention must be paid to the time at which the caller left the message. The reason for this relates to the indicated amount of time promised that the call will be returned on the voice mail message callers hear. For example, if the voice mail message indicates that calls will be returned within 30 minutes, the caller should expect a callback within that period of time. Not following through with this could leave the caller feeling frustrated and angry with the service provided. An example of a voice mail message callers will hear when telephoning the office during office hours when all lines are busy may be the following: "Thank you for calling Dr. Smith's Dental office. Currently all of our lines are busy because we are assisting other callers. Please leave your name, phone number, and a brief message, and your call will be returned within 30 minutes. We apologize for any inconvenience this may cause and thank you for your patience."

> **checkPOINT**
>
> 2. What role does effective management of the voice mailbox play in communication with patients?

SPEAKING ON THE TELEPHONE

Each time the telephone is answered in the dental office, an impression is being made on the caller. The dental office administrator is the person responsible for creating a positive and professional image of the dental practice and this is accomplished by effectively communicating the intended message. Therefore, the lack of nonverbal cues in telephone communication, such as those discussed in Chapter 5, makes the dental administrator's verbal communication skills all the more important when speaking on the phone. The use of the words chosen, how they are pronounced, the expression used when speaking, and whether or not the office administrator cares about what the patient has to say are all part of the impression made by the office administrator, and these factors are the subject of this section. In addition to the phone-specific points made below, keep in mind the guidelines for general communication from the previous chapter, which contribute to effective telephone communication, particularly regarding having a good attitude.

Showing Respect for Patients

When speaking with patients either on the phone or in person, an effective communication technique to incorporate into everyday dialogue is to use manners and smile. This is a simple and effective method for communicating successfully with any person you encounter in the dental office whether the person is a staff member, patient, or salesperson. Consciously using manners when communicating with people is a welcomed gesture that conveys respect and concern. During busy times it can be easy to forget to say "please" and "thank you" and smile while you assist patients, since you are focused on completing many tasks within a limited time frame. However, using an abrupt approach with a patient just once can undo a lot of relationship building, and it may be difficult for the patient to overcome, unless the disrespect is acknowledged and an apology offered.

Integrating manners into everyday communication creates a pleasant and professional working atmosphere. Incorporating manners into conversation on the telephone is just as imperative for developing professional relationships as using them in face-to-face encounters with people. The following suggestions for using manners in the workplace are helpful when dealing with patients, colleagues, and outside contacts.

Address the person you are speaking to. When speaking to someone for the first time, always make sure you will be addressing him or her correctly, that is, the way in which the caller prefers to be addressed. For example, if the caller tells you that his name is John Smith, you would address him as "Mr. Smith" until he advises you otherwise. In addition to this, clarify the correct spelling of the caller's name if you are speaking to a first-time caller so as not to make any errors while recording his or her information. If you are speaking face to face with a patient or colleague, incorporate nonverbal techniques such as eye contact and smiling.

Give positive feedback whenever you can. Building relationships with patients and colleagues allows for opportunities to provide compliments and praise. For example, if a colleague provides assistance to you by helping you with some of your daily tasks, a positive remark to the colleague regarding the effort made in helping you provides acknowledgment and appreciation, which is an appropriate response for maintaining a professional relationship. A compliment should not be exaggerated or given out of context since it may be viewed as insincere and create suspicion. Therefore, compliments should be direct and succinct.

Say "Thank You". Being polite goes a long way in the development of relationships. Saying thank you to a patient in the dental office can be very easily integrated in the office administrator vocabulary since there are many opportunities to say thank you. Answering the telephone yields an opportunity to thank a caller for calling the office. Box 6-2 provides some examples to use when answering the telephone. In addition, saying thank you to the caller can be done at the end of the telephone conversation. For example, when a patient calls to schedule an appointment, at the end of the phone call just before saying good-bye, interjecting with "Thank you for calling" can evoke an equally polite response from the caller such as "you're welcome," which leaves the caller feeling as if the telephone call to the dental office was sincerely appreciated. Using the phrase "thank you" can be very effective in maintaining professional relationships. Be careful

checkPOINT

3. Give an example of how you can use manners in the workplace. Explain why it is helpful.

BOX 6-2
Phrases to Use When Answering the Telephone

"Thank you for calling Peach Avenue Dental. This is Tracey. How may I help you?"

"Good Morning and Thank you for calling Dr. Smith's office. This is Tracey speaking."

"Good Afternoon. Dr. Smith's office. Tracey speaking."

not to use the more casual form "thanks" when the phrase "thank you" is more appropriate; doing so does not impart the same level of sincerity and can hinder the development of the professional relationship.

Speaking Clearly

Speaking clearly on the telephone is a factor of effective telephone communication that is often taken for granted. That is, people often assume that they do speak clearly and pronounce words distinctly so that they are understood, when they actually do not. Imagine speaking to someone on the phone who has the mouthpiece of the phone on her chin. Can you hear her clearly? Likely not—-the person would probably sound muffled or far away, and, as a result, you would strain to hear her. This muffled sound can also be a result of placing the telephone receiver on your shoulder and holding it with your chin while you speak. Eating or chewing gum while speaking can also distort speech on the phone. Likewise, speaking too quickly can cause the person you are talking with to focus more on trying to keep up with your words instead of trying to understand the conversation. Allow time for the person you are speaking with to respond to questions or comments by pausing for a moment after you have spoken. Alternatively, if you are having difficulty hearing a patient because he or she is speaking very quietly, always begin by adjusting the volume on your phone. This often solves the problem. If the difficulty persists, let the patient know you have difficulty hearing what is being said and request that the person speaks a little louder in order that you can hear him or her.

Therefore, to ensure that your words are clear and easy to understand, hold the phone receiver directly over your mouth and approximately 1 inch away. This allows the speaker to clearly hear what you are saying without interference. Holding the mouthpiece too close to your mouth creates distracting sounds that interfere with the communication. The correct pronunciation of words and the tone of your voice also influence the clarity of your voice; both of these components are discussed in the upcoming sections. There are different types of phone varieties that will facilitate keeping the phone mouthpiece at an acceptable distance away while talking. One of these is the use of a headset, either wired or wireless. Most phone systems have a headset in place or have the capability to be equipped with one. A wireless headset gives the office administrator freedom to access other areas of the dental office while talking on the phone and minimizes the frequency of placing callers on hold to obtain information out of reach. For example, accessing a patient's paper chart can be easily done while using a wireless headset to answer telephone calls. With the technology available today, most headsets provide a higher degree of clarity in the phone, which also assists in communicating in a clear voice with callers.

Pronunciation and Word Choice

The correct pronunciation of words facilitates understanding when speaking with patients, particularly in regard to dental terminology with which the patient may not be familiar. If you are not clear on the pronunciation of a word, consult a dictionary or ask a coworker for assistance.

TABLE 6-1 Words to Avoid Using With Callers

Avoid	Replace With
Hi	Hello
Bye	Goodbye
Yah	Yes
Just a sec	One moment please
Hold please	Would you mind holding?
What?	I'm sorry I didn't quite hear you.

Moreover, your choice of words can also affect the patient's understanding. Although it is important to use accurate, proper terminology when speaking with patients, you should also, wherever possible, use terms with which they will be familiar. For example, a patient will likely be more familiar with the term "TMJ" than with the term "temporomandibular joint." Although they are both the same in meaning, TMJ is a term that most people recognize and understand. Using terminology that is unfamiliar to a patient when discussing his or her treatment can be confusing and create frustration. Some patients may interpret your use of the terminology as either condescending or having negative connotations for the type of treatment involved. Table 6-1 supplies some examples of words to avoid using while on the telephone and their recommended replacements.

Confidence and Voice Tone

Although nonverbal cues will obviously not be directly evident in phone communication, they can influence you to speak with more confidence. For example, try smiling while you are speaking to someone on the phone. Your voice will sound lifted, and you will speak at a higher volume. If you are seated, focus on correct posture, with shoulders back, abdominals tucked in, and neck straight, and you will find that your voice will project confidence (Fig. 6-4). Sometimes, standing up while speaking can also help you communicate confidently.

The tone of your voice greatly influences the impression you make while on the telephone. The pitch, volume, tone, and rhythm are all factors that assist in conveying the spoken message while on the phone. These elements act as the nonverbal components of communication on the telephone. For example, if you raise your voice while speaking, depending on the tone used you can communicate either a happy, cheerful message, or one of frustration and anger. A person who is angry may use a higher pitched tone that communicates a sense of anger to the caller. In other words, your voice reflects emotion through inflection. That is, if you are happy, you will likely speak at a higher tone or volume and will vary your inflection more; using a monotone voice can communicate indifference or laziness. Vary your inflection and avoid speaking in a monotone voice while on the phone. The person who answers the telephone in the dental office represents the personality of the office. Always project a cheerful, positive expression when you answer the phone, to project the image of a professional who is genuinely concerned about the patient calling the office.

checkPOINT

4. Explain how voice tone and inflection influence the nonverbal message you send while on the phone to patients.

Using a consistent rhythm when speaking on the telephone is necessary to communicate effectively. Speaking too quickly or too slowly can be distracting and frustrating for the patients as they attempt to interpret what you are saying. Speaking quickly may send the message that you are too busy or impatient with the caller. Speaking too slowly may imply that you are bored or unsure of the information you

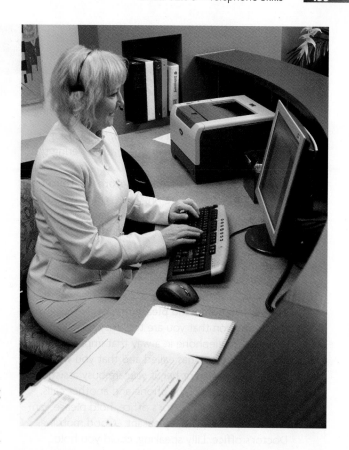

FIGURE 6-4 Using correct posture while on the phone.

are giving to the patient. Use an evenly paced rhythm and allow time for the caller to respond by leaving momentary pauses when necessary.

Undivided Attention

Despite the busyness and noise of the dental office, it is critical that you provide your undivided attention to the patient you are speaking to on the phone. This means that you must block out environmental noises, such as people talking around you, telephone ringing, and extraneous noise. Attentively listening means that you are responding to the patients while they are speaking or that you are providing verbal cues that you are listening to them. Conveying the message to patients that they are important and that you are willing to help by addressing questions and concerns assists in developing positive, long-term relationships. While you are speaking with patients on the telephone, make sure that you have the opportunity to speak with them without interruptions. If the patient is calling at a busy time, politely inform the person that you are currently completing a few tasks that require immediate attention and agree to a specific time to return the call. Alternatively, you could place the caller on hold, go to a quiet place, and complete the phone call without interruption.

> ✓ **checkPOINT**
>
> 5. What does it mean to provide a patient with your undivided attention on the phone?

MANAGING MULTIPLE PATIENT INTERACTIONS

The telephone ringing while you are completing paperwork or are on the other line can be bothersome. It is natural to feel frustration when you are focused on a task and an interruption occurs. However, remember that patients calling the dental office are unaware that they are interrupting your work. To treat them rudely in such situations comes as a shock to them and could lead them to take their business elsewhere. Box 6-3 outlines five general rules for answering the telephone in the dental

BOX 6-3
Guidelines for Telephone Answering

Points to remember for effective telephone answering

1. **Give the caller your full attention.** Stop eating, talking, or doing any activity before answering the phone.
2. **Always answer the telephone before the third ring.** Listening to a telephone ring more than three times when you are the caller intimates that the dental office employees are not concerned with answering the phone or with the person who is calling. New patients may hang up and call another office, and current patients will express their dissatisfaction by voicing their concerns or transferring elsewhere.
3. **Answer in a polite and pleasant tone.** Never give the impression that you are too busy to talk. Always answer the telephone in a way that implies you are happy the person has called and that you would like to talk to him or her. If you are busy assisting another patient on the phone and another calls, instead of saying "Doctor's office, hold please," answer the phone with a pleasant, "Good morning, Doctor's office, Lilly speaking, could you hold please?" If you need to, explain to the patient that you are currently assisting a patient on the phone and you would be happy to help him or her when the call is completed. Offer the patient the option of calling back.
4. **Always identify who you are to the caller.** It is annoying for callers to have to guess or outright ask who they are talking to. Identifying yourself will help build rapport with the patient and influence his or her impression of you and the office, as the patient is able to address you directly.
5. **Respond to questions in an enthusiastic manner.**
6. **Have writing utensils ready to jot down information from the caller.**
7. **Never put patients on hold for long periods of time.** If you tell a caller, "I will be with you in a minute," make sure that you get back to her before that "minute" is up! If you need more time than you had originally thought, check back in with her and ask whether she would rather wait another minute (or other specified amount of time) or be called back. If she prefers to be called back, give her a time frame within which to expect your call such as "I will call you back within 30 minutes." Then, be sure to call her back within the time frame promised. Keeping the patient waiting too long on hold could result in losing that patient.
8. **Never transfer a call to the wrong person.** If you must transfer a call to another person in the office, make sure that the person is in the office to accept calls; otherwise, offer the caller the option of leaving a message either with you or on voice mail. Do not transfer a patient just because you are busy and would like to get rid of the call. Transferring a call to the wrong person or to someone who is not in the office may lead the patient to think that you are incompetent in your job or that you do not care and can be very frustrating for the caller. Ensure that the patient gets connected with the correct person, or provide a direct number she can call if the line is busy. Ask the patient to call you directly if she has trouble reaching the person she needs.

office, which will assist you in mastering the skill of effectively communicating with patients over the phone.

When you are on the telephone with a patient and the other telephone line is ringing, ask the caller you are speaking with if he or she would hold for a few moments so that you can answer the other ringing line. Callers are often understanding of this situation and are willing to hold. When you answer the other line, ask the new caller if he or she could please hold for 1 minute while you complete a call on your other line. The time frame you provide to the caller is very important. Use the second hand on your watch or a small hourglass timer to keep track of the time while you finish your call. Of utmost importance is that you return to the second caller in the time promised. If after the minute you have not completed your first phone call, return to the second caller and ask whether he or she would like to continue holding or to be called back. Always allow the patient to provide an answer before placing him or her on hold. If the patient does not like to hold, tell him or her that you will call back as soon as you are available; it is good manners to provide a time frame for this also. Usually 30 minutes is acceptable.

Providing patients with the option of speaking with another staff member to address their reason for calling could also be helpful in avoiding patients feeling disrespected. If a patient is calling to book an appointment or discuss treatment and another staff member is available to help, ask whether he or she would mind assisting the patient. Working together as a team is especially important during busy times.

Another challenge is assisting patients on the phone while also assisting patients in the office. Although there are no hard-and-fast rules for managing such situations, there are some general guidelines to keep in mind. If you are on the telephone, a patient arrives at the front desk, and you are close to completing the call, you should complete the call before assisting the patient who has arrived at the desk. However, you should acknowledge the patient in the office right away by looking up and smiling, while continuing the phone conversation; do not wait to hang up the phone to acknowledge the patient. On the other hand, if the call has just begun or will take a little while, ask the caller to hold and address the patient in front of you. If the transaction takes a small amount of time, proceed with it. If the transaction requires a few minutes, ask if the patient will mind waiting in the reception area while you complete the call you had begun. Managing these situations will require tact and skill, and if you need to, ask another staff member to assist you in handling the situation. The goal is to manage the situation effectively and competently.

> **✓ checkPOINT**
>
> 6. What is the best way to acknowledge a patient who arrives at the dental office while you are on the telephone with another patient?

There are some phone calls that require your immediate attention, regardless of what you are in the midst of doing or how many calls you have waiting. These include emergency calls, calls from other dentists or physicians to the dentist in the office, and any personal emergency calls to staff members. In situations in which you must take messages for the dentist or other members of the dental team, be sure to follow the preferred message-taking system in the office.

TAKING MESSAGES

Regardless of the size of the dental office, you will likely receive calls for some or all of the staff at some point that will require that you take a telephone message. Figure 6-5 is an example of what a telephone message pad looks like. The information requested on the message pad helps you obtain pertinent information from the caller to be delivered to the receiver of the message. The date and time of the call as well as the name and phone number of the person calling are the most important pieces of information to provide to the recipient. The message left by the caller must be written in the body of the message sheet and be as detailed and legible as possible. Procedure 6-1 provides steps to follow for taking an accurate phone message.

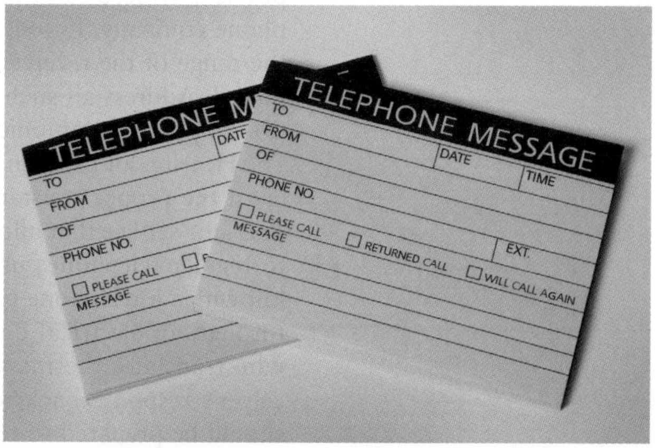

FIGURE 6-5
Telephone message pad.

PROCEDURE 6-1 Taking an Accurate Telephone Message

1. Ask the caller to spell his or her name for you if you are unsure of the spelling.
2. Ask the caller for the phone number at which he or she wishes to be called. Record the number. Repeat the number back to the caller for confirmation.
3. Ask the caller if the call is urgent.
4. Ask the caller if there is a detailed message for the person he or she is calling. If so, record the message and repeat it back to the caller.
5. Assure the caller that you will deliver the message to the staff member he or she is calling for.

PERSONAL PHONE CALLS

Because the telephone is the lifeline for the dental practice, it should be kept available for business-related calls at all times. This means that personal calls should be restricted to emergency calls only on the office phone. Some offices may dedicate one line of the multiline phone for use by the staff members, and if this is the case, only that line should be used for personal calls. In any case, it is still recommended that personal calls on the office phone be limited to emergency calls. The use of personal cell phones should be restricted to staff areas, such as the lunch room, or outside of the office.

checkPOINT

7. When should you use the dental office phone for personal calls?

Even when using your own phone to make personal calls in the office, keep them to a minimum and keep them short. Keeping your cell phone at the front desk for use is not suggested.

BARRIERS TO PHONE COMMUNICATION

As discussed in the previous chapter, the environment can create barriers in the communication process. Loud background noise, such as music or talking, can make a conversation on the telephone frustrating for both the caller and the person answering the phone, as the messages being sent can be difficult to decipher. Keep the background noise level to a minimum when talking on the phone by moving to a conference room or other quiet place, if possible. Also, as an office policy, it could be established that talking among the staff should be minimal in the front desk area, to maintain a quiet, distraction-free environment.

Technical difficulties with the telephone can also create barriers to effective telephone communication. A telephone line that has technical interference, such as static or crossed lines, can also lead to miscommunication. In such cases, a telephone may need to be replaced or the problem may need to be reported to the local phone company. If you are using a cordless phone, make sure that you are within the range of the receiver and that the battery does not need to be recharged or replaced. Address all such problems as soon as possible to avoid prolonged interruption to phone communication in the office.

Hearing and speech impairments on the part of the caller can also create barriers if the proper assistance is not in place. **Telecommunications relay service** is an operator service that allows people with hearing and speech disabilities to place calls to regular telephones using a **telecommunications device for the deaf (TDD)**, also known as a telephone typewriter (TTY). The TDD is used to send typed messages through an electrical communications channel over the telephone to an operator, who translates the message to speech for the receiver and then translates the receiver's response back to text for the caller. As a dental office administrator, you should be prepared to receive such operator-assisted calls. Moreover, if you receive

BOX 6-4
Tips for Communicating With Patients With Disabilities Over the Telephone

Speech Impairments

A person calling the office who has a speech impairment may stutter, slur his or her words, or have unintelligible speech. Use the following tips when communicating with someone who has a speech impairment:

- Listen patiently and give the person time to speak. Avoid rushing the person by attempting to guess what he or she is trying to say.
- Always repeat back your understanding of what the person has said to you.
- Ask questions that require short answers in response.
- Allow additional time for the person to communicate if a communication aid, such as a synthesized speaker, is being used.
- If you are having a lot of difficulty understanding the person, ask for an interpreter or recruit another staff member to assist you.

Vision Impairments

Patients who have a vision impairment may require the use of equipment that enables to communicate via a computer, such as software used to speak information from the computer, or screen magnification software. Keep the following tips in mind during your telephone communication:

- The screen reading software supplies the information to the person using a synthesized computer voice. Injection inflection in your tone will not be communicated.
- If you are directing a patient to a Web page, the information he or she views using this software may be distorted.

Hearing Impairments

Patients with hearing impairments may have a variation of some or total hearing loss. When communicating over the telephone with people who are deaf or hard of hearing, keep in mind the following:

- Raising your voice may be effective for persons with mild hearing loss.
- If the person you are communicating with wears a hearing aid, it may not be necessary to raise your voice or use any special communication devices. However, a hearing aid can sometimes create feedback noise while on the phone in the form of a high-pitched tone. Let the patient know this is occurring and this allows them to make adjustments to minimize the feedback.
- Patients who are severely hard of hearing may use a relay service, which is a 24-hour, 7-day-a-week telephone assistance. To use a relay service, an individual uses his or her TTY to contact a relay operator who also has a TTY. The operator then calls the dental office and acts as an interpreter. When using the relay system, the relay operator types everything you say so it is important to speak as if you are speaking to the hearing-impaired person and not someone else.

checkPOINT

8. What are some barriers to phone communication in the dental office?

calls from patients with hearing or speech disabilities who might benefit from such service, you can mention the service to them and direct them to proper sources to learn more about it, such as the Web site of the Federal Communications Commission (www.fcc.gov/cgb/dro/trs.html).

Box 6-4 outlines tips to keep in mind when communicating over the telephone with persons who have disabilities such as hearing impairments and visual or speech impairments.

TYPES OF INCOMING CALLS

Over the course of a day, the dental office administrator will routinely handle certain types of incoming telephone calls. Whether the calls are from established patients or prospective patients, they should be handled professionally and courteously. A good practice to keep in mind is to treat each caller as if he or she were in the office in person making his or her inquiry. This will help you focus on treating the patient with respect and courtesy throughout the phone call and providing each

PROCEDURE 6-2 *Steps to Follow in Answering the Telephone in a Dental Office*

1. Smile.
2. Provide an appropriate greeting for the time of day. Identify the name of the dental office and who you are. Example: "Good morning, Dr. Girtel's office, Lilly speaking."
3. Always finish the call with the phrase "Thank you for calling."
4. Once you have completed the call, allow the caller to hang up first.

patient with the same courtesy. Procedure 6-2 outlines general steps to follow in answering the telephone in a dental office that are applicable to all types of calls. Of the many phone calls made to the dental office each day, most are regarding appointment scheduling, account inquiries, dental emergencies, and service inquiries. Each of these types is briefly presented below. Note that tasks related to many of these calls, such as appointment scheduling and dental emergencies, are covered in detail in later chapters of the book.

Appointment Scheduling

Many calls you will receive will be from established patients calling to schedule an appointment for treatment such as recare appointments for teeth cleanings or other treatment recommended by the dentist. New patients will also call to schedule appointments in order to see the doctor or hygienist.

Account Inquiries

Patients who have received a statement from the dental office may require an explanation for the cost of the services they received. In some offices, the dental administrator is responsible for handling account inquiry calls. If such is the case in your office, you will need to provide the information. If there is an office manager or other individual responsible for this area of patient services, pass the caller on to that person. Attempting to provide an explanation in an area that is outside your scope of responsibility could create frustrations. Inform the caller that you will direct him or her to the appropriate staff member.

Dental Emergencies

A dental emergency is a situation in which the patient calls and reports pain, swelling, or bleeding in the mouth. Dental emergencies are given priority when presented by the patient. The office you work in will have a policy regarding the determination of emergencies and how to address the situation. Make sure that you are aware of what the office policy is in this regard. The topic of dental emergencies and how to handle this type of telephone call effectively are covered in greater detail in a later chapter.

Treatment Inquiries

On occasion, existing or potential new patients will call inquiring about the cost of treatments offered. Most dental offices have a policy of not quoting prices over the phone. Often, this policy is in place because the cost of performing the same dental treatment for two different patients can vary. The recommended approach is to provide a ballpark figure for the person, with an explanation that the exact amount will be determined on examination. For example, if a caller inquires about the cost of a teeth cleaning, depending on the office policy, you may need to inform the caller that an exact quote is not possible without first having a consultation with the dental hygienist or dentist. This is because each person's dental treatment requirements are different and cannot be determined without a clinical evaluation. Providing a cost estimate will vary from state to state and between dental offices.

Challenging Calls

The dental office administrator is the member of the dental team who handles all incoming calls. Unfortunately, not all of the incoming phone calls are pleasant telephone calls to handle. There are some calls that require some assertiveness and some inquiry to categorize and then effectively handle the call.

Upset Patients

Some patients may call the dental office because they are upset with a statement of account they have received or because of a service they received. When a patient telephones the office because he or she is upset, consider the following points in effectively handling the call:

- Ask the patient to explain the reason for being upset.
- Speak calmly and never raise your voice.
- Assure the patient that you want to help.
- Go to a quieter area of the office, where concentrating on the issue at hand will be much easier.
- Listen to the patient, using verbal cues to demonstrate that you are listening.
- If the patient is upset about account charges, explain him or her if you can.
- If the patient becomes irate or belligerent, tell the patient that you will have to call him or her back, or have the office manager do so.
- Take notes throughout the telephone call.
- Follow through with any promises made to the patient, such as returning the call.
- Record the telephone call information in the patient chart.
- Inform the dentist or office manager of the call.

checkPOINT

9. What are three things you should do when dealing with an upset caller?

Telemarketers, Solicitors, and Unidentified Callers

From time to time, callers will ask to speak with the dentist or other clinician in the dental office but will not identify themselves. In many cases, such calls are from telemarketers and solicitors. The dentist will inform you, or the office policy manual will outline, what the preference is regarding callers who wish to speak with clinicians in the office. General policies in this regard are as follows:

- Inform the caller that the dentist cannot be disturbed while with a patient and that you would be happy to give the dentist a message.
- If the caller still refuses to identify himself or herself for the dentist to return the call but wishes to call back, inform the caller that the best way to make contact is to leave information for the dentist and that the call will be returned when the dentist has time available.
- Inform the dentist that a caller is trying to reach the dentist but does not wish to leave a name.

legal TIP

Recording the telephone call in the patient chart is an important part of the patient's history in the dental office. If the patient has a concern about any aspect of his or her experience in the dental office, it must be recorded in his or her chart. Further to this, there must also be documentation describing how this concern was addressed. Maintaining a thorough and complete patient chart includes all communication with the patient.

Legitimate callers who are trying to reach the dentist will typically leave a message and provide their information for the dentist to call them back. As the dental office manager, one of your responsibilities is to tactfully and professionally manage these types of calls. If the caller becomes persistent and begins to take up a greater amount of time than required on a frequent basis, ask the office manager to handle the call, or encourage the dentist to allow you to provide the caller with a response to his or her inquiry.

BOX 6-5
Guidelines for Making Telephone Calls

1. **Always identify yourself and the reason for your call at the beginning of the call.** When you are calling a patient, an insurance company, or a pharmacy, always begin the call when answered with "Good morning/afternoon, this is Lilly from Dr. Smith's office calling to ... (provide reason) ...." This provides the caller with everything he or she needs to know right away to direct your call to the proper person. Once you have provided this information, you can then ask who you are speaking with.
2. **Allow the person responding to you to provide or ask information without interruption.** Showing respect and being courteous to the person you are calling is important, as you are projecting an image of the dental office and the staff members through the impression you are making on the person receiving the call.
3. **Be prepared to provide information.** Have information ready to give to the person you are calling. If you are calling another dental office or pharmacy, you may have to provide information regarding a patient. You may want to have the patient's chart ready.

TYPES OF OUTGOING CALLS

In addition to handling incoming calls, you will also be responsible for contacting various external agencies by telephone on a daily basis. Making calls to other dental offices to refer patients, phoning pharmacies to provide prescription information for patients, calling insurance companies for benefit inquiries, and phoning patients for appointment confirmations are just some of the more common types of outgoing calls in a dental office. Box 6-5 provides you with three general rules to keep in mind when making outgoing calls.

Referrals

In a general dentist office, the dentist may feel that it is necessary to refer a patient to a specialist for treatment. In this case, it will be the duty of the dental administrator to contact the specialist's office and arrange an appointment for the patient. To facilitate a patient's dental treatment, a specialist such as an orthodontist or oral surgeon may be required to complete a part of the treatment. The dentist and the specialist then work as a team, providing the necessary treatment for the patient, to achieve the desired outcome.

> *legal TIP*
>
> Leaving personal patient information on a recording, such as voice mail, is considered a violation of a patient's privacy. The information you leave for a patient on a voice mail message should be limited to the date and time of the appointment. Information such as the reason for the appointment must not be left on the answering machine. If the patient would prefer that you did leave this information for them, have them provide a written request before making this change.

Prescriptions Called in/Renewed

Patients who require prescription medication from the dentist may obtain a written prescription (Fig. 6-6) from the dental office, or a prescription may be called in directly to the pharmacy. Procedure 6-3 outlines the method used to call in a prescription for a patient. A prescription for a patient can be called in only after the dentist has written or renewed the prescription. The dentist is the only staff member in the office who has the authority to renew or write a new prescription for a patient.

Patient Confirmation

Phoning patients the day prior to their scheduled appointment is a policy employed in most dental offices. Confirming patient appointments helps the dental office administrator keep the schedule under control and maintain a steady of flow of

Dr. Guy S. Girtel - Family Dentistry

Dr. Guy Girtel (02553)
#204, 7125-109 Street
Edmonton, AB
T6G 1B9

Tel: (780)4355300

Patient: Dawna Hawkes DOB: Aug/8/62

Address: 11022 - 64 Avenue
Edmonton, AB T6H 1T5
Tel: (780)43479

Rx: Amoxil 500 mg Capsules Dispense: 30

Sig: Take 1 capsule every 8 hours until finished

Refills: 0

Note: (Amoxil 500 ten days)

Dr. Guy Girtel Date: 25-Feb-09

☐ Substitution Permissible

FIGURE 6-6 Prescription.

patients in the dental office. The telephone call to the patient usually involves a short statement such as "Good morning Mrs. Jones, this is Dr. Smith's office calling to confirm your appointment with our hygienist tomorrow afternoon at 2 PM. We're looking forward to seeing you then. Please call our office to confirm this appointment." The call should be short and to the point. Confirming appointments in the dental office is a proactive way to decrease the number of patients who do not make the scheduled appointment or cancel with little notice. Telephoning patients and speaking to them directly 1 or 2 days prior to the appointment allow time for you to fill a cancelled appointment spot and eliminate the frustration that can occur when a patient does not show up for the appointment time.

Some patients may prefer to be contacted via e-mails to confirm their scheduled appointment. This is a much more efficient way to confirm appointments for some patients, particularly if they are not near a phone, yet can access their e-mails.

PROCEDURE 6-3 *Calling in a Prescription for a Patient*

1. Ensure that you have all the necessary items to complete the call: the patient's chart, correct spelling of the patient's name, prescription from the dentist, and the name and phone number of the pharmacy.
2. Call the pharmacy. You will be asked to provide the name of the patient, the name and phone number of the prescribing doctor, and the prescription (as written by the doctor). You must read the prescription exactly as written.
3. Record the information in the patient's chart.
4. You may follow up and call the patient to inform him or her that the prescription has been called in to the pharmacy.

Chapter Summary

The telephone etiquette you display while communicating with patients provides a representation of the dental office. This image of the dental practice is representative of every staff member in the office. To succeed as a dental administrator, you will need to master the skill of speaking effectively on the telephone and be consistent in showing respect to patients. Likewise, you will need to develop tact and skill in effectively communicating with patients in the dental office and responding to telephone calls simultaneously. Taking phone messages accurately and managing challenging calls such as emergencies and those from upset patients are other critical skills that are developed through practice in the dental office.

Review Questions

Multiple Choice

1. **In the dental office, you may have to manage all but the following types of calls:**
   a. account inquiries.
   b. appointment scheduling.
   c. dental emergencies.
   d. staff emergencies.
2. **Outgoing calls in the dental office do not include**
   a. referrals to specialists.
   b. prescription renewals.
   c. hospital deliveries.
   d. patient confirmation.
3. **The TDD is used to send typed messages through an electrical communications channel over the telephone**
   a. true
   b. false
4. **An efficient way to have a telephone conversation with a patient is to**
   a. use the speaker phone feature of the phone to talk with the patient and address paperwork at the same time.
   b. allow the voice mail message to answer the phone and respond to the inquiry afterward.
   c. actively listen to the patient and minimize distractors while on the phone.
   d. ask the patients if they would prefer an e-mail confirmation for their appointment.
5. **An example of using positive feedback with a patient is**
   a. saying please and thank you when you can.
   b. complimenting the patient.
   c. thanking the patient for being loyal to the practice.
   d. holding the door open for a patient using a wheelchair.
6. **Which is the best example of providing undivided attention to a patient?**
   a. using direct eye contact when speaking to a patient
   b. asking the patient to hold while you finish another call
   c. going to a quiet area to speak with the patient on the phone
   d. asking all other patients in the waiting room to refrain from speaking while you are on the phone
7. **Only the office manager can phone in prescriptions for patients to the pharmacy.**
   a. true
   b. false
   c. Only the dentist can phone in prescriptions.
   d. Only the office administrator can phone in prescriptions.
8. **A patient's condition is considered a dental emergency when**
   a. swelling is present.
   b. bleeding is present.
   c. the patient is in pain.
   d. any of the above are occurring.
9. **Patient concerns should be written in the patient chart**
   a. only if the concern was addressed.
   b. when they occur.
   c. if the office manager allows it.
   d. never.
10. **What would be an appropriate response to a patient with whom you are having trouble hearing on the telephone?**
    a. "please call me back at a later time when your phone is working properly."
    b. "turn up the volume on your phone, I cannot hear you."
    c. "I am having difficulty hearing you, could you speak up please?"
    d. "You need to speak a lot louder if you want me to hear you!"

Critical Thinking

1. A patient with obvious swelling in the upper right anterior area of his or her mouth has arrived at the dental clinic. The patient demands to see the dentist and would like some pain relievers immediately. What do you say to this patient?
2. The daily schedule is full, and the dentist is 15 minutes behind schedule. A patient calls and is very upset about a filling that was placed that morning. The patient demands to talk with the dentist and insists on waiting on the phone. What would you say to calm the patient down?
3. Line 2 is ringing. You are finishing a call on line 3, and Mr. Jones is standing in front of you waiting to settle his account. How do you handle this situation? Who would you give priority to, and why?
4. Describe how you would encourage a caller to leave a message for the dentist when he or she does not want to leave information, but would like to call back.

HANDS-ON ACTIVITY

1. Develop a dental emergency procedure policy for the dental office you work in that guides the staff on how to respond to a patient calling or walking in with a request for immediate treatment. This policy should define what constitutes a dental emergency and provide clear, step-by-step instructions on how to respond to the patient. Include the questions that should be asked of all patients. Keep your policy to one page.
2. You have been asked to create a personalized telephone message pad for the dental office in which you have just been hired. Include as much information for detail as you can while keeping the message sheet to an acceptable size.
3. Create a voice mail message for Jones Street dental office. You work Monday-Thursday 8 AM–5 PM. The office will be closed for the July 4 holiday weekend and will return on the next business day. The dentist is out of town, so she is not available to see emergencies. It has been arranged with Dr. Smith's office to accept emergencies, that phone number is 991-887-2500.
4. Write a script of how you would address a caller who has just called the dental office and you have asked her to hold because you are completing a call with another patient. The patient does not want to hold but would like her question answered immediately.

Reference

Molle E, Durham L. Administrative medical assisting. Baltimore, MD: Lippincott Williams & Wilkins, 2004.

Web Sites

Telecommunications for the Deaf
http://www.tdi-online.org/

Americans with Disabilities Act
http://www.usdoj.gov/crt/ada/

Telecommunications Relay Service
http://www.fcc.gov/cgb/dro/trs.html

U.S. Department of Labor, Office of Disability Employment, Effective Interaction
http://www.dol.gov/odep/pubs/fact/effectiveinteraction.htm

Pronunciation Dictionary
http://www.cooldictionary.com/

chapter SEVEN

Written Communication

OBJECTIVES

After completing this chapter, you should be able to do the following:

- Spell and define key terms
- Identify the characteristics of effective sentences and recognize common sentence errors
- Discuss guidelines for choosing appropriate words when writing
- List the major marks of punctuation and explain their uses
- Demonstrate proper use of capitalization, abbreviations, numbers, and spelling
- List and explain the components of a business letter
- Describe the different types of letter formats
- Identify and explain the steps to writing an effective letter
- Discuss ways of sending written communication in the dental office
- Perform the steps involved in sorting incoming mail in the dental office

KEY TERMS

- declarative sentence
- interrogative sentence
- imperative sentence
- exclamatory sentence
- simple sentence
- compound sentence
- complex sentence
- compound-complex sentence
- letterhead
- heading
- inside address
- subject line
- salutation
- body
- closing
- signature line
- enclosure
- margins

In the dental office, written communication occurs on a daily basis and consists of many different types of documentation: letters to dental specialists, letters to insurance companies, patient communication and incident reports, and staff meeting agendas and minutes. You have a responsibility as the dental office administrator for ensuring that all outgoing written communication is correct and that the message intended is clear in the correspondence. Moreover, you are responsible for managing the flow of incoming

OUTLINE

written communication in the office. In other words, your ability to correctly interpret correspondence and direct the correspondence to the correct staff member or respond appropriately to it is a vital skill for success in your role. Thus, this chapter provides you with the tools you need to effectively write, send, and manage business correspondence.

To this purpose, the chapter begins with a review of some writing basics, such as sentence structure and common sentence errors, word choice, punctuation, and other style issues. It then covers the components and formats of the business letter, along with guidelines on how to write effective letters. Methods of sending written communication are presented next, followed by a discussion of how to manage incoming mail in the dental office.

WRITING BASICS

Written correspondence in the dental office is an essential part of the business transactions occurring in the dental practice. As an office administrator, your role will include developing, responding to, and sending various types of written correspondence. Box 7-1 provides a list of most of the written correspondence you will encounter in some aspect of your role. Written correspondence can be sent in various ways such as through the postal service, by fax, or by electronic mail. Each of these methods will be discussed in this chapter.

Corresponding with patients and organizations by using a business letter presents a professional image of the dental office. To develop written communication that is easily understood and provides pertinent information, you must be able to write effectively. The basics of effective writing involves the understanding and mastery of the fundamentals of effective sentence structure, word choice, punctuation, capitalization, abbreviations, numbers, and spelling. Although thorough coverage of these topics is beyond the scope of this book, a brief review of them is provided below.

Effective Sentences

A sentence is a group of words that expresses a complete thought. A sentence always begins with an initial capital letter in the first word and ends a period, exclamation mark, or question mark. As sentences are a fundamental component of language, you must learn how to effectively use them to communicate successfully. In the dental office, you will be required to use sentences in your written correspondence that are succinct and have purpose. As you compose written documents in the dental office, writing sentences may seem the most difficult part of the composition. Often, sentences seem either too long or too short and incomplete. Effective writing requires the use of sentences of varying length and complexity. For this reason,

BOX 7-1
Written Correspondence Sent and Received in the Dental Office

- Practice newsletter
- New patient information letter
- Recare appointment and reminder cards
- Thank you card
- Welcome letter
- Dental laboratory orders
- Overdue account notices
- Letters from specialist office
- Occasional cards (birthday, sympathy)
- Insurance company treatment information letter
- Reactivation letter to patient

knowing the distinction between types of sentence will assist you in the correct usage of sentences in your writing skills.

Sentences are used in different ways, for example, to make a statement, ask a question, issue a command, or make an exclamation. In other words, sentences can be classified according to the purpose they are meant to serve. There are four main types of sentences classified according to their purpose.

A **declarative sentence** is used for making a statement. A declarative sentence can make either a positive or negative statement and is always punctuated with a period. Examples of declarative sentences are:

The office is closed on weekends.
The phone rang five times before it was answered.

An **interrogative sentence** is used for asking questions. An interrogative sentence is always punctuated with a question mark. Here are some examples:

Would you like to make an appointment for Thursday morning?
Do you have dental insurance?

An **imperative sentence** is used when issuing a command. An imperative sentence is distinguished by its use of words, and not the punctuation, such as with the previous types of sentences. The imperative sentence gives a direct command to someone. It can be punctuated with either a period or an exclamation mark. For example,

Stop it.
Go away!

An **exclamatory sentence** is a declarative sentence marked with an exclamation point. For example,

The dentist told me I was caries free!
I made my appointment for Thursday!

Sentences can also be classified according to their structure. That is, how the sentence is made up of clauses. A sentence must contain at least one independent clause and can also contain more than one dependent clauses. Review Box 7-2 for information on clauses. As you compose written documents in the dental office, writing sentences may seem the most difficult part of the composition. Often, sentences seem either too long or too short and incomplete. Effective writing requires the use of sentences of varying length and complexity. Four types of sentences are commonly used in the English language: simple, compound, complex, and compound-complex. These are described below.

A **simple sentence** is an independent clause without any dependent clauses.

Example: *The woman was reading a magazine.*

A **compound sentence** contains two or more independent clauses joined together.

BOX 7-2 Clauses

There are two types of clauses used in sentences: independent and dependent.

An independent, or main, clause is the part of the sentence that can stand alone.

A dependent, or subordinate, clause is a part of the sentence that cannot stand alone and that must be attached to an independent clause.

Example:

Independent clause: *Jane gets a pen and some paper.*

Dependent clause: *before she answers the phone*

Example: *The woman was reading a magazine, and the patient sat down in the chair.*

A **complex sentence** contains a single independent clause and one or more dependent clauses.

Example: *The woman was reading a magazine because she was interested in the article.*

A **compound-complex sentence** contains two or more independent clauses and one or more dependent clauses.

Example: *The woman was reading a magazine and the patient sat down in the chair because they were waiting for the dentist.*

Varying the sentence type in writing is an effective way to maintain the readers' interest. Using simple sentences only may create a sense of detachment for the reader, whereas the exclusive use of longer, complex sentences may provide the reader with too much information to absorb at once. The following is an example of effective use of the various sentence types together:

> The patient was late. When she arrived, I explained to her that she would have to reschedule because the dentist does not see patients who are 30 minutes or more late. She yelled at me that that was not fair and slammed her fist on the counter, I went and got the dentist, and he escorted her out of the office. She is no longer a patient at our office.

checkPOINT

1. Why should you be able to distinguish between different types of sentences?

As sentences are a fundamental component of language, you must learn how to effectively use them in order to communicate successfully. Specifically, you must understand how thoughts are organized within a sentence and how to avoid common sentence errors.

Avoiding Common Errors

Becoming proficient in written communication requires practice and familiarity with the terminology preferred for use in the correspondence. Common errors in written correspondence occur in such areas as sentence fragments, run-on sentences, and comma splices. All of these common errors are addressed next.

Sentence Fragments A sentence fragment is a group of words that cannot stand alone because it is not a complete sentence.

Fragment: *Because the dentist is running behind schedule.*
Complete sentence: *You will need to reschedule your appointment because the dentist is running behind schedule.*

To recognize when a sentence is a fragment, try using the following tip: If you place the phrase "I realize" in front of the sentence and it still sounds fine, the sentence is correct. If the sentence sounds unusual, it is probably a fragment and should be corrected. Table 7-1 demonstrates examples of this tip and how to use it. Almost every fragment is meant to be a part of the sentence that appears right before it. To easily fix the fragment, the period at the end of the sentence right before the fragment should be deleted and replaced with a comma. For example,

Fragments: *I walked quickly. Because the bus was waiting.*
Corrected: *I walked quickly because the bus was waiting.*

Run-On Sentences A run-on sentence joins two independent clauses together without any punctuation. When a run-on sentence is used, the writer is making a punctuation error. That is, two independent clauses are fused together when they should be separated with a comma and coordinating conjunction, semicolon, or period.

TABLE 7-1 Identifying Fragments

Complete Sentence	Sounds Fine
The door was locked.	*I realize* the door was locked.
It was windy.	*I realize* it was windy.
Fragment	**Sounds Unusual**
After the party.	*I realize* after the party.
Maybe.	*I realize* maybe.

Run-on sentence: *The schedule today is full it will be a busy day.*
Corrected: *The schedule today is full. It will be a busy day.*

To fix a run-on sentence, try one of the following:

- Use a period to separate the clauses into two sentences.
- Join the clauses with a coordinating conjunction, depending on their relation to one another.
- Join the clauses with a semicolon.

Comma Splices A comma splice refers to a sentence in which two independent clauses are incorrectly joined using a comma. One way to recognize that this error has occurred is to read the sentence and determine whether the you can place a period in the sentence and develop two complete sentences. If this can be done, then you cannot use just a comma to separate the two sentences, and you must also add a coordinating conjunction to the comma or use a semicolon.

Comma splice: *The patients waited for an hour, the hygienist was very late.*
Two sentences: *The patients waited for an hour. The hygienist was very late.*

If you can determine that the sentence in question is a comma splice, you can correct the error by doing the following:

- Divide the sentence into two sentences by using a period.
- Separate the two clauses using a comma and a coordinating conjunction.
- Separate the clauses using a semicolon.

The most common way to correct a comma splice is to maintain the comma and add a coordinating conjunction. Review the coordinating conjunctions in Box 7-3.

checkPOINT

2. How do you recognize that a sentence is a comma splice?

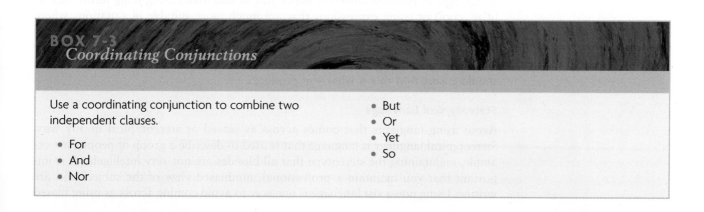

BOX 7-3
Coordinating Conjunctions

Use a coordinating conjunction to combine two independent clauses.

- For
- And
- Nor
- But
- Or
- Yet
- So

Word Choice

To develop you skill of writing effectively, it will be necessary for you to use language that is appropriate for the audience you are writing for and, specifically, to fulfill your intended purpose. Not paying attention to the language you are using can result in inappropriate use of words, which can negatively affect your representation of the dentist, the dental team, and yourself. Focusing on the level of language formality to incorporate in your letters, avoiding slang terms and expressions, avoiding stereotypical language, and minimizing the use of contractions will facilitate the presentation of a professional, well-written business letter.

Level of Formality

Writing in a style that your audience expects and also fits your purpose is key for producing an effective written communication. There are many different levels of formality. When you write a letter to a patient or an insurance company, you will use a formal style of writing, and when you write to friends and family members, you would use an informal style. There is a range associated with formality. That is, there are varying levels of formality that are used in the dental office. The following examples provide instances of when the various levels of formality are used.

- **Formal.** A letter written to a patient, insurance company, or other outside agency; generally, the audience is not very well known or is not known at all.

Writing sample (patient letter): Thank you for contacting our office last week to arrange your appointment for a new patient examination on January 18, 2009. Enclosed are the information forms you will need to complete prior to your appointment. If you have any questions, please contact our office at (555) 818-5300 prior to your appointment.

- **Semiformal.** A letter written to a well-known individual. This can include a staff member or a family member.

Writing sample (staff memo): I hope everyone enjoyed the long weekend! It is nice to see you back and refreshed! Just a reminder that our staff parking will be limited for the next week as construction is completed on the parking lot. Please use the side road for parking; the parking lot next door is also available. Please contact the Office Manager if you have any concerns.

- **Informal.** This style of writing should never be used in the dental office for written communication. Informal writing conveys disrespect and an unprofessional attitude.

Writing sample (patient sympathy card): Hi Mr. Smith, we all heard the bad news and we feel really sad about it! Try to stay positive! We'll see you next year!

Slang Terms and Expressions

In any type of business correspondence you should avoid using slang terms such as (y'all, cool) or using expressions that are much more suitable in situations where you are talking with friends or family members, such as "add fuel to the fire" or "make my day." Slang terms create a level of informality in a written piece. If your intended audience expects a more formal approach to the written document, you should ensure that this is what you produce.

Stereotypical Language

Avoid using language that comes across as biased or stereotypical in any way. Stereotypical language is language that is used to describe a group of people, for example, maintaining the stereotype that all blondes are not very intelligent. It is important that you maintain a professional, nonbiased view of the subject you are writing. Using nonsexist language is one way to avoid coming across as using biased language in your writing. For example, using generic terminology such as "postal worker" instead of "mailman" or "nurse" instead of "male nurse."

Contractions

Using contractions in our everyday vocabulary can create confusion when it comes to whether or not contractions should be used in written correspondence. A contraction occurs when one word is created by joining two words together with an apostrophe. For example, "I am" becomes "I'm" or "cannot" becomes "can't." The use of the apostrophe can also add to confusion to show possessiveness and, when used incorrectly, can change the meaning.

The level of formality being used in your written communication must be determined before writing. With the increasing use of e-mail in the dental office between employees, patients, and other outside agencies, a less formal approach can be seen in the style of writing in some communication. Using contractions is not something that is completely discouraged, as long as the format is right for it. That is, if you are writing to a patient via e-mail to inform him or her that there is not an appointment available at the time he or she requested, a formal way to word your correspondence would be "The appointment time you requested for Thursday is not available at this time. There is availability on Wednesday, would you be able to attend that day?" A less formal response may be "The appointment time you requested for Thursday isn't available. How does Wednesday sound?" The use of the contraction in the correspondence relaxes the tone of the letter and comes across as unprofessional. When you are trying to make a point or want to maintain professional relationships, try to avoid using contractions.

> **checkPOINT**
>
> 3. Why should you pay attention to word choice when writing business correspondence?

Punctuation Review

Punctuation serves the following purposes in written communication:

- represents ideas clearly
- shows how ideas are related
- separates items in a series
- indicates where thoughts begin and end
- expresses time, quantities, and measurements

Correct use of punctuation is an important detail to pay attention to in written communication. Incorrect use of punctuation marks can change the intent of the message. The following sentences provide an example of incorrectly using a question mark:

- Incorrect: *The mandibular right lateral incisor shows incipient caries?*
- Correct: *The mandibular right lateral incisor shows incipient caries.*

Incorrect use of punctuation in the first sentence changes the statement to a question. Punctuation placed in the wrong part of the sentence, or incorrect punctuation used in a sentence, can change the meaning of the message. In the earlier example, this type of error in a letter sent to an insurance company or legal office changes the message as a result of poor punctuation use.

Below is an overview of the major marks of punctuation: period, comma, semicolon, colon, question mark, exclamation point, apostrophe, quotation marks, and dash.

Period

The period is used at the end of all sentences, except for questions and exclamations. The period signifies that a complete thought has been expressed. Additionally, periods are used in abbreviations. The following are examples of period use.

- Statement: *The patient has made an appointment for Wednesday.*
- Command: *Answer the phone immediately.*
- Request: *Please tell the dentist the patient has arrived.*

Periods are sometimes used in acronyms, abbreviations in which each letter represents a separate word, or other abbreviations, for example, U.S.A., etc., Ph.D., acct. However, there are instances where abbreviations are used and the period is not required, such as YMCA, ADAA, and AMA.

Periods are also used in currency to show dollars and cents ($25.54).

Correct placement and use of the period in sentences was discussed earlier in this chapter.

Comma

The comma is the most commonly used punctuation mark. Commas are used in the following circumstances:

- to separate items in a series
- to coordinate grammatical structures (joining two independent clauses)
- to set off nonrestrictive phrases and clauses
- to prevent misreading
- to create emphasis

The comma is often misused in written communication. Paying attention to its proper use and consulting a grammar reference will help minimize errors. The following guidelines outline the main areas to pay attention regarding comma usage.

1. Use commas to separate independent clauses when they are joined by a coordinating conjunction.
   Her appointment was rescheduled, but she remained in the waiting area.
2. Use commas before introductory clauses, phrases, or words, which come before the main clause.
   While the patient waited, the hygienist readied the operatory for use.
   However, the patient was early and did not mind waiting.
3. Use a pair of commas in the middle of a sentence to set off clause, phrases, and words that are not essential to the meaning of the sentence.
   *Next Wednesday, **which is my wedding anniversary,** is the only day I am available.*
4. Do not use commas to set off essential elements of a sentence, such as clauses that begin with "that."
   *The car **that** is running is burning a lot of oil.*
5. Use commas to set off three or more words, phrases, or clauses written in a series.
   The patient was informed she would need a crown, a bridge, and root canal therapy.
6. Use commas to set off names, dates, addresses, and titles.
   He was born on July 13, 1970, and she will always remember.
7. Use commas to shift between the main topic and a quotation.
   She replied to the dentist through tears, "I'm not that scared."

Semicolon

A semicolon represents a break between clauses that is stronger than that indicated by a comma, but not as strong as that of a period or colon. Semicolons are also used to separate items in a series when the items contain punctuation. You will usually use a semicolon to link independent clauses that are not joined with a conjunction. Pay attention to only joining independent clauses that are closely related in meaning. Examples of correct semicolon use follow:

Example: *Brushing and flossing help to prevent caries; rinsing with a mouth rinse is also important.*

Example: *The hygienist recommended three monthly recall appointments; however, the patient has only attended once this year.*

You can also use a semicolon where you would use a period. However, when punctuating a list or series of items, you should use semicolons instead of commas. For example:

The dental assistant called the dental supply company and placed a large order, which consisted of toothbrushes; sterilization supplies; paper products; masks; and hygiene instruments.

Colon

The colon represents a break in a sentence. The break is more complete than that of a semicolon, but not a complete stop, as with a period. Colons are used to introduce a series or list after a sentence, introduce a question or related statement, and express time using numbers. The following are examples of correct colon use:

Introducing a series or list: *The patient was given three options: extract the tooth, restore the tooth, or do nothing.*

Related statement: *The dental administrator was concerned with one thing: How was the patient going to pay for this treatment?*

Quotation Marks

Quotation marks are used to enclose a direct quote of someone's words. You should use double quotation marks immediately before (") and directly after (") quoted material or dialogue. Quotations are also used to reference titles of shorter works, such as poems, play, and essays. Longer works such as movies and books are placed in italics. Quotations are also used to set off some words, referred to as terms.

General rules for punctuation and quotation marks are as follows:

- Commas and periods are placed inside the closing quotation mark.
  The patient said, "Finally, I can afford to pay for my crown."
- Semicolons and colons are placed outside quotation marks.
  The dentist discussed the poem "The Road Less Traveled," a poem she was not fond of.
- Question marks and exclamation points are placed only inside the quotation marks if they are part of the original quotation.
  The patient telephoned and said, "Why did I get this bill?"
- Single quotes are used to show a quote within a quote.
  I heard her saying, "The patient then said 'Why can't I have this done for free?'"

Exclamation Point

Expressing emotion or a sense of urgency can be accomplished in a sentence by using an exclamation point. Both imperative sentences and statements can be punctuated with an exclamation point. In formal business writing, the exclamation point is not often used.

Example: *I can't believe how many patients came in today!*

Apostrophe

An apostrophe is used to form a possessive case of a noun, or to show that you have left out letters to form a contraction. As previously noted, using contractions in formal business correspondence is not recommended.

Example: *The enamel's luster has been worn off from aggressive brushing.*
Example: *I haven't heard back from that patient.*

To form a possessive form of a plural noun ending in "s," the noun remains the same with an apostrophe added after the "s."

Example: *She has two bridges' that must be replaced.*

Note that the possessive form of "it" is "its" without an apostrophe. "It's" is the contraction for "it is."

Dash

Using a dash is acceptable when you want to set off a phrase in a sentence that would be too lengthy to set off using commas. Dashes are also used to show an abrupt interruption in thought.

> Example: *You can select either treatment plan—from the ones attached to this letter—or return to the office for an in-depth consultation.*

Dashes can also be used to showcase a list of elements.

> Example: *Crowns, bridges, veneers—all types of cosmetic dentistry are performed in our office.*

Capitalization

Always capitalize the first word in any sentence. Additionally, capitalize the following words:

- the personal pronoun *I*
- the names of persons, businesses, government agencies, and institutions
- both names in a hyphenated name
- nationalities, races, and languages
- the names of religions and denominations
- academic degrees and personal titles used as part of people's names
- historic periods and events, as wells as holidays and other recognized special days
- calendar days, months, and seasons

what IF ?

You are given notes from the office manager to create a letter to an insurance company but are unsure of the capitalization rules. What would you do?

Always have a dictionary and grammar resource available for use when you are unsure about capitalization, abbreviation, number rules, or grammatical rules. An up-to-date dictionary is an invaluable resource. The Internet can also be of help in deciding, for example, how to abbreviate a term or how to apply the correct rule of grammar. Use of such resources may be necessary sometimes to properly write a letter. Do not mail a letter that you feel unsure about regarding the grammar, punctuation, or spelling. Have a coworker or the dentist review the letter prior to its being mailed out to ensure accuracy.

Abbreviations

Whenever possible, avoid unnecessary and nonstandard abbreviations. Most importantly, be consistent throughout the letter. For example, if you are going to abbreviate using periods (Ph.D.), then do so throughout the letter. General guidelines for abbreviations are as follows:

- Abbreviations that use periods (Ph.D., B.C.) should have no space after the first period.
- Abbreviated names that use periods should have a space after each period (H. G. Wells)
- Always check with the person or business about the correct way to abbreviate if you are in doubt about the abbreviation they use.
- Avoid abbreviating given names.
- Abbreviating titles before and after names is acceptable.

Numbers

Deciding whether to spell out a number or use figures can be easily determined by using the "rule of ten." In the "rule of ten," any number under 10 should be spelled out (five, nine) as well as any number divisible by 10 (ten, twenty, ninety). All other numbers more than 10 should be presented in Arabic numerals (21, 43, 99). Using this rule can help you be consistent in your writing. In the dental environment, teeth numbers in written correspondence would be exempt from the "rule of ten."

BOX 7-4
Common Types of Letters Written in the Dental Office

- Welcome letters to new patients
- Letters to referring dentists
- Letters to patients regarding an overdue account
- Treatment explanation or request for payment of treatment to insurance companies
- Thank you letter to a staff member, patient, or service provider
- Letters of information regarding changes in policies or additions to the staff in the office

THE BUSINESS LETTER

One of the most important documents you will be responsible for writing as a dental administrator is the business letter. You will be expected to write many different types of letters for different reasons. Box 7-4 lists the different letters seen in the dental office. To effectively write such letters, you need to understand the basic components of a letter, primary letter formats, and guidelines for letter writing.

Components

The typical business letter may be broken down into standard components. Figure 7-1 shows these components, which are explained below.

A business letter is always written on **letterhead** paper. Letterhead is the paper used by businesses that has the preprinted name and address and other contact information located at the top, and sometimes at the bottom, of the page. The letterhead page will include the name of the dentist and dental office, the address, phone number, fax number, and e-mail address. If the office has a logo or slogan associated with it, this will also be on the letterhead page. Matching envelopes and business cards are also used to establish a corporate identity.

The **heading** of a letter includes the address of the person sending the letter and the date the letter is written. When letterhead is used, there is no need to type the dentist's name and address on the page, as this has been preprinted. The date the letter is written must be typed, should include the day, month, and year, and must not be abbreviated. It should be typed as follows: May 28, 2006. If the dentist has a preferred date format, follow it. The date should be typed approximately two to four lines from the top of the page.

The **inside address** of the letter includes the name and address of the receiver of the letter. This is found four to seven lines below the date of the letter. Make sure that the address of the person to whom the letter is being sent is typed completely and that no abbreviations are made. If there are any incomplete portions of the address, such as an unknown apartment number or postal code, find this information before completing the letter. This information can be found by phoning the person or business or accessing a postal code directory or phone book. The title of the person who is receiving the letter should never be abbreviated, nor should any part of the address. The following example shows an incorrect addressing of the inside address on a letter:

Dr. Jane Smith
Smith Dental Studio & Associates
127 Parkland Ave.
Springfield, MI
12345

5572 Wilcox Ave
New Leeds, OH 32470
December 10, 2010

Heading
Includes the sender's address and the date

[*Four to seven spaces*]

Mr. Robert Bailey
10134 Blake Street
New Leeds, OH 32470

Inside address
Includes the name and address of the recipient

Subject line

Re: Staff Changes

[*Double space*]
Dear Mr. Bailey:

Salutation
Typically starts with "dear" and includes a colon at the end

[*Double space*]
Some staff changes are occurring at Downy Dental, and we wanted to let you know about them. Rest assured, however, that providing quality dental care for you remains our mission.

Body
Includes two or three paragraphs, typically. The first paragraph states the purpose of the letter. The other paragraphs provide the details.

[*Double space between paragraphs*]
First, we are happy to notify you that a new dentist, Dr. Julie Chang, DDS, will be joining us at Downy Dental. Dr. Chang has practiced dentistry for 12 years in Cashockton, OH, specializes in cosmetic dentistry, and graduated from the University of North Carolina School of Dentistry in 1998. Please give Dr. Chang a warm welcome the next time you are in the office.

Second, we are sad to announce that, Dr. Brian Mellon, DDS, will be retiring at the end of this year. Dr. Mellon co-founded Downy Dental in 1979 and has provided excellent dental care for thousands of patients since then and entertained them with his quirky sense of humor. Please join us in wishing Dr. Mellon well in his retirement. Of course, Drs. Washington and Trevor will continue to be available to serve your dental needs.

[*Double space*]
Sincerely yours,

Closing

[*Four spaces*]

Brenda Manning
Dental Office Administrator

Signature line
Includes sender's signature in blue or black ink, followed by the sender's name typed.

Dictator's/writer's initials

BW/bm

Enclosure line

Encl.

FIGURE 7-1 Main components of a business letter.

Done correctly, this address would read as follows:

Dr. Jane Smith & Associates
Smith Dental Studio
127 Parkland Avenue
Springfield, MI
12345-6789

Note that the state abbreviation did not change. Two-letter state abbreviations that are recognized by the postal service are listed in the appendices. When addressing a letter to more than one person, type the first and last names of both people on separate lines. The woman's name would be typed first; otherwise, use the rule of alphabetical order. When addressing a letter to a person at a business address, type the name, followed by the position title, on the same line.

Type the **subject line** two spaces below the inside address. A subject line briefly describes the purpose or content of the letter. Not all letters will have a subject line. If the letter does have a subject line, it is begun with the abbreviation "Re:." An example of a subject line is, "Re: Orthodontic Consultation."

The **salutation** is a greeting to the reader: i.e., "Dear Mrs. Ross:." The salutation is typed two lines below the subject line. Always use a colon at the end of the salutation and capitalize the name and title of the person being addressed. Use the following guidelines when typing salutations:

- If the gender of the recipient is known, use "Mr." or "Mrs." as appropriate, followed by the last name; for example: Dear Mrs. Smith
- If the gender is not known, use the person's first name in the salutation; for example, "Dear Pat Smith:"
- If the letter is addressed to two people type, include the appropriate title before each last name; for example, "Dear Mrs. Smith and Mr. Fox:"
- If the letter is addressed to a dentist, include "Doctor" as the title; for example, "Dear Doctor Smith:"
- Never address the receiver as "Sir," "Madam," or "To Whom It May Concern"

The **body** of the letter is the portion of the letter that conveys the message. The message can be one or more paragraphs in length. Use these tips to write a letter that looks professional and organized.

- Use letterhead for the first page only. If the letter is more than one page in length, use paper of the same color and weight as the letterhead for subsequent pages. There must be identifying information at the top of the page for the reader should the pages get separated. For example, the line at the top of the second page should have the receiver's name and the date typed underneath it. Two lines underneath, continue the letter.
- Use page numbers if the letter is more than one page long.
- Never continue a sentence onto the next page. Finish the page with a complete sentence and then start a new sentence on the next page.
- E-mail addresses and Web site addresses should be placed on one line and not continued onto the next line or page.
- A table or graph should appear only on one page.

The **closing** of the letter must be placed two lines below the final paragraph of the letter. Closings must be professional and convey sincerity to the receiver. Standard closings include the following: "Sincerely yours," "Best regards," and "Respectfully." The closing should be followed by a comma and then four lines left for the signature line. The **signature line** is the space left for the signature of the person from whom the letter is to be sent. If the letter is from the dentist, the dentist's signature must appear above his or her typed name. The dentist may have a preference as to the format of this portion of the letter. The typed name portion may read: Dr. J. Smith, or Dr. Jane Smith, or Jane Smith, DDS. Be aware of the dentist's preference for the signature line. If you are instructed to sign the letter on behalf of the dentist, sign your name and in front of the typed signature line, write "for."

Two lines below the signature line, the initials indicating the dictator and writer of the letter can be found. This is optional information and appears as follows: JS/rd. The capitalized letters are the initials of the person who dictated the letter. The lowercase letters are the initials of the person who typed the letter.

You may on occasion include additional information in a letter, such as a photocopy or a radiograph. In this situation, you would need to make note of the enclosure on the letter. Anything that you include with the letter is considered an **enclosure**. Two lines below the dictator and writer initials, the abbreviation "Encl." or "Encls." is typed to indicate that there is something included with the letter. Two lines below the enclosure line, the abbreviation for "carbon copy" would appear. If the letter is also being sent to another person who is not addressed in the address line, this would be indicated at this point in the letter. For example, if the letter is being sent to Dr. Jane Smith, who is the medical doctor of the patient the dentist is treating, a copy of the letter may be sent to the patient. The line would be typed as follows: "cc: John Andrews." The doctor reading the letter would then be aware that the patient has received a duplicate copy of the letter.

checkPOINT

4. What are the parts of the business letter?
5. Why would you use the abbreviation "Encls." at the end of a letter?

Letter Formats

The most common types of letter formats used in the dental office are full block, block, and semiblock styles. Figure 7-2 shows an example of a full block letter. A full-block letter has all lines starting flush left from the margin in every section of the letter. This creates a uniform look to the letter. A block style letter, shown in Figure 7-3, has all lines flush left with the margin, with the exception of the date, address, closing, and

5572 Wilcox Ave
New Leeds, OH 32470
December 10, 2010

Mr. Robert Bailey
10134 Blake Street
New Leeds, OH 32470

Re: Staff Changes

Dear Mr. Bailey:

Some staff changes are occurring at Downy Dental, and we wanted to let you know about them. Rest assured, however, that providing quality dental care for you remains our mission.

First, we are happy to notify you that a new dentist, Dr. Julie Chang, DDS, will be joining us at Downy Dental. Dr. Chang has practiced dentistry for 12 years in Cashockton, OH, specializes in cosmetic dentistry, and graduated from the University of North Carolina School of Dentistry in 1998. Please give Dr. Chang a warm welcome the next time you are in the office.

Second, we are sad to announce that, Dr. Brian Mellon, DDS, will be retiring at the end of this year. Dr. Mellon co-founded Downy Dental in 1979 and has provided excellent dental care for thousands of patients since then and entertained them with his quirky sense of humor. Please join us in wishing Dr. Mellon well in his retirement. Of course, Drs. Washington and Trevor will continue to be available to serve your dental needs.

Sincerely yours,

Brenda Manning
Dental Office Administrator

BW/bm

Encl.

FIGURE 7-2 Full-block letter format.

5572 Wilcox Ave
New Leeds, OH 32470
December 10, 2010

Mr. Robert Bailey
10134 Blake Street
New Leeds, OH 32470

Re: Staff Changes

Dear Mr. Bailey:

Some staff changes are occurring at Downy Dental, and we wanted to let you know about them. Rest assured, however, that providing quality dental care for you remains our mission.

First, we are happy to notify you that a new dentist, Dr. Julie Chang, DDS, will be joining us at Downy Dental. Dr. Chang has practiced dentistry for 12 years in Cashockton, OH, specializes in cosmetic dentistry, and graduated from the University of North Carolina School of Dentistry in 1998. Please give Dr. Chang a warm welcome the next time you are in the office.

Second, we are sad to announce that, Dr. Brian Mellon, DDS, will be retiring at the end of this year. Dr. Mellon co-founded Downy Dental in 1979 and has provided excellent dental care for thousands of patients since then and entertained them with his quirky sense of humor. Please join us in wishing Dr. Mellon well in his retirement. Of course, Drs. Washington and Trevor will continue to be available to serve your dental needs.

Sincerely yours,

Brenda Manning
Dental Office Administrator

BW/bm

Encl.

FIGURE 7-3 Block letter format.

signature lines, which are all flush right. A semiblock letter is a combination of the full-block and block letter formats. The semiblock letter also begins each paragraph with an indented, or tabbed, first line. Figure 7-4 is an example of a semiblock letter.

Writing an Effective Letter

Writing an effective letter is a necessary skill for the dental office administrator. Throughout your career you will become familiar with the many types of letters in the dental office. You will write letters to patients, insurance companies, referring doctors, and employees. There are five main steps necessary to prepare for and develop an effective letter:

1. Identify the purpose
2. Organize the facts
3. Know your audience
4. Choose an appropriate template
5. Proof a sample copy for spelling and accuracy

Identify the Purpose

Consider why you are writing the letter. Ask yourself what I am trying to achieve by writing this letter. What is the outcome I would like to achieve? In the dental office, writing a letter to a patient regarding an overdue account may have a goal of collecting monies owing. A letter to a referring doctor may have a goal of providing information to facilitate a patient's future treatment. Consideration of the desired outcome of the letter is important when writing, particularly if you are developing a letter from scratch. If you are given notes from which to develop a letter, knowing the outcome will help you understand the notes.

5572 Wilcox Ave
New Leeds, OH 32470
December 10, 2010

Mr. Robert Bailey
10134 Blake Street
New Leeds, OH 32470

Re: Staff Changes

Dear Mr. Bailey:

Some staff changes are occurring at Downy Dental, and we wanted to let you know about them. Rest assured, however, that providing quality dental care for you remains our mission.

First, we are happy to notify you that a new dentist, Dr. Julie Chang, DDS, will be joining us at Downy Dental. Dr. Chang has practiced dentistry for 12 years in Cashockton, OH, specializes in cosmetic dentistry, and graduated from the University of North Carolina School of Dentistry in 1998. Please give Dr. Chang a warm welcome the next time you are in the office.

Second, we are sad to announce that, Dr. Brian Mellon, DDS, will be retiring at the end of this year. Dr. Mellon co-founded Downy Dental in 1979 and has provided excellent dental care for thousands of patients since then and entertained them with his quirky sense of humor. Please join us in wishing Dr. Mellon well in his retirement. Of course, Drs. Washington and Trevor will continue to be available to serve your dental needs.

Sincerely yours,

Brenda Manning
Dental Office Administrator

BW/bm

Encl.

FIGURE 7-4 Semiblock letter format.

Organize the Facts

Organization of information in the letter is just as important as correctly stating the facts. In other words, make sure that you have your facts straight and that you write about them as they occurred. If you are writing a letter to a referring doctor's office and you are informing him or her that the patient did not return to the office for follow-up treatment as required, do not write, "Mrs. Jones finally attended her appointment 3 months after the initial appointment was scheduled." In this case, the reader requires additional information to fully understand what has happened. A better way to write this would be as follows: "Mrs. Jones was scheduled to return to our office on June 14, 2006. She rescheduled her appointment on two occasions and presented to our office on September 10, 2006." This provides the facts of the situation in this letter, which are pertinent regarding the patient's treatment plan. Accuracy and correctness are very important in letters of a medical nature. Once the letter is written, it may become a part of the patient's legal chart.

Make sure that the letter is clear and concise and does not leave any room for doubt when it is read. For example, closing a letter with a request that a patient contact you is unclear. How would you like to be contacted and when? Be specific: Ask the patient to contact you by phone on January 7, 2006. Alternatively, you may also inform the patient that you will be contacting him or her by telephone on that date. In conjunction with a clear message, you must also keep your message to the point. Using direct, short sentences may be more effective than wordy ones.

Know Your Audience

Knowing the gender of the person receiving your letter is important so that the recipient can be properly addressed. Also, consider the comprehension level of the reader. Letters to doctors will likely use more dental terminology, whereas letters to patients will likely require layman's terms to get the message across. Try to phrase the letter in a way that will not leave the information open to interpretation; that is, be specific! Have a colleague read the letter and interpret it so that you can get an idea of its comprehensiveness.

Choose an Appropriate Template

Unless the dentist has a preferred letter template, you will need to choose such a template. A template provides you with the layout, or format, of the letter, in which the main elements of the letter are already predetermined for you and some standard text may already be typed. If you use a computer program that provides you with step-by-step instructions in developing and formatting a letter, such as a letter wizard, your task will be much easier. For example, all professional letters use **margins.** The use of margins in a letter provides space on the right and left sides and top and bottom of the letter pages. Margins are necessary for the proper alignment of the components of the letter, such as the address, body, and closing. Selecting a template in a letter wizard program on the computer will set margins for you.

Although not a major element in letter writing, attention should be paid to the type of font used. A font is a typeface or style of type. The font size and type should be selected prior to letter writing as they can affect how the letter is read. Using an Arial font in a 13- or 14-point size is more appropriate for cards, for example. The standard acceptable font and size for a professional letter are Times New Roman and 12 point size.

Proof a Sample Copy for Spelling and Accuracy

Pay attention to detail concerning spelling and accuracy of written communication in the dental office. Such accuracy is important because once a copy of the letter is placed in the patient's chart, it becomes part of the patient's record, which is a legal document. In most cases, the dentist will provide you with the information you will be writing about. In some situations, you will be responsible for drafting the letter from scratch. Correctly transferring information into a letter form is a key responsibility of the dental office administrator. Question the dentist or other team member regarding any words or phrases that are not clear or understandable to ensure an accurate and concise letter. The following are examples of errors that can occur in written correspondence in the dental office:

- The letter you wrote stated: "Dave Smith presented in our office today and tooth 35 was extracted under general anesthesia." The notes from the dentist read: "Tooth 53 was extracted under general anesthesia." The transposed numbers of the tooth make the difference between a primary tooth extraction and a permanent tooth extraction.
- The dentist provided notes to you that read, "Mrs. Jones will not require prophylactic antibiotics prior to dental treatment." The letter you wrote stated, "Mrs. Jones will require prophylactic antibiotics prior to dental treatment." The error of omitting the word "not" from the letter can make an impact on the dental treatment and health of this patient.
- The dentist provided you with notes, part of which stated, "Patient did not take antibiotics." When you typed the letter, you wrote, "The patient did not take antibiotics prescribed for him by Dr. Jones." Although this may be true, be careful about adding to, taking away from, or rearranging the phrases provided in the dentist's notes without the permission of the dentist. Such changes can alter the meaning of the message.

BOX 7-5
How to Develop an Effective Letter?

Use the guidelines below to develop an effective letter:

1. Define your purpose
   Before you begin writing a business letter, ask yourself:
   - Why am I writing this letter—what has led up to it?
   - What information do I need to provide? For example, dates of previous letters, reference, or account numbers.
   - What arguments do I need to use?
2. The first paragraph
   - The first paragraph of the letter should introduce the subject matter and either state or imply your purpose in writing.
3. The body of the letter: The body of the letter should consist of one or more paragraphs. It should develop clearly and logically the argument and facts of the case. If there is more than one paragraph, each paragraph should focus on a separate aspect of the subject matter and there should be clear links between paragraphs.
4. The final paragraph: The final paragraph should leave the reader in no doubt about your attitude toward the subject of the letter.
5. Achieve the right tone: Although the reader of your letter may be unknown to you, it is important to achieve a suitable tone in your writing and not to be too casual or too formal. So, as far as possible:

   Avoid Jargon whenever possible.
   Use shorter sentences rather than longer ones.
   Be clear and to the point, but don't be too blunt.

The inaccuracy of information as a result of carelessness in written correspondence can lead to situations in the dental office in which patients' health could be put at risk or dentists' practice could be held legally responsible. In most cases, all written correspondence going out of the practice, such as letters, will be signed by the dentist or office manager and should be approved by either of them before sending them out. In some cases, the office administrator will be responsible for writing and approving the correspondence. In these situations, follow the tips provided in Box 7-5 on steps to ensuring letter accuracy, before sending the letter out.

In any case, always print out and read at least one copy of the letter. Reading a letter on the computer screen after you have spent some time writing it is different from seeing the letter on paper. After you write the letter, print out a copy, read it, and then leave the letter for a few minutes or longer. Go back and read the letter again. Using spell-check on the computer will aid in minimizing spelling and grammar errors but not the comprehensiveness of the letter. At this step of the process, your goal is to make sure that you have provided the facts in an organized fashion and you have included the main points of the letter. Constructive criticism from a colleague should be seen as helpful, and an opportunity to enhance your writing.

checkPOINT

6. What are the five steps necessary for writing an effective letter?

Editing your letter for spelling errors and proofreading for grammatical errors are two critical steps in finalizing your letter. At this final stage, you should be critiquing the following items when reviewing the letter:

- grammar
- spelling
- capitalization
- accuracy of facts
- conciseness
- organization

Finding and making corrections is a valuable exercise in developing letter writing skills.

After corrections have been made in the letter document, print another copy of it to proof. As was pointed out earlier, leave the letter for a few minutes and then return to it for a review before finalizing.

OTHER TYPES OF WRITTEN DOCUMENTS

As the dental administrator, you will be responsible for ensuring that the terminology used in the correspondence leaving the dental office is correct and suitable for the audience it is intended. You will need to be aware of all types of written documents used for correspondence in the dental office and have the ability to manage these documents as they come in and go out of the dental practice. Examples of different types of written documentation include patient correspondence, letters between dentists, mail promotions, and employee memos.

Patient Correspondence

There are many types of patient letters you will be responsible for sending out to patients. Some of these are as follows:

- *Financial arrangement letter:* The patient who requires financial arrangement for treatment is sent a letter that outlines the arrangement and gives the patient the opportunity to make a decision before starting treatment.
- *Welcome letter:* New patients coming in to the practice are sent information letters that provide them with the particulars of the office such as hours of operation, financial policies, dental insurance policies, and treatment information.
- *Abandonment letter:* A patient who is consistently noncompliant may receive a letter from the dental office requesting that he or she seek an alternate office for his or her dental treatment.
- *Notice of collection letter:* Providing the patient with reasonable notice that their delinquent account will be forwarded to collection is a courteous and professional way to manage this type of patient.
- *Treatment letter:* Before beginning treatment, a patient will be supplied with a written estimate of his or her treatment options.
- *Referral letter:* Patients who are being referred to a dental specialist will have a letter sent on their behalf from or to the referring dentist with the particular information about their treatment.
- *Special occasion letter:* Patients who are celebrating a birthday or anniversary or are suffering from illness or loss may be recognized with a personalized letter.
- *Thank you letter:* Thanking a patient for his or her loyalty, referral or kind act can be done with a personalized letter from the staff.

The dental office you work in will have a template of some or all of these letters for you to work with when required.

Letters Between Dentists

When a patient is referred to a dental specialist for treatment, the dentist and the specialist work together to facilitate the dental care of the patient. This is done through written correspondence of treatment recommended and completed. All information received remains in the patient chart.

Mail Promotions

Occasionally the dental office may have information that is to be mailed out to patients because it concerns a new type of treatment that most patients may be interested in accepting, for example, a new teeth-whitening formula or other type of cosmetic dentistry.

checkPOINT

7. Why would you send a patient a special occasion letter?

Employee Memos

Correspondence between staff members occurs regularly in the dental office. Memos can be sent by written letter and distributed to all staff members or they can be sent via e-mail. More commonly, e-mail is used to distribute employee memos. Employee

PROCEDURE 7-1 *How to Fold a Letter for a No. 10 Envelope?*

1. Make sure that the letter is properly signed.
2. Compare the inside address on the letter with the address on the envelope to be sure they correspond.
3. Place the letter face-up on the desk.
4. Fold slightly less than one third of the letter up toward the top edge of the sheet.
5. With the edges even at the sides, crease the fold.
6. Fold the top downward so that the top edge of the letterhead is within $\frac{1}{2}$ inch of the bottom fold. With the edges even at the sides, crease the fold.
7. Insert into the envelope with the last crease toward the bottom of the envelope.

memos consist of general information that all staff must be aware of, such as upcoming events, office closures, birthdays. Employee memos can also be used to inform employees individually of meetings with the manager.

METHODS OF SENDING WRITTEN COMMUNICATION

There are many options available today for sending written communication. As technology progresses, our options expand. In the dental office, the following methods can be used for sending written communication:

- postal delivery
- courier
- facsimile
- electronic mail

Preparing for Postal Delivery

Once the letter has been written and proofread, it is then ready for the signature. Have the person who you are writing the letter for sign the document. After it has been signed, remember to make a photocopy of the letter for the chart or file. The letter must be folded into thirds before inserting it into the envelope. A standard business letter is written on 8½ × 11 size paper. When folded into thirds, this size fits into a standard business envelope, or a No. 10 envelope.

Review Procedure 7-1 for steps on folding a letter for a No. 10 envelope. If you are using a window envelope, follow the steps in Procedure 7-2 to do this correctly. Often a window envelope is used for sending account statements and checks. These forms often have perforated or marked areas for folding the paper so that the recipient address shows properly in the window.

The following points should be considered before sending the letter to ensure confidentiality of the receiver:

- Use security envelopes when mailing account statements. Security envelopes prevent the information of the contents of the envelope from being identified from the outside.

PROCEDURE 7-2 *How to Fold a Letter for a No. 10 Window Envelope?*

1. Place the sheet facedown, top toward you.
2. Fold the upper third down toward you.
3. Fold the lower third of the sheet up so that the address will be on the outside.
4. Insert the sheet in the envelope with the last crease at the bottom so the inside address shows through the window.
5. Check to see that the ZIP code or postal code shows through the window.

- If you are mailing checks or receipts that are smaller than the envelope, place the item in a piece of paper that has been folded in thirds. This will provide the security needed, particularly if you are not using a security envelope.
- Make sure that the address you are sending the documentation to is a current address. If you are unsure, contact the receiver before sending the letter to confirm the address.

Before sealing the envelope, make sure that the front of the envelope has a proper recipient address and a return address. Figure 7-5 shows the recommended layout of a properly addressed envelope. The U.S. Postal Service has a recommended address format that should be used to ensure that mail is properly sorted. The return address is placed on the top left-hand side of the envelope and has a margin of $^{1}/_{2}$ inch. The return address should not be longer than five lines. The return address on business envelopes in the dental office is often preprinted on the envelope.

The recipient's address is typed four spaces to the left of the return address and 12 spaces down from the top of the envelope and centered. Make sure not to use abbreviations in the address. The only acceptable abbreviation in an address is the state or province. Postal codes and ZIP codes must be complete. That is, the ZIP code should consist of nine digits and postal code should include six digits. Whenever possible, type the recipient's address on the envelope. A handwritten business envelope does not portray the professional image desired. Using a label with the address printed on it is an acceptable alternative and useful when addressing the same recipient routinely, such as an insurance company.

If there is a notation that must be placed on the envelope such as "personal," "confidential," or "x-rays enclosed," place this on the left-hand side of the envelope two lines below the return address. Be careful not to write anything in the lower right-hand area of the envelope, as this part of the envelope is used by the post office for bar-code purposes. The post office places a bar-code sequence to be read by computers that sort the mail for efficient delivery.

Keep the following points in mind when preparing the envelope:

- Use an 8-point font for the recipient's address and any other information on the envelope.
- Do not use an envelope that is dark in color, as it creates difficulty in reading the information typed on it. Light-colored envelopes with black ink are preferred.
- Do not use a font that is difficult to read quickly.
- If you are using a window envelope, there should be at least a 1/8-inch margin around the address.

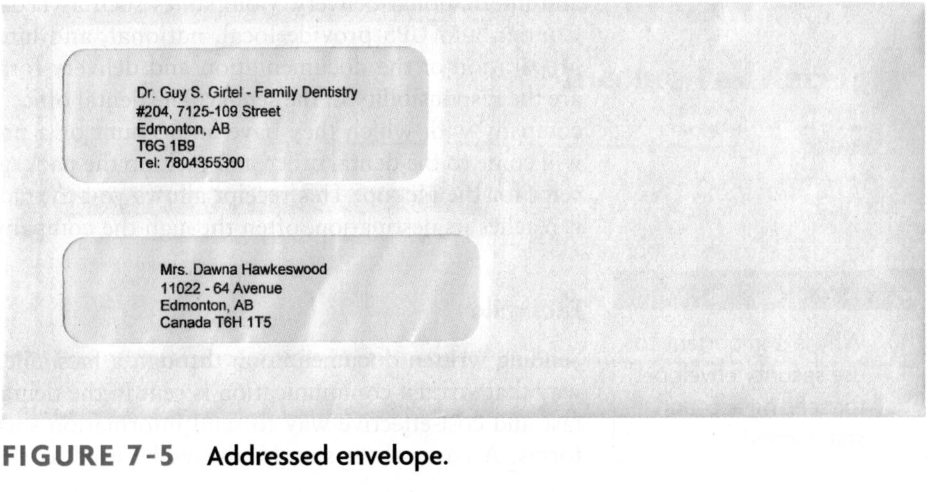

FIGURE 7-5 Addressed envelope.

Postage

Postage must be put on the envelope in the form of a stamp or permit imprint. Some dental offices have postage meter machines. These machines have a prepaid amount of postage and imprint the postage stamp directly onto the envelope. There are variations of postage meters available, and depending on the volume of mail sent out of the office, the amount of prepaid postage in the machine will vary. Refilling the postage meter machine when it depletes its postage is done by paying the post office for the postage and receiving a code to enter into the machine, which reloads the machine with postage.

There are many ways in which mail can be sent out of the dental office other than via the post office. From time to time, it may be necessary to have documentation or other items sent by courier. This decision is generally made on the basis of the urgency and value of the item, such as an item that must be received by the recipient by a certain date that cannot be guaranteed by the post office or an item that is of substantial monetary value to the sender or recipient. The post office does offer the following types of postal services for mailing:

- *Express mail:* This type of mail is guaranteed to arrive at its destination within 1–2 business days.
- *Priority mail:* This type of service offers delivery of the document within 2–5 business days.
- *First class mail:* This is the most commonly used type of mailing by both businesses and individuals for sending standard letters and mail.
- *Standard mail:* This is the service used to send packages and parcels.
- *Registered mail:* This service provides protection for items or documents that are considered valuable by the sender. A registered letter or parcel requires the signature of the receiver.
- *Certified mail:* This type of service is designed to provide a receipt for the sender that the receiver has received the mail. The receipt provided to the sender is designed to provide proof of receipt of the item.

checkPOINT

8. What is the most common method used to mail documents from the dental office?
9. When is standard mail used?

Keep in mind that postage rates do change from time to time. Sending a letter or package using insufficient postage amounts will result in the item being returned to the sender for more postage. A greater amount of postage is required for mailing items internationally. Your post office, or postal Web site, can provide you with rates for international mailing.

Courier

There are many businesses that provide delivery service of documents and items. Some courier companies provide local deliveries only, whereas others provide local and international delivery. Companies such as Federal Express (FedEx), Purolator Courier, and UPS provide local, national, and international courier service. The preparation of the documentation and delivery forms for these courier companies are the responsibility of the sender. The dental office you work in may have a courier company with which they have an account or a preference. The courier company will come to the dental office and pick up the package or envelope and provide a receipt for the pickup. This receipt allows you to track the package and know when it reaches its destination, often through the company's Web site.

checkPOINT

10. Why is it important to use security envelopes for sending account statements?

Facsimile

Sending written documentation through a facsimile, or fax machine, is a common way that written communication is sent in the dental office. A fax machine offers a fast and cost-effective way to send information such as letters, records, and order forms. A cover sheet should always be used as the first page of the fax you are

Downy Dental Office
5572 Wilcox Ave
New Leeds, OH 32470
501-279-8809 Fax: 501-279-8810

FACSIMILE COVER PAGE

DATE: __________
FROM: __________
TO: __________
Re: __________
PAGES: __________

NOTES:

Confidentiality Disclosure
This fax may contain confidential information belonging to the sender and may be used only for the purpose for which it was requested or intended. Permission to use or disclose this information has been granted by law or the patient. Further use or disclosure without additional patient authorization or as otherwise permitted by law is prohibited. Please notify the sender at the number above if you believe you have received this fax in error. Thank you

FIGURE 7-6 Fax cover page.

transmitting. Figure 7-6 is an example of a fax cover page. Note the bottom of the page is where you will find the confidentiality statement. Most dental offices have fax cover pages preprinted, which can be accessed easily. Computer software programs also provide templates for fax cover pages, where the information can be typed in and the completed page printed off for use. The information found on a fax cover page includes the following:

- Name of the sender and receiver (and company name)
- Date
- Subject line
- Fax number and phone number of receiver
- Number of pages being transmitted
- Confidentiality statement

Electronic Mail

In the dental office, you may be in contact with patients or other staff members through e-mail. In later chapters we will discuss electronic communication in more detail. As a general rule, make sure that a copy of all communication with patients

legal TIP

Ensuring the confidentiality of patient information is mandated through HIPAA and as such, every precaution to do so must be taken. The confidentiality statement should be a part of all documentation that is transmitted electronically or by fax in the dental office. A sample confidentially statement for a dental office may be as follows:

"The documents accompanying this transmission contain confidential health information that is legally privileged. This information is intended only for the use of the individual or entity named above. The authorized recipient of this information is prohibited from disclosing this information to any other party unless required to do so by law or regulation and is required to destroy the information after its stated need has been fulfilled. If you are not the intended recipient, you are hereby notified that any disclosure, copying, distribution, or action taken in reliance on the contents of these documents is strictly prohibited. If you have received this information in error, please notify the sender immediately and arrange for the return or destruction of these documents."

through e-mail is printed off and placed in the patient's chart. E-mail between staff members should be kept to business-related subjects and not be personal.

Use the following guidelines when sending electronic mail to any person.

Personalize the Letter

Always use the recipient's name in the salutation of the correspondence. This will personalize the letter and provides the recipient with the confidence that the letter was intended for him or her and not an automatically generated e-mail. Never send an e-mail that may be deemed generic by the recipient. Most generic e-mails get deleted before they are opened.

Use a Relevant Subject Line

Never send an e-mail without a subject or with a generic subject line. The recipient may delete the e-mail before opening it as it can be construed as a virus. Make the subject line specific, such as "Your dental appointment Monday June 5" or "Follow up to your phone call."

Never Use All Capital Letters

Using all capital letters in any correspondence is considered shouting. Use a 12-point font size to maintain an easy-to-read, professional feel to the letter. Be aware of how the recipient may be interpreting your letter. Use formal working to avoid any miscommunication.

Spell Check

Most e-mail programs come equipped with a spell-check function. Always spell check your correspondence before sending it. Spelling errors make an negative impression on the recipient that you do not care.

Provide Your Information in the E-mail

Make sure that your name, phone number, mailing address, and e-mail address are present on the correspondence.

Phone Whenever You Can

Telephoning a patient or outside agency is always much more effective form of communication than writing. It allows you to provide the patient with your undivided attention and in most cases the response is much quicker!

checkPOINT

11. Name four ways to send written communication.

MANAGING INCOMING MAIL

While working in the dental office, you will encounter several different types of mail:

- Letters from other dentists
- Invoices from suppliers
- Payments from patients and insurance companies
- Magazines for the waiting room
- Newsletters and flyers
- Samples

- Mail addressed as personal and confidential to the dentist
- Mail addressed to other clinical team members from suppliers
- Professional journals
- Radiographs from other dental offices and insurance companies

Sorting these many different types of mail is the responsibility of the dental office administrator. The dentist or office manager will explain the process of sorting mail and the preference, if any, that the dentist has for how the mail should be sorted. In most situations, a lot of the mail will be the responsibility of either the dental office administrator or the office manager. If you are ever unsure as to the nature of the mail and whether or not it should be passed on or opened by you, check with the office manager or the dentist. You do not want to open mail that is not intended for your eyes. All mail should be opened using a letter opener. Tearing the envelope open could tear the contents inside. Some office policies dictate that all mail is stamped with a date stamp when it is received. If there is more than one piece of documentation in the envelope, use a paper-clip to keep the papers together. Stapling the papers together could damage original documentation.

Follow the following general rules when sorting mail:

- Separate mail into two piles: envelopes and magazines/samples/promotional materials
- Using the letter opener, open all envelopes and check for any enclosures or letters with more than one page. Paper-clip these items together.
- Date stamp each item (if required)
- Place all checks in one pile or folder in preparation for recording them.
- Correspondence from other dentists regarding patients should be placed in the patient's chart for the dentist's review.
- Throw away any advertising that the dentist has requested be disposed of
- Distribute mail to the appropriate staff members: office manager, clinical staff, and dentist.

Chapter Summary

Dental office administrators need to be well versed in the area of written communication. Writing skills, good grammar, punctuation, and attention to detail are all necessary for developing effective written documents in the dental office. The goal of all written documentation is to provide a message that is clear and accurate. Your responsibility is to ensure that this goal is met. Following the preferences of the dentist in composing and distributing documentation in the dental office will help create the professional image that should be imparted. Ensuring that correct spelling and grammar in letters can be done by using the computer spell-check, proofreading your work, and asking other staff members to critique the letter helps achieve the professional image an accurate, concise business letter imparts.

Review Questions

Multiple Choice

1. **Punctuation serves all of the following purposes except that**
   a. it shows how ideas are related.
   b. it separates items in a series.
   c. it expresses time and quantity.
   d. it adds humor to the sentence.

2. **An exclamatory sentence is**
   a. a simple sentence with an exclamation mark.
   b. a declarative sentence marked with an exclamation point.
   c. an imperative sentence marked with an exclamation point.
   d. two independent clauses separated with a period.

3. **Level of formality in letter writing refers to**
   a. style suitable for the audience.
   b. a formal style of writing.
   c. informal writing.
   d. none of the above.

4. **Types of letter formats include all but**
   a. full block.
   b. part block.
   c. semiblock.
   d. block.

5. **A sample copy of a letter is the stage of writing where you critique all except**
   a. grammar.
   b. spelling.
   c. accuracy of facts.
   d. why you are writing.

6. **Which of the following is the most commonly used punctuation mark?**
   a. period
   b. dash
   c. comma
   d. question mark

7. **The inside address on the business letter includes**
   a. the name and address of the sender
   b. the name and address of the receiver
   c. the address, not the name, of the sender
   d. the address, not the name, of the receiver

8. **Consideration of the outcome of letter is part of which step in developing a letter?**
   a. organizing facts
   b. identifying the purpose
   c. knowing the audience
   d. proofing a sample copy

9. **What should you always do before having the letter signed before mailing?**
   a. Spell check the document
   b. print and read at least one copy
   c. e-mail a copy to the office manager
   d. add a personal note of your own

10. **HIPPA mandates that which of the following is included in facsimile correspondence?**
    a. address and phone number of the sender
    b. confidentiality statement
    c. patient information
    d. receiver address

Critical Thinking

1. The dentist has handed some notes to you to type a letter regarding a patient. You are having trouble deciphering the handwriting. How do you handle this?
2. A coworker has asked you to proofread a letter she wrote. There are a large number of spelling, punctuation, and grammatical errors. What advice do you provide your coworker regarding resources available to minimize errors?

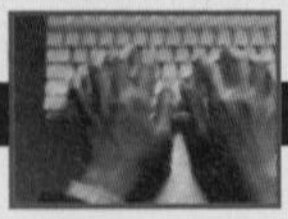

HANDS-ON ACTIVITY

1. Design a fax cover page for the office you are working in.
2. Write a letter to a new patient, thanking him or her for the referral to the practice. Use the semiblock format.
3. Prepare a letter for an insurance company of your choice, asking it to send payment for a claim that you are attaching. Prepare the letter for folding into an envelope by showing marks on the letter to indicate the folds, and address the proper size envelopes for mailing.

Bibliography

Lester M, Beason L. McGraw-Hill handbook of English grammar and usage. New York, NY: McGraw-Hill, 2004.

Web Sites

American Health Information Management Association
http://library.ahima.org

U.S. Postal Service
http://www.usps.com

Canada Post
www.canadapost.ca

part THREE

Dental Office *Management*

chapter EIGHT

Patient Record *Management*

OUTLINE

OBJECTIVES

After completing this chapter, you should be able to do the following:

- Spell and define key terms
- Identify the contents of the dental chart
- Identify documentation forms found in the dental chart, such as the patient demographic form, health and dental history form, clinical charting form, progress notes form, and treatment plan form
- Document patient information in the dental chart, following guidelines provided
- Describe the types of information documented in the patient dental chart
- Explain the purpose of an incident report, when it is used, and the information found on it
- Describe and show how to prepare a dental chart for a new patient, emergency patient, and returning patient in the dental office

KEY TERMS

- patient chart
- paperless office
- health and dental history form
- infective endocarditis
- prophylactic antibiotics
- clinical chart forms
- progress notes
- treatment plan
- incident report

The **patient chart** in the dental office is a legal document that contains the dental and medical history of the patient, along with demographic information. It plays an important role in ensuring that patients receive the dental treatment they require. All members of the dental team are responsible for ensuring that accurate information is contained in the chart. Furthermore, as discussed in Chapter 2, legal, moral, and ethical standards regarding patient records must be adhered to in order to avoid a possible breach of contract between the dentist and patient.

Many types of patient charts are available, and the preference of the dentist regarding the organization of patient information is the deciding factor regarding what type of chart is used. Figure 8-1 provides an example of a patient chart. The patient chart should provide accurate, thorough, and up-to-date information on the patient's dental treatment. All correspondence, treatment recommendations, and evaluations must be recorded in the chart.

To prepare you to properly manage patient charts, this chapter introduces you to the contents of and types of forms included in patient charts, how to record patient communication, when and how to write up an incident report, and how to prepare a patient chart for new, emergency, and returning patients.

Some dental offices may maintain a "paperless" chart system. This means that the patients' dental treatment, evaluation, and history are maintained through computerized means. Most dental offices still maintain a paper chart system. Regardless of the system used, effective maintenance of the patient chart involves ensuring that the chart is complete, legible, accurate, and easily retrievable by the dental staff members. The same contents will be found in each patient chart whether it is a computerized or paper chart. Figure 8-2 shows an example of one type of computerized patient chart. Although there are many different types of computerized dental practice management software programs available, the essential patient chart information is similar for each program. As you read through each of the remaining chapters, you will see examples of computerized patient chart information using the DENTRIX practice management software.

> ✓ *check*POINT
>
> 1. Regardless of the type of patient chart system used in the dental office, what are the components necessary for effective maintenance of patient charts?

PATIENT CHART CONTENTS AND FORMS

The patient chart contains not only dental patients' dental history, but their medical history and demographic information, as well. The medical history of the patient is limited to what the patient tells the dentist. That is, the dentist receives information about the patient's medical history from the health history forms that patient

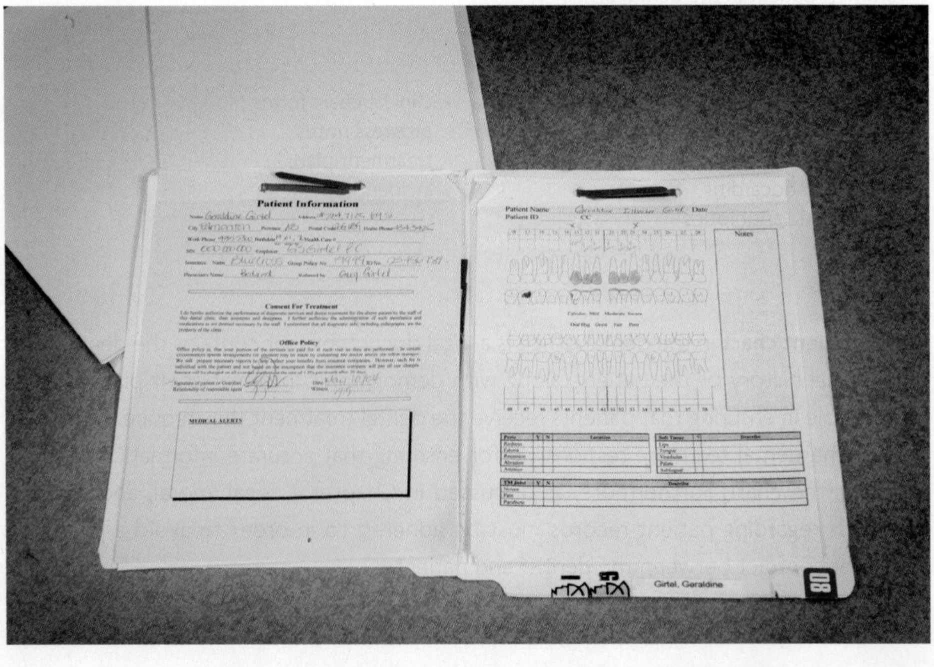

FIGURE 8-1 Patient chart.

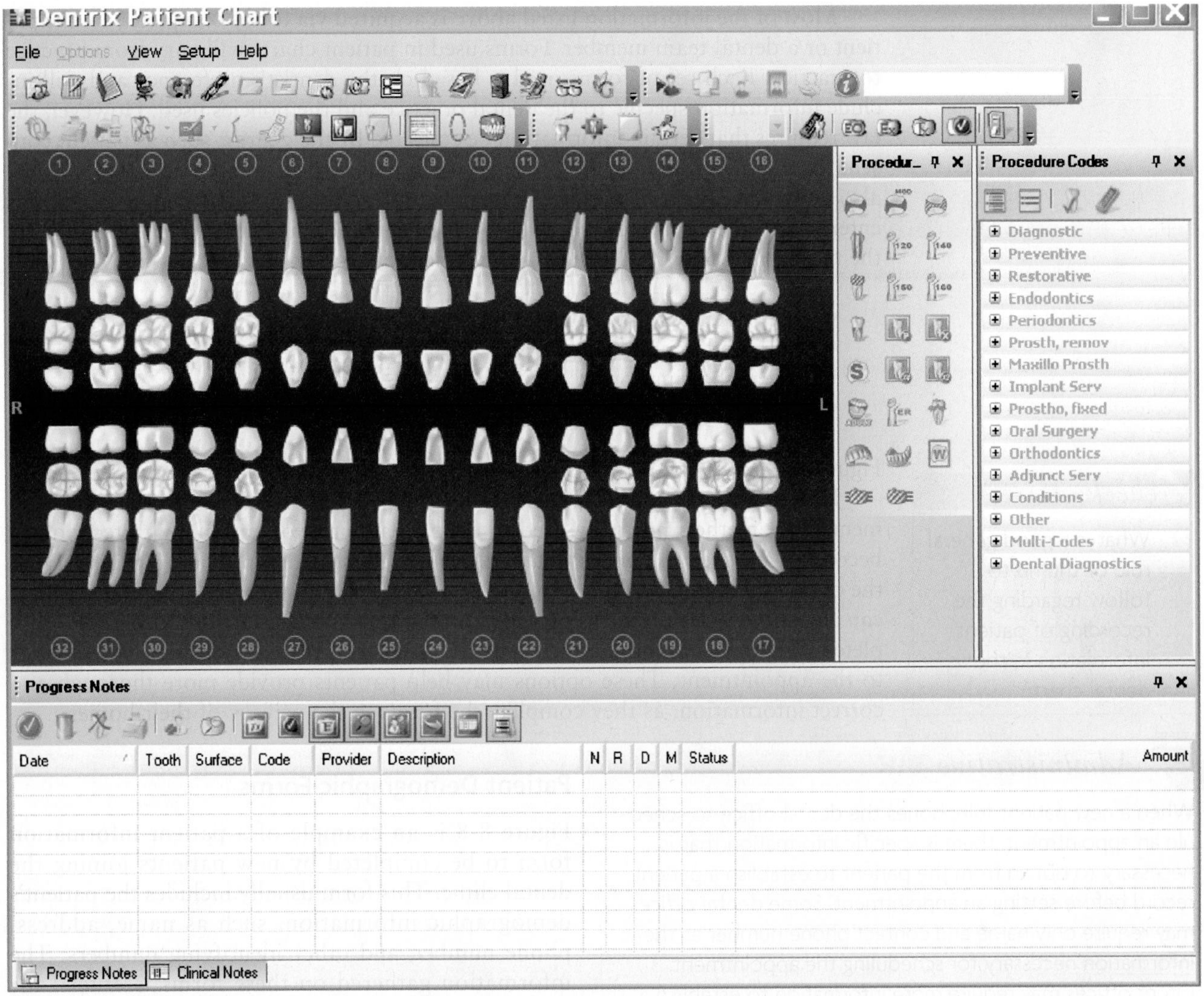

FIGURE 8-2 Computerized patient chart. DENTRIX image courtesy of Henry Schein Practice Solutions, American Fork, UT.

complete and any verbal information received from the patient. Specifically, a patient chart must include the following:

- name, address, and phone number
- social security number and date of birth
- current employment information
- Healthcare/Medicare number
- dental insurance information
- medical and dental history
- radiographs
- dental treatment plans, recommendations, and treatment completed
- dentists' and hygienists' progress notes
- correspondence from, to, and about the patient
- letters and information from outside agencies regarding the patient (doctors and insurance companies)

There may be other types of information that are found in the patient chart, depending on the preference of the dentist. A general rule of thumb to follow regarding patient information in the chart is that if it has to do with the patient, it should be documented or copied and placed in the patient chart.

Most of the information listed above is acquired via forms completed by the patient or a dental team member. Forms used in patient charts will vary from practice to practice. Each set of forms used is based on the dentist's preference and will include information specific to the dental practice and the policies used. However, the law requires that certain information be collected by the dentist, such as patient consent for treatment. In a dental office in which patient records are entirely electronic, also known as a **paperless office,** the patient still signs a form but the information is entered into the computerized chart by the dental administrator. The following are the most commonly used forms in the patient chart:

- patient demographic form
- health and dental history form
- clinical charting form
- progress notes form

Figures 8-3 to 8-6 show examples of each of these types of forms.

Having patients complete their forms in the dental office prior to their appointment is the method normally used to collect patient information. With technology becoming an integral part of dental patient appointments, providing patients with the option of completing the forms prior to their visit has become common. Patients can access information forms provided on the clinic's Web site and bring them completed to their dental appointment, or the forms can be mailed to the patient prior to the appointment. These options may help patients provide more thorough and correct information, as they complete the forms in the privacy of their homes.

*check*POINT

2. What is a good general rule of thumb to follow regarding the recording of patient information in the dental chart?

Administrative TIP

When a new patient telephones the dental office to schedule an appointment, there is specific information that is necessary to obtain from the patient to establish a patient record before setting an appointment. Some dental offices may require only name and contact phone number as the information necessary for scheduling the appointment. Other offices may require more information to establish a patient record. A new patient telephone call information sheet is a very useful tool in establishing a patient record. This is a form that is kept in an accessible place to collect the necessary patient information, such as name, address, phone number, date of birth, and insurance information. Having this information prior to the patient appointment allows you to mail the proper forms to the patient for completion prior to the appointment and verify insurance information. The form can also be used to collect information such as the referral source of the patient. If a current patient has referred a new patient, this is an opportunity to send a thank you card or other acknowledgment to the referring patient. Finally, documenting when the new patient demographic and health history forms were sent can also be verified on this form. When the patient arrives for the scheduled appointment, the form can then be filed in the patient chart, as it is written documentation of the initial contact with the patient. Figure 8-7 is an example of what the new patient telephone call information sheet may look like. This form can be modified to fit the requirements of the dental office.

Patient Demographic Forms

Figure 8-8 is an example of a patient information form to be completed by new patients joining the dental clinic. This form usually includes the patient's demographic information, such as name, address, phone number, and other identifying numbers. The information gathered on these forms is crucial for the development of the patient chart. Usually the patients' social security number is part of the information asked for on this form as well as employment and dental insurance coverage information. These are important pieces of the patient chart regarding the collection and maintenance of the financial component of the patient account. Failing to collect this information can result in difficulties collecting payment for treatment. This is particularly true when a patient has dental insurance since the insurance carrier often requires such personal information as unique identifiers for the policyholder and family members. Additionally, having this information is important in situations where the patient refuses to pay for treatment and the account must be sent to a collection agency.

The patient demographic form is also a way to gather information that is helpful in determining the general dental concerns of the patient. Following are examples of questions that can be used on a patient demographic form that allows the patient to specify the concerns.

Patient Information

Name______________________________ Address______________________________

City ____________________ Province__________ Postal Code__________ Home Phone__________

Work Phone______________ Birthdate___/___/___ (DAY MTH YR) Health Care #____________________

SIN____________________ Employer______________________________

Insurance: Name____________________ Group Policy No____________ ID No.____________

Physician's Name ________________________ Referred by ________________________

Consent For Treatment

I do hereby authorize the performance of diagnostic services and dental treatment for the above patient by the staff of this dental clinic, their assistants and designees. I further authorize the administration of such anesthetics and medications as are deemed necessary by the staff. I understand that all diagnostic aids, including radiographs, are the property of the clinic.

Office Policy

Office policy is, that your portion of the services are paid for at each visit as they are performed. In certain circumstances special arrangements for payment may be made by consulting the doctor and\or the office manager. We will prepare necessary reports to help collect your benefits from insuance companies. However, each fee is individual with the patient and not based on the assumption that the insurance company will pay all our charges. Interest will be charged on all overdue accounts at the rate of 1.8% per month after 30 days.

Signature of patient or Guardian ____________________ Date ____________________

Relationship of responsible agent ____________________ Witness____________________

MEDICAL ALERTS

FIGURE 8-3 Patient demographic form.

Dental History

Reason for Today's Visit ____________ Date of last dental care ____________

Former Dentist ____________ Date of last dental X-rays ____________

Address ____________

Check (✓) if you have had problems with any of the following:

☐ Bad breath	☐ Grinding teeth	☐ Sensitivity to hot
☐ Bleeding gums	☐ Loose teeth or broken fillings	☐ Sensitivity to sweets
☐ Clicking or popping jaw	☐ Periodontal treatment	☐ Sensitivity when biting
☐ Food collection between teeth	☐ Sensitivity to cold	☐ Sores or growths in your mouth

How often do you floss? ____________ How often do you brush? ____________

Medical History

Physician's Name ____________ Date of Last Visit ____________

Have you ever taken any of the group of drugs collectively referred to as "fen-phen?" These include combinations of Ionimin, Adipex, Fastin (brand names of phentermine), Pondimin (fenfluramine) and Redux (dexfenfluramine). ☐ Yes ☐ No

Have you had any serious illnesses or operations? ☐ Yes ☐ No If yes, describe ____________

Have you ever had a blood transfusion? ☐ Yes ☐ No If yes, give approximate dates ____________

(Women) Are you pregnant? ☐ Yes ☐ No Nursing? ☐ Yes ☐ No Taking birth control pills? ☐ Yes ☐ No

Check (✓) if you have or have had any of the following:

☐ Anemia	☐ Cortisone Treatments	☐ Hepatitis	☐ Scarlet Fever
☐ Arthritis, Rheumatism	☐ Cough, Persistent	☐ High Blood Pressure	☐ Shortness of Breath
☐ Artificial Heart Valves	☐ Cough up Blood	☐ HIV/AIDS	☐ Skin Rash
☐ Artificial Joints	☐ Diabetes	☐ Jaw Pain	☐ Stroke
☐ Asthma	☐ Epilepsy	☐ Kidney Disease	☐ Swelling of Feet or Ankles
☐ Back Problems	☐ Fainting	☐ Liver Disease	☐ Thyroid Problems
☐ Blood Disease	☐ Glaucoma	☐ Mitral Valve Prolapse	☐ Tobacco Habit
☐ Cancer	☐ Headaches	☐ Pacemaker	☐ Tonsillitis
☐ Chemical Dependency	☐ Heart Murmur	☐ Radiation Treatment	☐ Tuberculosis
☐ Chemotherapy	☐ Heart Problems	☐ Respiratory Disease	☐ Ulcer
☐ Circulatory Problems	☐ Hemophilia	☐ Rheumatic Fever	☐ Venereal Disease

MEDICATIONS
List medications you are currently taking:
____
____

ALLERGIES
____
____

Authorization

I certify that I, and/or my dependent(s), have insurance coverage with ____________ and assign directly to
Name of Insurance Company(ies)

Dr. ____________ all insurance benefits, if any, otherwise payable to me for services rendered. I understand that I am financially responsible for all charges whether or not paid by insurance. I authorize the use of my signature on all insurance submissions.

The above-named dentist may use my health care information and may disclose such information to the above-named Insurance Company(ies) and their agents for the purpose of obtaining payment for services and determining insurance benefits or the benefits payable for related services. This consent will end when my current treatment plan is completed or one year from the date signed below.

____________ Signature of Patient, Parent, Guardian or Personal Representative ____________ Date

____________ Please print name of Patient, Parent, Guardian or Personal Representative ____________ Relationship to Patient

Payment is due in full at time of treatment unless prior arrangements have been approved.

FIGURE 8-4 Health and dental history form. Courtesy of Nathan Henderson, DDS.

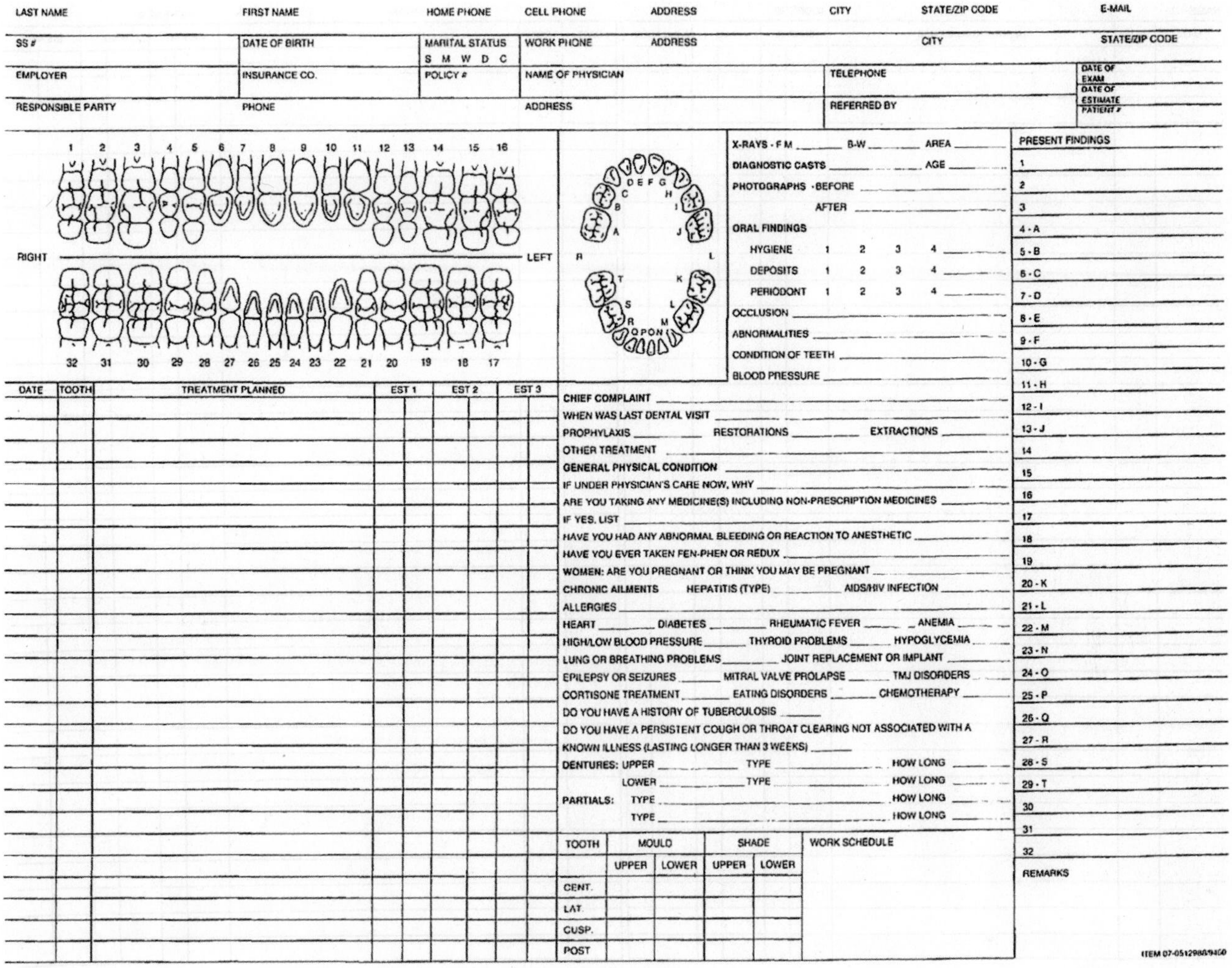

LAST NAME | FIRST NAME | HOME PHONE | CELL PHONE | ADDRESS | CITY | STATE/ZIP CODE | E-MAIL

SS # | DATE OF BIRTH | MARITAL STATUS S M W D C | WORK PHONE | ADDRESS | CITY | STATE/ZIP CODE

EMPLOYER | INSURANCE CO. | POLICY # | NAME OF PHYSICIAN | TELEPHONE | DATE OF EXAM | DATE OF ESTIMATE | PATIENT #

RESPONSIBLE PARTY | PHONE | ADDRESS | REFERRED BY

1 2 3 4 5 6 7 8 9 10 11 12 13 14 15 16

RIGHT — LEFT

32 31 30 29 28 27 26 25 24 23 22 21 20 19 18 17

A B C D E F G H I J / T S R Q P O N M L K

R L

X-RAYS - F M ____ B-W ____ AREA ____
DIAGNOSTIC CASTS ____ AGE ____
PHOTOGRAPHS - BEFORE ____
AFTER ____
ORAL FINDINGS
HYGIENE 1 2 3 4 ____
DEPOSITS 1 2 3 4 ____
PERIODONT 1 2 3 4 ____
OCCLUSION ____
ABNORMALITIES ____
CONDITION OF TEETH ____
BLOOD PRESSURE ____

DATE	TOOTH	TREATMENT PLANNED	EST 1	EST 2	EST 3

CHIEF COMPLAINT ____
WHEN WAS LAST DENTAL VISIT ____
PROPHYLAXIS ____ RESTORATIONS ____ EXTRACTIONS ____
OTHER TREATMENT ____
GENERAL PHYSICAL CONDITION ____
IF UNDER PHYSICIAN'S CARE NOW, WHY ____
ARE YOU TAKING ANY MEDICINE(S) INCLUDING NON-PRESCRIPTION MEDICINES ____
IF YES, LIST ____
HAVE YOU HAD ANY ABNORMAL BLEEDING OR REACTION TO ANESTHETIC ____
HAVE YOU EVER TAKEN FEN-PHEN OR REDUX ____
WOMEN: ARE YOU PREGNANT OR THINK YOU MAY BE PREGNANT ____
CHRONIC AILMENTS HEPATITIS (TYPE) ____ AIDS/HIV INFECTION ____
ALLERGIES ____
HEART ____ DIABETES ____ RHEUMATIC FEVER ____ ANEMIA ____
HIGH/LOW BLOOD PRESSURE ____ THYROID PROBLEMS ____ HYPOGLYCEMIA ____
LUNG OR BREATHING PROBLEMS ____ JOINT REPLACEMENT OR IMPLANT ____
EPILEPSY OR SEIZURES ____ MITRAL VALVE PROLAPSE ____ TMJ DISORDERS ____
CORTISONE TREATMENT ____ EATING DISORDERS ____ CHEMOTHERAPY ____
DO YOU HAVE A HISTORY OF TUBERCULOSIS ____
DO YOU HAVE A PERSISTENT COUGH OR THROAT CLEARING NOT ASSOCIATED WITH A KNOWN ILLNESS (LASTING LONGER THAN 3 WEEKS) ____
DENTURES: UPPER ____ TYPE ____ HOW LONG ____
LOWER ____ TYPE ____ HOW LONG ____
PARTIALS: TYPE ____ HOW LONG ____
TYPE ____ HOW LONG ____

TOOTH	MOULD		SHADE		WORK SCHEDULE
	UPPER	LOWER	UPPER	LOWER	
CENT.					
LAT.					
CUSP.					
POST					

PRESENT FINDINGS
1
2
3
4 - A
5 - B
6 - C
7 - D
8 - E
9 - F
10 - G
11 - H
12 - I
13 - J
14
15
16
17
18
19
20 - K
21 - L
22 - M
23 - N
24 - O
25 - P
26 - Q
27 - R
28 - S
29 - T
30
31
32
REMARKS

ITEM 07-0512988/9400

FIGURE 8-5 Clinical charting form. Courtesy of Nathan Henderson, DDS.

So that we may better assist you with identifying your dental concerns, please rank the following items in order of importance to you. (Rank using 1–4; 1 being most important.)

___Health preservation/keeping your teeth for life, eliminating disease
___Comfort and function/Does discomfort with your teeth limit your food choices?
___Esthetics/Are you happy with how your smile looks?
___Other______________________________

If you have had dental treatment recommended in the past and did not complete it, what factors prevented you from starting or completing treatment?

___Treatment was costly
___Did not have dental insurance
___Fear of pain/dental treatment
___Tooth did not hurt/Felt treatment was not required
___No time to schedule treatment
___Other______________________________

Determining the concerns and identifying barriers to dental treatment perceived by the patient allows you to address the concern early on in the relationship and overcome the barriers. For example, the dentist and hygienist can address issues that surround the comfort, esthetics, and health of a patient's dentition. If a patient is

NAME			ADDRESS					PHONE	PATIENT #		
DATE	TOOTH	TREATMENT RENDERED	CHARGE	PAID	BALANCE	DATE	TOOTH	TREATMENT RENDERED	CHARGE	PAID	BALANCE

FIGURE 8-6 **Progress notes.** Courtesy of Nathan Henderson, DDS.

New Patient Telephone Call Information Sheet

Date and Time of Call *December 4th, 2008 - 10:30am*

Name of Patient *Joan Smith*

Date of Birth *September 07, 1980*

Address *127 Oak St., New Haven, CT 99003*

Phone Number *Home: 222-987-6543* *Cell: 222-432-5678*

Insurance Information

Policy Holder *Dave Smith (spouse)*

Insurance Company *Blue Cross*

Policy Number/ID *Policy 12345, ID 334455-09*

Date of Birth *October 5, 1978*

Referred by *Andy Anderson (patient here)*

Appointment Date *January 19/08 @ 4:30pm*

Forms Mailed Date *December 4th, 2008*

FIGURE 8-7 **New patient telephone call information sheet.**

Welcome

We are pleased to welcome you to our practice. Please take a few minutes to fill out this form as completely as you can. If you have questions we'll be glad to help you. We look forward to working with you in maintaining your dental health.

Patient Information

Date ________ Home Phone (____)________ Cell Phone (____)________

Name ________ (Last Name) ________ (First Name) ________ (Middle Initial) SS/HIC/Patient ID # ________

Address ________ E-mail ________

City ________ State ________ Zip ________

Sex ☐ M ☐ F Age ____ Birthdate ________ ☐ Married ☐ Widowed ☐ Single ☐ Minor

☐ Separated ☐ Divorced ☐ Partnered for ____ years

Patient Employer/School ________ Occupation ________

Employer/School Address ________ Employer/School Phone (____)________

Whom may we thank for referring you? ________

In case of emergency who should be notified? ________ Phone (____)________

Primary Insurance

Person Responsible for Account ________ (Last Name) ________ (First Name) ________ (Middle Initial)

Relation to Patient ________ Birthdate ________ ID#/Soc. Sec. # ________

Address (If different from patient's) ________ Phone (____)________

City ________ State ________ Zip ________

Person Responsible Employed By ________ Occupation ________

Business Address ________ Business Phone (____)________

Insurance Company ________

Contract # ________ Group # ________ Subscriber # ________

Names of other dependents covered under this plan ________

Additional Insurance

Is patient covered by additional insurance? ☐ Yes ☐ No

Subscriber Name ________ Relation to Patient ________ Birthdate ________

Address (If different from patient's) ________ Phone (____)________

City ________ State ________ Zip ________

Subscriber Employed by ________ Business Phone (____)________

Insurance Company ________ Soc. Sec. # ________

Contract # ________ Group # ________ Subscriber # ________

Names of other dependents covered under this plan ________

Please Complete Both Sides

(Vers.D2S5504)

FIGURE 8-8 New patient demographic form. Courtesy of Nathan Henderson, DDS.

concerned with comfort and function, more than esthetics, the dentist would focus on achieving that goal with the patient. Questions such as the one above allow the patient to identify what their goal is for being in the dental office at the appointment. As the relationship develops with the dental office and regular dental visits are followed, the patient goal may evolve to include other services offered in dentistry.

As the dental office administrator, being aware of the patients' history regarding treatment, particularly any barriers that prevented treatment, is helpful for anticipating future concerns that the patient may have. For example, if the patient chose not to complete previous dental treatment due to cost issues, addressing the cost of treatment and examining payment plan options before scheduling treatment should be addressed early with the patient. Knowledge of a patient's past negative experience in a dental office because they are fearful, or dental treatment creates anxiety for them, allows you and the rest of the dental team to provide the patient with extra attention and allow for extra treatment time when the patient is in the clinic. For example, a patient who is very anxious may request a sedative prior to treatment. In situations such as this, your responsibility is to ensure that the patient has a ride home after the procedure, by a friend or family member. Patients who are very anxious may require extra time scheduled at the appointment so that the dental team can take extra time in comforting the patient throughout the procedure.

It is important that you pay special attention to patients who have the same name. For example, if there are two patients with the name John Smith, ask one patient to provide a middle name in order to distinguish between the two patients. Place an alert on the patient chart and in the computerized system that will inform users that they must check to ensure they have the correct patient chart prior to treatment or communication with the patient. You can confirm that you are speaking with the correct patient by asking the patient to verify the address that is filed for him or her or confirm the date of birth on file and the patient's address before speaking with him or her. In Chapter 12, where we discuss filing systems, other identifying factors for patients with the same name will be discussed.

✓ checkPOINT

3. Why should you be aware of a patient's dental treatment history and the barriers they perceived?

Health and Dental History Forms

Health and dental history forms are used to collect information regarding a patient's medical and dental history. The questions asked on the form are designed to gather specific information about the health of a patient. The information the patient provides will play a part in the treatment process and the recommendations the dentist provides for the patient. The health history is an invaluable tool for the dentist in the diagnosis and treatment of patients. Patients who know their health status and are totally honest in reporting it provide a good foundation for the planning of their dental treatment.

One vital piece of information that a medical history can provide is the presence of an infectious disease in the patient. Disclosure of such information by the patient can help the dental staff protect themselves and other patients appropriately. However, you and other dental team members must not rely solely on patients' disclosures in the health history form to protect yourself or others. It is not uncommon for patients to not know if they are carriers of hepatitis viruses, human immunodeficiency virus, or tuberculosis virus. Also, some patients do not reveal all the information they should when they complete a health questionnaire, for personal reasons. As a result, the dental team cannot rely on the accuracy of the information in a health history with regard to infectious disease status of the patient. As we discussed in Chapter 3, dental office personnel must assume that everyone is potentially infectious and universal precautions must be used for every patient.

The medical history provided by the patient also provides information regarding allergies (i.e., to latex or antibiotics), medications currently taken (i.e., blood thinners, birth control pills), and current medical conditions (i.e., epilepsy, pacemaker). This information is necessary for the dentist to provide effective dental care

what IF ?

What if a new patient tells you that he or she may have an allergy to a particular antibiotic but did not provide the information on his or her health history form because he or she felt it was "no big deal." What should you say to encourage the patient to provide the information?

It is important to inform the patient and educate him or her on the necessity of disclosing as much information as he or she can about his health and history. Knowing that a patient has an allergy to certain types of antibiotics will alert the dentist to not prescribe those antibiotics. An awareness of the medications the patient is currently taking also provides information for the dentist when making treatment decisions, which include prescribing medications that could create an adverse reaction with current medications. Finally, knowledge of current medical conditions will keep the staff members in tune with the behavior of the patient while in the clinic. Should a patient be prone to seizures, the staff members must watch for signs of seizure occurrences and respond appropriately.

to patients. For example, awareness of a latex allergy will alert the staff to use non-latex products while the patient is receiving treatment in order not to aggravate the sensitivity.

The health history form a patient must complete prior to the first dental appointment provides a detailed account of existing and past medical conditions, medications currently being taken, and allergies. Some patients may feel that certain medical conditions they may have or have had in the past are not relevant to dental treatment. Although most dental treatment is completed without any adverse occurrences, the patients' health condition can influence the outcome of the procedure. If the dentist is aware of the medical conditions of the patient, the preparation and approach used for the procedure can be changed to avoid a negative outcome. Many medical conditions such as cardiac problems, allergic reactions to materials, and taking certain prescription and nonprescription medications can affect the outcome of treatment if the dentist is not made aware.

Some dental procedures, such as oral surgery and periodontal procedures, can cause bleeding. For this reason the dentist needs to know that the patients' blood will clot normally. Many medical conditions can affect how quickly blood will clot, for example, a patient with hemophilia or liver diseases. In addition, medications that affect clotting factors of the blood such as aspirin and warfarin should be disclosed in the health history. Further, a patient who takes medications to treat a chronic illness such as diabetes or bowel disease may have a weakened immune system and informing the dentist of these facts will allow the dentist to take a different approach when treating dental infections. Many patients need to take preventive antibiotics before dental procedures are performed. For example, some patients with an artificial heart valve, or an artificial hip or knee, may need to take an antibiotic prior to certain treatments to help prevent a serious infection such as **infective endocarditis** from occurring. Infective endocarditis is an infection of the heart's inner lining or valves that can destroy the heart valves. When certain bacteria are introduced into the bloodstream of a patient who has abnormal heart valves or damaged heart tissue, the risk for developing infective endocarditis is greatest. Some dental procedures can cause a brief bacteremia in susceptible patients, and it is recommended by the American Heart Association that these patients follow an antibiotic regimen prior to and after the dental procedure. This is referred to as **prophylactic antibiotics**, because the antibiotics are taken to help prevent the infection. Box 8-1 outlines the prophylactic antibiotic guidelines recommended for dental professionals by the American Heart Association and outlined by the American Dental Association. Your role as a dental office administrator includes being knowledgeable of the guidelines involved with prophylactic antibiotic recommendations. Patients may not realize the importance of informing the clinical staff of their medical conditions. For example, you may find that the patient will mention a medical condition that he or she has in conversation with you, yet the patient will neglect to inform the dentist. Your responsibility is to inform the dentist of this information and to encourage the patient to tell the dentist everything about their heath history. As you develop relationships with patients, your role may broaden to include discussions with patients about the necessity of taking prophylactic antibiotics prior to dental treatment, and provide education on this topic.

Allergies that a patient may have such as to certain foods, materials, chemicals, or medications are an important part of the health history. A patient who has an allergy to latex materials can experience life-threatening reactions if exposed to the material. In the dental office, latex can be found in the gloves that are worn by the clinical staff and rubber dam material for restorative work. Knowledge of patient's allergies to medications is also necessary when the dentist is prescribing medications. This knowledge allows the dentist to consider alternative medications for patients.

The initial health history completed by a new patient in the dental office is a detailed account of the patients' past and present health history. Some patients may

BOX 8-1 Prophylactic Antibiotic Guidelines for Dental Procedures

The new guidelines are aimed at patients who would have the greatest danger of a bad outcome if they developed a heart infection.

Preventive antibiotics prior to a dental procedure are advised for patients with the following conditions:

1. Artificial heart valves
2. A history of infective endocarditis
3. Certain specific, serious congenital (present from birth) heart conditions, including unrepaired or incompletely repaired cyanotic congenital heart disease, including those with palliative shunts and conduits
4. A completely repaired congenital heart defect with prosthetic material or device, whether placed by surgery or by catheter intervention, during the first six months after the procedure
5. Any repaired congenital heart defect with residual defect at the site or adjacent to the site of a prosthetic patch or a prosthetic device
6. A cardiac transplant that develops a problem in a heart valve

The new recommendations apply to many dental procedures, including teeth cleaning and extractions. Patients with congenital heart disease can have complicated circumstances. They should check with their cardiologist if there is any question at all as to the category that best fits their needs.

Adapted from the Journal of the American Dental Association (2007).

inform you that they are unsure of how to answer a specific question on the health history form. In this situation, you should inform the patient that he or she will have the opportunity to review the question with the dentist and provide the information at that time. You must then inform the dentist, or the dental assistant, about the patient's inquiry before the dentist or the dental assistant sees the patient. The health of a patient can change over time and for that reason an annual health history update should be completed by the patient, and the patient should be encouraged to inform the dentist of any changes to their health history as they occur.

Creating as complete a picture as possible of the patient involves both dental and medical history information.

checkPOINT

4. Why should the dentist be made aware of patient medical conditions?

checkPOINT

5. What is infective endocarditis?

checkPOINT

6. Why should you be knowledgeable about why a patient needs prophylactic antibiotics?

Clinical Chart Forms

Every patient chart includes a **clinical chart form.** This form provides an illustrated representation of the dental treatment a patient has or will receive.

Charting is essential to record information on health and/or disease of the dentition in a form that can be used now and later. At the least, clinical charts are needed for medical and legal protection reasons, to know what teeth and pathology was present before treatment was started. Moreover, the success or failure of treatments is impossible to gauge over time without gathering the proper information at initial treatment.

One method of charting used in the clinical environment is the SOAP method. This method provides a written sequential outline of the patients' dental concern and the approach to be taken for treatment. The acronym SOAP represents the following:

- S—Subjective—This is the information provided by the patient regarding the concern.
- O—Objective—This is the information gathered by the dentist based on what is observed when the examination is completed.
- A—Assessment—This is the diagnosis that the dentist makes.
- P—Plan—This is the treatment plan, which the dentist recommends and the treatment completed regarding the particular concern.

legal TIP

The health and dental history of a patient must be kept confidential is a part of doctor-patient confidentiality. This means it must not be discussed with any person outside of the dentists' office without the prior permission of the patient. There may be situations where the dentist must speak to the patients' medical doctor regarding the patients' condition, or medications and in this case the dentist will contact the other healthcare provider once permission from the patient is given. This permission can be given verbally or in writing.

checkPOINT

7. What is the purpose of the clinical charting form?

Understanding the SOAP method of charting used by practitioners on the dental team allows you to easily follow the sequence of events leading up to an appointment being scheduled for the patient. It also provides a documentation of the communication and treatment between the patient and dentist.

Example SOAP charting note:

S: Patient complains of "swelling around tooth" and "bad taste" in mouth, some pain in same area of swelling (tooth #1–#3)
O: Dr. Smith completed specific examination of oral cavity, percussion and ice test performed, radiographs taken
A: Dr. Smith diagnosed tooth #2 as requiring root canal therapy
P: Two appointments for root canal therapy to be scheduled 1 week apart

A periodontal screening examination form is also a part of the patients' clinical record. The dental hygienist places a great amount of focus on the patients' periodontal health and to achieve optimal dental health the dental hygienist will often begin the patient appointment by assessing the current state of the patients' periodontal health. Part of the comprehensive hygiene examination involves the assessment of oral health using a periodontal screening form. To assess the condition of the patient's gums, the hygienist will use a measuring probe instrument, which is placed between the tooth and the gum to measure the distance, or depth, between the gums and the tooth. This is a very important screening tool used by the dental hygienist. In order for the dentist to proceed with comprehensive restorative treatment, such as fixed prosthodontics, the patient must have healthy periodontal conditions to adequately support the restorations. Figure 8-9 is an example of a computerized periodontal screening form.

Various chart forms and systems for charting are available. Chapter 4 outlined the tooth numbering systems and the surface abbreviations used when charting teeth.

The following two guidelines apply to clinical charting of teeth conditions:

- Chart existing restorations and conditions that do not require treatment using one color, for example, the color blue.
- Chart caries and conditions that require treatment using a different color, for example, the color red.

Using two different colors on the clinical chart form allows the dental staff to view, at a glance, the treatment that is required and the treatment that has been completed. Using one color to show both treatment completed and treatment required would not provide accurate charting information. Figure 8-10A is an example of how a patient's clinical chart would appear using a computerized charting system.

Table 8-1 provides abbreviations used in clinical charting of teeth conditions. This table is designed to provide you with examples used in the dental office when charting certain procedures or treatments and to provide you with an opportunity to familiarize yourself with abbreviations used in some, but not all, dental offices. The dental office you work in may have charting abbreviations that are preferred by the dentist and clinical staff, and may not be found on this list. Figure 8-10B is an example of some of these charting notations using a computerized charting system.

Progress Notes Forms

The **progress notes form** is the section of the chart in which a narrative documentation of patient care and communication may be recorded chronologically. Figure 8-6 is an example of a progress notes form found in a patient chart. Some dental clinics may use a lined piece of paper separated into three or more columns. Each column represents a different part of the communication with the patient. Starting on the left-hand side of the page, the first column contains the date that the communication or treatment took place. The second column provides the details of the

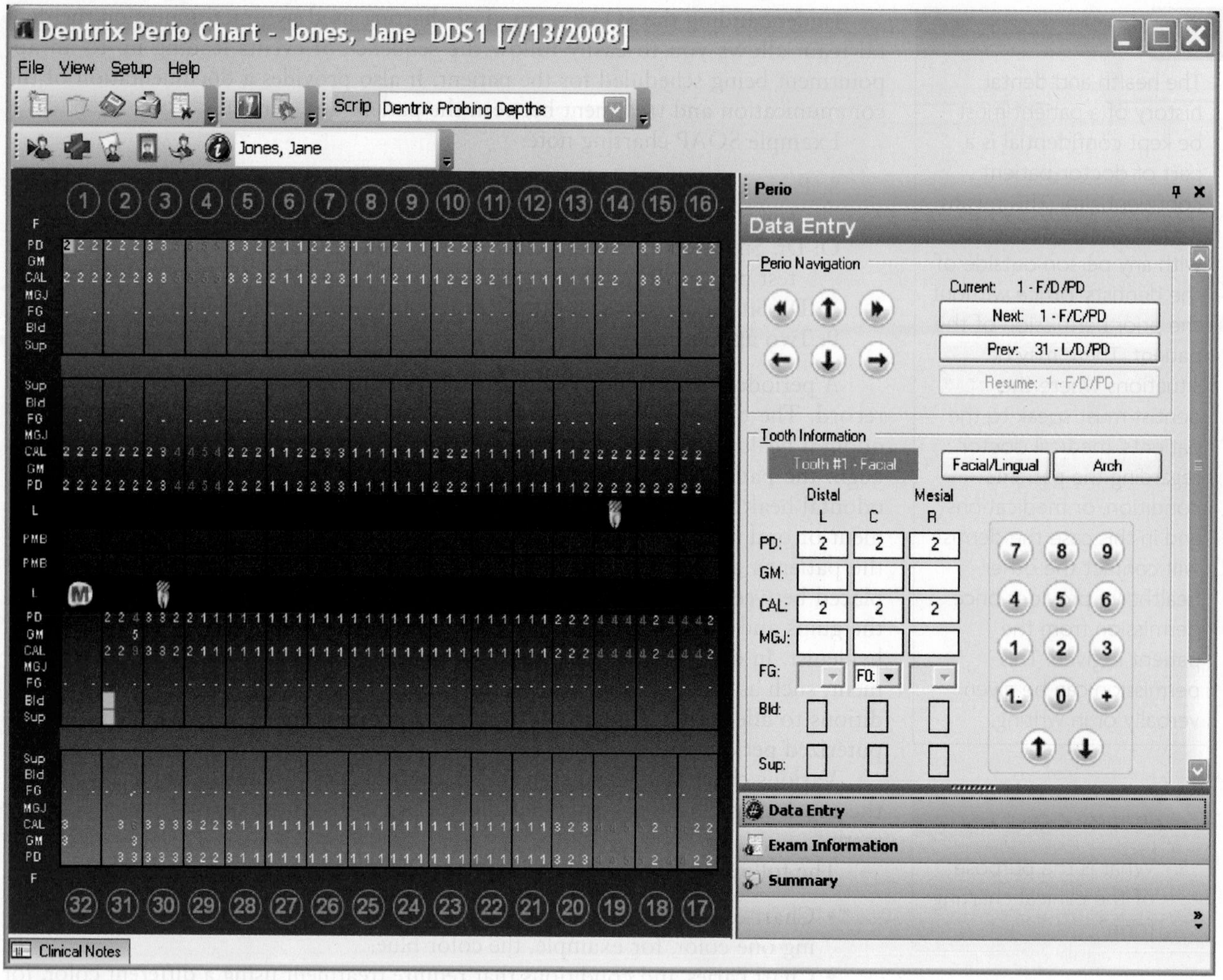

FIGURE 8-9 Computerized periodontal screening form. DENTRIX image courtesy of Henry Schein Practice Solutions, American Fork, UT.

treatment or communication, and the third column provides the patient's response to treatment or follow-up care of the treatment. The dentist in the clinic will have a preference regarding the layout of the form used. Some dental offices may use a plain piece of paper to record the information. Regardless of the style of form used, information regarding patient treatment and communication must include the date and details of the treatment or communication and the name or initials of the staff member responsible for documenting the information.

Where a computerized practice management program is used, the progress notes are recorded into the patient's chart on the computer. The clinical staff and administrative staff have access to the form in both the operatory and administrative areas of the office. Figure 8-11 is an example of progress notes used in a computerized patient chart.

Treatment Plan Forms

Each time a patient visits the dental office to see either the dentist or hygienist, a treatment plan is discussed with the patient. If a patient has seen the dentist for an annual checkup and the dentist has not found any teeth that require restoring or other treatment, the patient is usually given a recommended treatment plan of

A

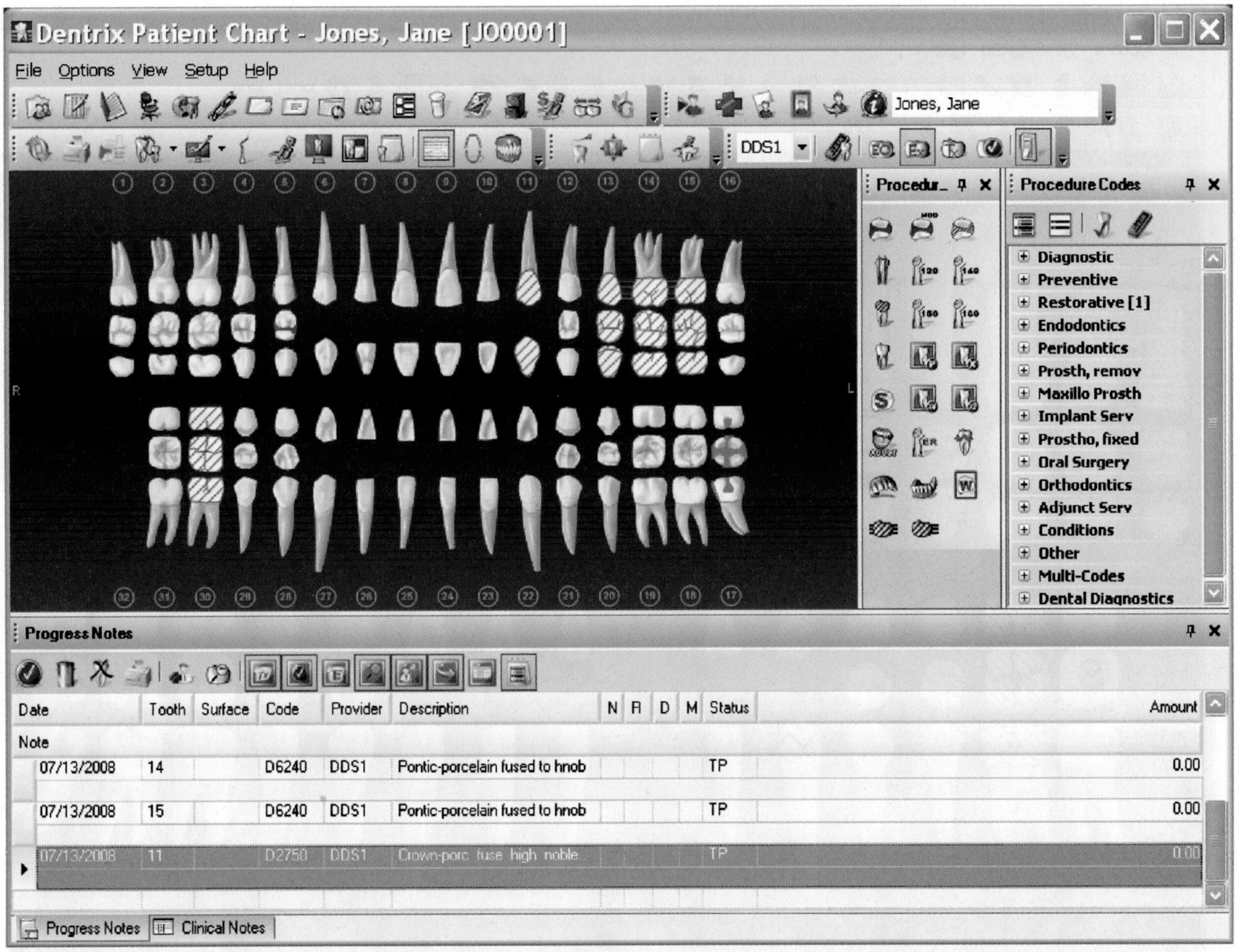

FIGURE 8-10 Clinical portion of patient chart, computerized. DENTRIX images courtesy of Henry Schein Practice Solutions, American Fork, UT. **(A)** Notice the colors used to distinguish between treatment completed by a previous provider (green), treatment completed by current provider (blue) and treatment, which is planned (red). **(B)** Clinical chart sample. Note the following treatments indicated in the chart:

Tooth #5: Restoration, MID
Tooth #7: Restoration, D
Tooth #9: Root canal therapy
Tooth #11: Crown
Tooth #13: Bridge abutment
Tooth #14: Bridge pontic
Tooth #15: Bridge abutment

Tooth #17: Restoration, MODBL
Tooth #21: Watch
Tooth #25: Extracted/missing
Tooth #27: Fractured
Tooth #30: Crown
Tooth #31: Sealant
Tooth #32: Extracted/missing

returning in 6 months to 1 year for an examination. In any case, each patient is asked to return to see the dentist or hygienist on a regularly scheduled basis. Figure 8-12 is an example of a **treatment plan** that is written up manually, and Figure 8-13 provides an example of what the treatment plan would look like when a computerized practice management program is used.

In the treatment plan, patients are given an itemized and prioritized list of the dental treatments that they require to achieve optimal oral health. The breakdown provides a description of the treatment and the cost of the treatment. If the insurance information is known, the treatment plan can also provide a breakdown of the patient responsibility for the cost and the amount the insurance company will pay toward the treatment cost. One of the advantages to using a computerized practice management program for providing patients with treatment plans is that it allows

> **checkPOINT**
>
> 8. What does a treatment plan form provide?

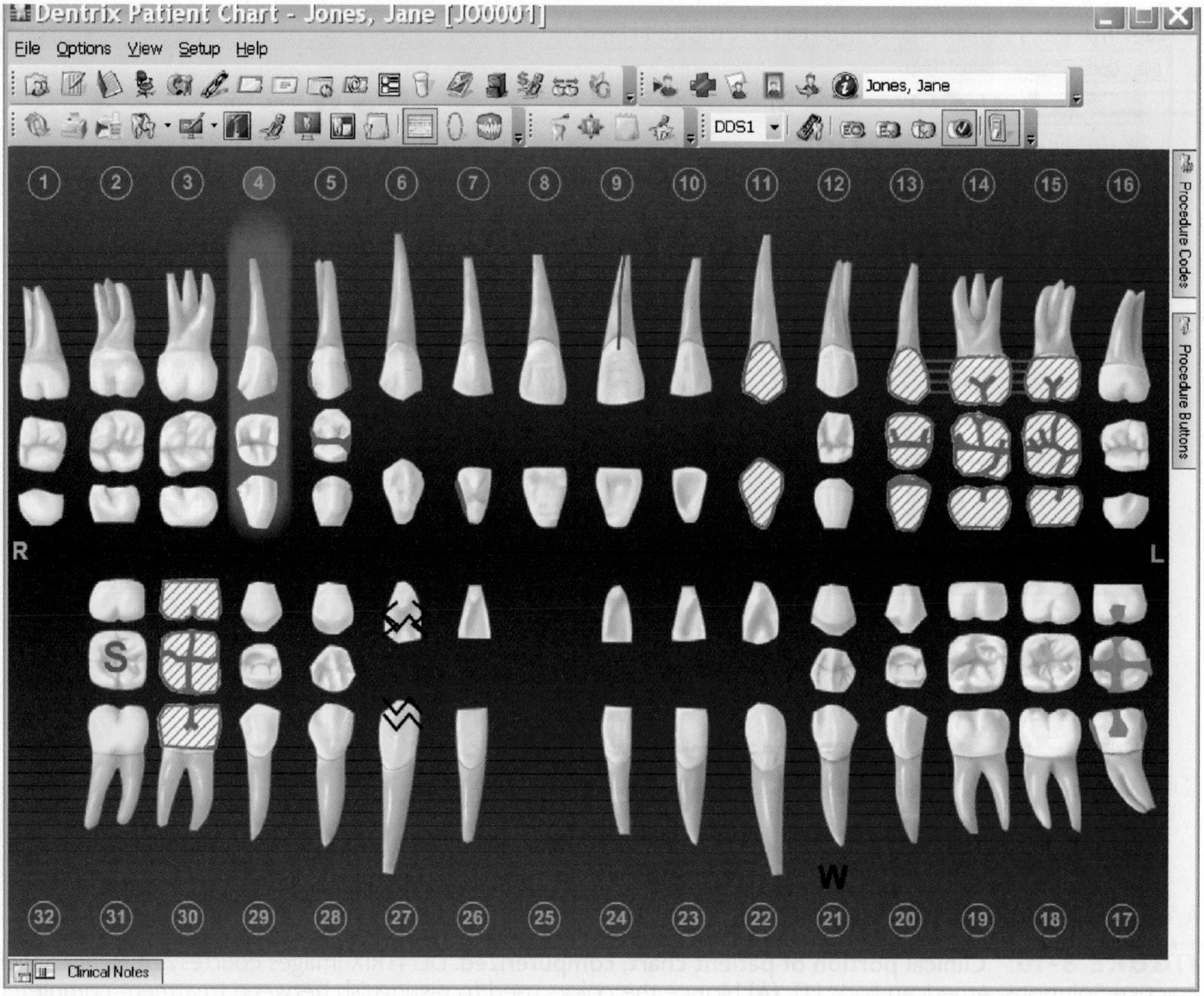

B

FIGURE 8-10 *(Continued)*

you to present the treatment plan to the patient using an educational tool. When presenting the treatment plan to the patient using a case presentation tool is useful for explaining the procedure to the patient and discussing alternatives. In Chapter 15, we will discuss patient billing and insurance company involvement in relation to treatment plans and the effective presentation of treatment plans.

RECORDING PATIENT COMMUNICATION

Providing efficient communication between the dentist and patient is another important role of the patient chart. The patient chart is also a legal document. For these reasons, all information recorded in the chart must be accurate. The accurate information recorded allows the dentist to communicate effectively with other dentists and physicians and provide continuity of care for the patient. Because the chart is a legal document, it can be subpoenaed in a malpractice suit. Ensuring that the information written in the chart is correct, recorded as it happened, and legible can help to win a malpractice suit or prevent one from occurring. All types of communication between patients and staff members must be documented by the staff member who is involved in the communication. The

TABLE 8-1 Abbreviations for Clinical Charting

Condition	Description	Abbreviation	Symbol
Missing tooth	Not present		Draw line through missing tooth
	Unerupted (impacted)	IMP	Circle tooth, write IMP below tooth
Fracture	Crown		Use line to denote fracture line
	Root		Draw "x" through missing portions of tooth
Restorations	Amalgam	Record surface(s) + A e.g., OA, MOA, MODLA	Outline shape of restoration on all tooth views as seen clinically; fill in with solid color
	Tooth colored - composite	Record surface(s) + -comp	Outline shape of restoration on all tooth views as seen clinically
	FIXED PARTIAL DENTURE (bridge)	FPD	Place blue "x" through roots of missing teeth
	Abutment - crown Pontic - replacement		Chart abutments using lines to fill in tooth
	COMPLETE DENTURE	CUD	Write above arch
	IMPLANT	IMPLANT	Write "implant"
Caries	Record all surfaces involved, including caries noted on radiographs		For primary, root, or recurrent caries, outline the carious area and fill in completely
	Overhangs	"OH"	Label defective area as "OH"
	Open margin	"open margin"	Chart the restoration and label defective area as "open margin"
	Fractured restoration	"fractured"	Chart area fractured
Extraction indicated	Erupted tooth		Place "x" over crown and root views
	Impacted tooth		Circle all views

following types of communication between the patient and dental team must be documented:

- treatment diagnosed and completed
- patient education
- patient concerns and complaints
- treatment plan acceptance and decline
- medical history changes

Keep in mind that there are specific areas of the chart that must only be written in by the clinical staff, such as the progress notes form or clinical chart form. As an office administrator, you are not likely to be present in the operatory when the treatment is being completed and patient instructions given. For this reason, the clinical team is responsible for recording this information.

Although each dental office may have a preferred style of documentation, the following general guidelines will provide you with a style that can easily be modified.

1. Check to make sure you have the correct patient chart.
2. Always record the date and time of entry first.

3. Print the information neatly in the chart. This will ensure that the information is easily legible by others who must read it. Never assume that everyone can read your cursive writing.
4. If you use abbreviations in your documentation, make sure they are accepted by the clinic, to avoid confusion. For example, using the abbreviation Ca for cavity could also be confused for the abbreviation for cancer if it is not a common abbreviation used in the clinic.
5. If you are documenting a conversation with the patient, use quotations when possible to identify the patient's exact words.
6. Document information as soon as possible after the communication; do not leave all the recording for the end of the day, as accuracy can be lost by doing this. Find a quiet place to document where distractions would be minimal.
7. All missed appointments and last minute cancellations should be recorded in the chart. Record the reason that the patient provided for the missed or cancelled appointment.
8. Record only the facts of the communication. Do not record information that is based on assumption or someone else's account. In other words, you must not record your assumptions of a situation. For example, if a patient had slurred speech while speaking to you, you would record that the patient "exhibited slurred speech" not that "the patient was intoxicated and had slurred speech." You can record only the facts as they are presented to you, not what you think may have occurred.
9. Never document for another person or have another person document for you. Documentation requires an accurate recording of the facts. If you were not involved directly or not present for the communication, you cannot provide accurate facts.
10. Information recorded in the dental chart must be written in pen and must never be erased, blacked out, whited out, or torn out of the chart. If you make an error, a single line must be drawn through it, with your initials placed at the end. The correct information must then be written.

checkPOINT

9. What information might be recorded in a patient chart by the dental office administrator?

All entries in a patient chart are done in chronological order. This is another reason, besides accuracy, why information must be recorded as it happens instead of a day or more later. A lack of chronological order among entries looks unprofessional and can create confusion when the chart is being reviewed to continue treatment.

Instructions for the patient from the dentist or hygienist must also be recorded in the chart. For example, if the dentist asks you to make follow-up contact with the patient after treatment was received, the request must be documented in the chart. The information you receive from the patient regarding the follow-up treatment must be recorded in the chart also. If you are unable to contact the patient, that is, they do not respond to your phone calls, this must also be documented. You must record the date and time of the call, the outcome, and any action you took, if required.

Printouts of any e-mails and transcribed phone messages from patients must be placed in the patient chart. Any responses to these forms of patient communication must also be placed in the chart. Patient charts may include special pockets or areas designated to hold certain types of correspondence, particularly for correspondence on paper smaller than an 8.5 × 11 in. paper, such as telephone messages,

***Administrative* TIP**

When a patient calls the dental office to inquire about treatment he or she has received or requires, politely place him or her on hold and retrieve him or her chart from the files. With the patient information in front of you, it will be much easier to reference information he or she is referring to and to record the information you are receiving. If the patient is providing you with a lengthy explanation, jot notes on a separate piece of paper and rewrite the information in a legible manner once the call is complete. Place the original piece of paper you used to make the notes in the chart once you have rewritten the information. If you ever need to refer to your original conversation with the patient, your original notes will remind you much more easily of the conversation than your rewritten notes.

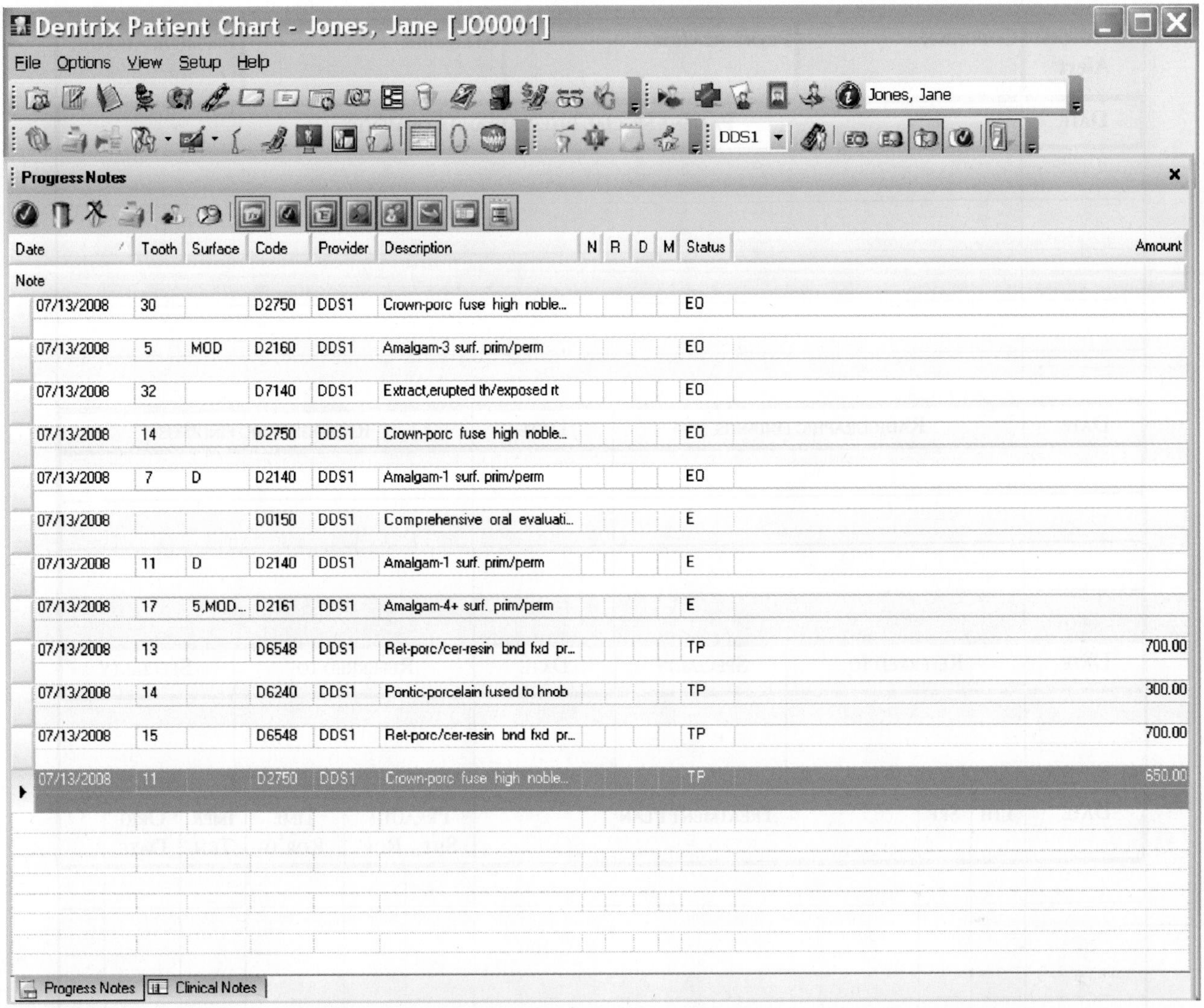

FIGURE 8-11 Progress notes, computerized. All types of treatment are listed in the progress notes. In this example, treatment that has been completed by another provider, the current provider, and treatment that is planned to be completed is listed in the progress notes. DENTRIX image courtesy of Henry Schein Practice Solutions, American Fork, UT.

prescriptions, and referral forms to other practitioners. Maintaining an accurate and up-to-date patient record includes keeping all documentation that occurs between the patient and the dental office in the patient chart.

INCIDENT REPORTS

In your role in the dental office, you may encounter situations in which you need to document incidences of patient or staff injury or medical emergency, negative behavior, or other unusual events of concern. **Incident reports**, or records of such incidences, are completed by a staff member who was involved in or who witnessed the incident. Each dental office may have a standard form that is used or may use a method that does not involve a form.

Once the form is completed, it is reviewed by the dentist or office manager and placed in a file that is usually kept separate from patient charts. A copy of the incident form may also be placed in the patient's chart. If there are injuries sustained by any of the persons involved, the dentist must be summoned immediately so that

Medical Alert	Condition	Premedication	Allergies	Premedication

Date	Patient Special Interests and Comments

Date	Radiographic findings	Date	Radiographic findings

Date	Referred to	Specialty	Date	Referred to	Specialty

Date	Tth	Srf	Treatment Plan	Preauth Snt	Preauth Rcv	Time Rqr'd	Impr Tkn	Orig Date	✓

FIGURE 8-12 Treatment plan.

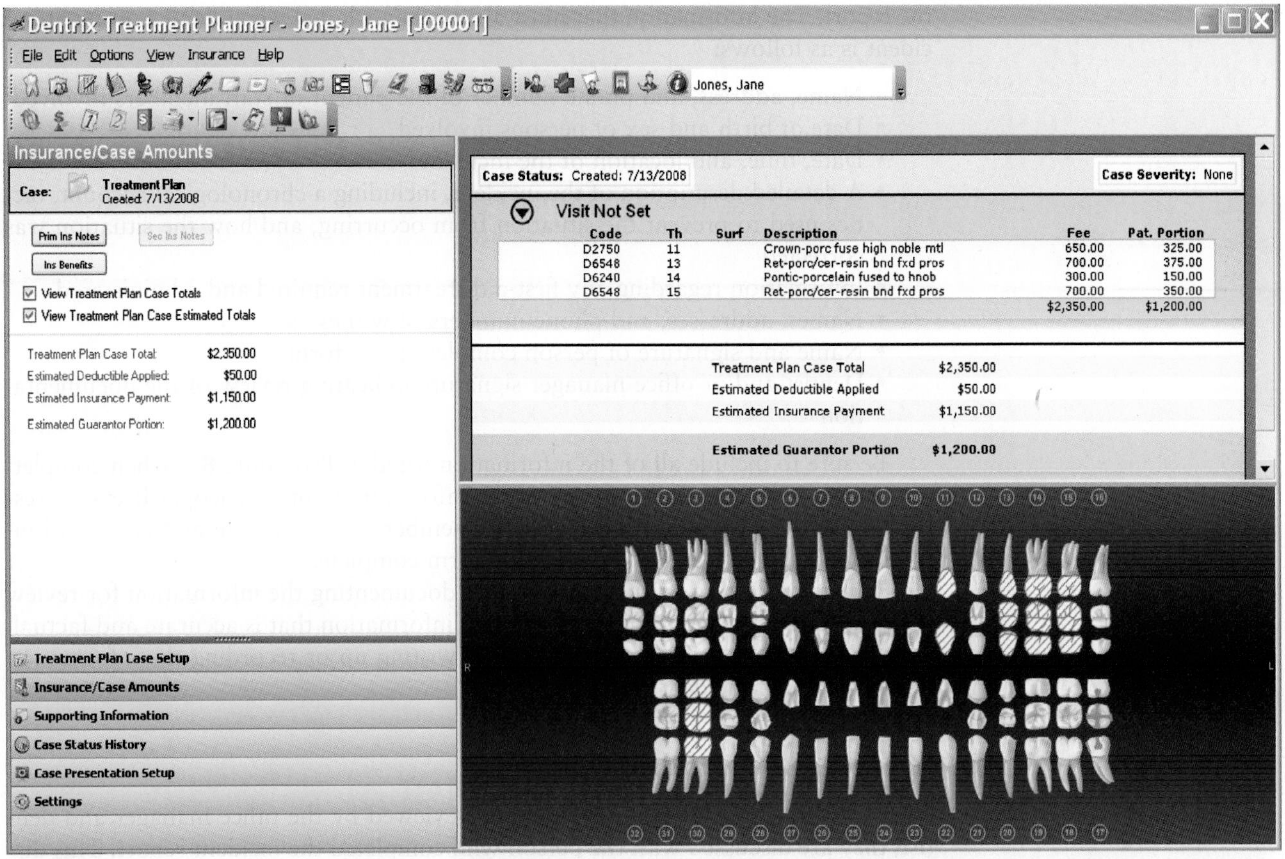

FIGURE 8-13 Treatment plan, computerized. DENTRIX image courtesy of Henry Schein Practice Solutions, American Fork, UT.

first-aid is properly administered. The dentist would then be required to document any findings and first-aid required.

When to Complete an Incident Report?

Incident reports are often required by insurance companies and legal representatives. For example, if a patient in the office is injured, the liability insurance the dentist has in place would provide any compensation to the patient or staff member, if required. Although injury-related incident reports in a dental office are rare, there are other situations that may occur that require the completion of an incident report. These situations include the following:

- a patient having an allergic reaction
- a patient being belligerent or showing aggressive behavior toward staff
- a staff member altercation with a patient or other staff member
- employee needlestick injuries
- a patient having a medical emergency
- a staff member having a medical emergency

When you are unsure about whether to write up an incident report, consult with the office manager or dentist. If you are unable to consult with either of these individuals, go ahead and write it up. It is safer to complete one than not.

What to Include in the Incident Report?

The dental office you work in may or may not have a formal incident report form. Instead, your office may only provide guidelines on what information to include in the report. The information that must always be included when documenting an incident is as follows:

- Name, address, and phone number of the patient or staff members involved
- Date of birth and sex of persons involved
- Date, time, and location of the incident
- A detailed description of the incident, including a chronological account, tactics used to prevent the situation from occurring, and how the situation was corrected
- Information regarding any first-aid treatment required and administered
- Names, addresses, and phone numbers of witnesses
- Name and signature of person completing the form
- Dentist and/or office manager signature indicating review of the documentation

Be sure to include all of the information listed in Procedure 8-1 when completing the incident form. Leaving any of the information out may jeopardize an investigation of the situation, if necessary. Remember to be accurate and ensure all information is correct and all areas of the form complete.

When completing an incident form or documenting the information for review for your office manager or dentist, provide information that is accurate and factual. Use the guidelines in Procedure 8-1 when writing up or recording the information to be used in an incident report.

Follow-Up to an Incident Report

After incident reports are completed and reviewed by the office manager and dentist, they are discussed with the person who completed the incident report. This discussion can include any or all of the following points:

- How the incident may have been prevented?
- How future incidents can be more effectively addressed?
- What areas of the office most incidents occur in?

PROCEDURE 8-1 *Guidelines for Completing an Incident Report*

1. State the facts of the incident clearly and succinctly. Do not add any of your personal thoughts, opinions, or assumptions in the recording. For example, if a patient was in the waiting room yelling loudly and name-calling another patient and you noticed the patient was slurring his words, you would not write: "Patient A was drunk and yelling loudly at patient B." Instead, you would write: "Patient A was slurring words and yelling loudly at Patient B."
2. Always document the incident using legible writing or a typewriter or computer. Never use script writing, as this may not be legible. Your name, title, and signature must appear at the end of the report.
3. Complete and submit the incident report to the office manager or dentist for review within 24 hours of the incident occurring. Complete it as soon as possible. The greater the lapse of time between the incident occurring and the documentation of it, the greater the risk of information being forgotten.
4. Address all areas of the report. That is, if there is a section that does not apply to the incident, such as no witnesses being present during the incident, write n/a in that area of the form or write "no witnesses were present," if documenting from guidelines.
5. Do not keep a copy of the incident report for your records. Once the report is completed, it is the property of the dental clinic and any copies that are removed from the clinic without permission of the dentist could be a violation of clinic policies.
6. Some dental offices may keep a copy of the incident report in the patient's chart, whereas others may keep all incident reports separate from the patient chart. Know the policies used in the office you are in and follow them.

- What topics, treatments, or situations most often lead to incidents occurring?
- How to avoid future incidents?

By achieving solutions to avoiding or effectively dealing with future incidents, staff members will develop confidence in effectively managing similar incidents in the future. A good rule of thumb to keep in mind is, if you are ever in a situation in the office in which the patient is upset or becoming threatening, request the assistance of the dentist or office manager in diffusing the situation. Attempting to manage a potentially dangerous situation on your own is not recommended, and since the incident will need to be documented afterward, having another person who can attest to your statement of facts can be helpful. Similar to a situation that is potentially threatening, a patient who is injured or having a medical emergency will also require the assistance of the dentist or other staff member trained to assist in medical emergencies. Never attempt to solve either of these types of situations on your own.

checkPOINT

10. What is the purpose of an incident report?

PREPARING A PATIENT CHART

Each time patients attend the dental office for an appointment, their charts must be prepared in some way. There are three types of patients who come into the dental office: new patients, emergency patients, and returning patients. Procedure 8-2 provides guidelines for preparing a dental chart that can be followed in any dental office. Use these guidelines to prepare patient charts in anticipation of the patient's visit.

New Patient

Each new patient in the dental office must complete a new patient form, health history form, and any office policy forms required by the clinic. Although a new patient may be new to the dental office, it is likely that the patient has been to see a dentist in the past. In situations where the patient is changing dentists, the patient will have information that they wish to have transferred over to the office where they will be attending. You may have to contact the dental office the patient previously attended to obtain information such as dental radiographs for the patient file. The patient will be responsible for contacting the previous dental office and requesting that the information be forwarded. Items that are most often requested

PROCEDURE 8-2 *Guidelines for Preparing a Patient Chart*

1. Make sure you have a chart folder and gather the forms you will need for a dental chart. These should include the following:
   - The completed patient forms
   - Completed health history forms
   - Clinical chart forms
   - Periodontal recording forms
   - Treatment services form
2. Place the chart forms in the chart in the order preferred by the dentist. This may include clinical information on one side of the chart and patient information forms on the other side. This is specific to the dental office and should be adhered to.
3. Get the necessary labels for the chart. If the last name is the recommended form of filing, select the labels that represent the patient's last name.
4. Type or print off the label for the patient's name. Place the last name labels or chart ID number labels along the edge of the chart in their appropriate place.
5. Place the year label along the top notch of the chart. This label will be replaced for each year the patient returns to the dental office. Do not replace the year label until the patient returns for the first visit in the year.
6. Apply any additional labels that are recommended for use in the dental office. This may include labels signifying allergies, medical alerts, or insurance type.

West Street Dental
123 West Street
Anytown, ST
USA
90000
(222) 234-5678

Patient Request for Information

Patient Information
Name ____________________
Address ____________________
____
Date of Birth ____________________

I ____________________ am requesting that the information contained in my patient chart be forwarded to the address below. Specifically, I would like the following information:
____
____
____

to be sent on my behalf to the following address:
____
____
____

Signed, this ________ day of ____________, 20_____ in the city/town of ____________
in the State of ____________________, USA.

Name (Printed)____________________

Name (Signed)____________________

FIGURE 8-14 Written request for patient information.

> **legal TIP**
>
> The patient information in the dental office is the property of the dentist. In situations where the patient is requesting that confidential information be forwarded to another dental office, it is important that the request be in writing. The patient must date and sign the request as well as itemize the information to be forwarded. Also, original copies must remain with the originating dental office. Figure 8-14 is an example of what a written request may look like.

by a patient who is transferring information to another dental office are radiographs. Both dental radiographs and dental impressions, or models, are part of the patient chart. Dental models are a diagnostic tool used by the dentist and are often kept in a box in another area of the dental office. A list of all patient diagnostic models is maintained to easily locate patient models when needed. Patient radiographs are often located in the dental chart, or on the computer chart, which can be easily duplicated. Original records should never be sent out of the dental office, duplicates of the requested information should be sent. Most importantly, familiarize yourself with the protocol followed in the dental office you work in regarding the forwarding of any patient information.

Each patient chart must be labeled using the label system in the office, and a patient name label must be placed on the chart. Keeping the labeling system consistent among all patient charts in the dental office is important when maintaining a professional and easy to organize filing system. There are many different labeling systems available; it will be your responsibility to ensure that the correct system is followed.

Emergency Patient

Emergency patients can be one-time patients in the dental office or become permanent patients. If the person is an emergency patient, use the emergency patient charts the dental office prefers. The emergency record is designed to provide a

legal TIP

Patient privacy in the dental office can be easily maintained by following the guidelines under Health Insurance Portability and Accountability Act (HIPAA). However, when a new patient is completing forms in the dental office, and you are compiling the chart and ensuring that everything that needs to be included in the chart is present, the issue of privacy can be inadvertently overlooked. Keep the following points in mind when compiling chart contents:

- Do not ask a patient specific information regarding health and medical history, when other patients may overhear.
- Keep the patient chart you are currently working on in a place where no other person can read the information contained.
- Keep labels concerning health and medication alerts contained to the inside of the chart.

smaller chart for one-time patients. The information included on it includes the patient information, health and dental history, an area for the dentist's notes, and a pocket for radiographs. This information is the immediate and necessary information needed by dental staff to assist a patient in an emergency situation. Usually the dental office will have financial policies concerning patients who come to the clinic for an emergency concern, such as payment in full for services rendered using specified forms of payment only. If the patient has dental insurance, the policy may require payment in full from the patient and the dental office will assist the patient in obtaining payment from their dental insurance carrier. Should the patient return to the dental office, they will need to complete the more detailed new patient registration form and familiarize themselves with the office policies and procedures, such as that shown in Figure 8-15.

Returning Patient

Patients who are returning to the dental office may be required to update their health and medical history. Depending on the policy of the dental office, updating the patients' dental clinical chart may be performed on a yearly basis. The health history of a patient should be updated on a regular basis as well. The health history

West Street Dental
123 West Street
Anytown, ST
USA
90001
(222) 234-4567

Office Policies

Appointment Scheduling
- We will make every effort to provide you with a convenient appointment time.
- We strive to keep our appointment schedule on time. If you are going to be late for your appointment, please telephone our office to let us know.
- Missed Appointments - unless canceled 24 hours in advance, our policy is to request a deposit from you prior to rescheduling your appointment. Your deposit will be put towards future services.

Financial
- Payment for professional services are due at the time dental treatment is provided. We accept cash, checks, ATM cards, Visa, MasterCard, Discover, and American Express. We offer an extended payment plan with prior credit approval.
- Payments are due within 10 days of receipt of your statement.

Dental Insurance
- Our office offers the courtesy of filing your dental claims electronically. You are responsible for any amounts not covered by your dental plan, due at the time of the appointment.

Please understand we file your claim for you as a courtesy. Your insurance is a contract between you and the insurance company. We are not familiar with your insurance plan.

FIGURE 8-15 Office policies.

update form and the clinical dental update form are typically placed into the chart of a patient returning after an extended absence.

Chapter Summary

The patient chart is a legal document of the dental office. Attention must be paid to the information placed and recorded in it. The contents of the patient chart are particular to the dental industry, and each helps provide optimal oral health for the patient. Care must be taken when recording information in the chart, and attention to detail is critical. Following the guidelines set out regarding the proper recording of information will ensure a properly maintained patient chart. Incidents that occur in the dental office that are out of the ordinary must be recorded using an incident report. Regardless of the preferred system in the dental clinic, all information that goes into the patient chart must be legible, accurate, and easily retrievable for all staff members.

Review Questions

Multiple Choice

1. **The patient chart does not include**
   a. date of birth.
   b. spouse's insurance information.
   c. radiographs from a previous dentist.
   d. patient's height and weight.

2. **This form provides an illustrated representation of the dental treatment a patient will receive**
   a. clinical chart form.
   b. health history form.
   c. progress notes form.
   d. incident report form.

3. **A periodontal screening form**
   a. is for the hygienists' use only.
   b. is an assessment tool used by the hygienist.
   c. provides a diagnosis for periodontal health.
   d. is for the dentists' use only.

4. **Progress notes**
   a. are recorded chronologically.
   b. can only be written by the dentist.
   c. are not part of the dental chart.
   d. are written on a yearly basis.

5. **Incident reports are completed by the**
   a. staff member involved in the incident.
   b. staff member who witnesses the incident.
   c. dentist.
   d. office manager.

6. **Using the SOAP method of charting, which statement best represents the Subjective portion?**
   a. "My tooth feels like it is really loose."
   b. "Your gums look fine to me, Mrs. Smith."
   c. "I recommend that you brush and floss at least twice a day."
   d. "I will schedule my appointment for next week."

7. **A narrative documentation of patient treatment and communication is known as**
   a. clinical notes.
   b. treatment plan.
   c. progress notes.
   d. incident report.

8. **Which of the following is not a type of communication to be documented in the patient chart?**
   a. Treatment diagnosed and completed
   b. Medical history changes
   c. Whether or not the patient can drive
   d. Patient concerns and complaints

9. **Which of the following situations requires the completion of an incident report?**
   a. Two staff members have a fistfight at lunch time in the staff room.
   b. A 7-year-old patient has an allergic reaction to the dental assistant's latex gloves.
   c. The hygienist accidentally pokes himself or herself with the needle he or she just used to give his or her patient local anesthetic.
   d. All of the above require incident reports to be written up.

10. **When a patient requests information from their chart be forwarded to another dental office which of the following actions must you take?**
    a. Photocopy the chart whether the patient requested it or not.
    b. Make sure the request is in writing before taking any action.
    c. Make sure the office manager will allow the transfer.
    d. Send a goodbye card to the patient.

Critical Thinking

1. Your coworker is in the habit of not recording information in the patient's chart when speaking with the patient on the phone. How will you explain to your coworker the importance of recording the information?

2. The new patient completing forms in the reception area has just informed you that he or she does not want to provide the dentist with answers to all of the health history questions because he or she is coming in only to have one tooth filled. How will you explain to the patient the necessity for this information?

3. Mrs. Jones has just received a treatment plan in the mail and is now phoning you because she has mistaken it for a bill for services and is quite upset. How do you explain to Mrs. Jones what the treatment plan is?

Hands-On Activity

1. You have been put in charge of creating a patient questionnaire that focuses on the past experiences the patient has had in dental offices. The office manager is trying to change the way things are performed in the office by offering services, which patients enjoy while at their dental appointment. Use questions which encourage the patient to provide as much information as possible regarding what they enjoyed and what they did not enjoy about their dental treatment, or what services they would like to see offered in the dental office.
2. Create a one-page information sheet to provide to patients about the necessity and importance of providing the dentist with as much health and dental history as possible.
3. You are the first office administrator in a brand-new dental practice. There are no incident forms available. Create one for use in the office.

Reference

P. B. Lockhart, B. Loven, M. T. Brennan, and P. C. Fox. The evidence base for the efficacy of antibiotic prophylaxis in dental practice. *J. Am. Dent. Assoc.* 2007; 138(4): 458–474.

Web Sites

American Dental Association
www.ada.org
American Heart Association
www.americanheart.org

DENTRIX
www.dentrix.com

chapter NINE

Patient Development *and* Maintenance

OUTLINE

OBJECTIVES

After completing this chapter, you should be able to do the following:

- List and explain guidelines for developing patient loyalty to the dental practice
- Explain the purpose of a recare system and name the primary types of recare systems
- Demonstrate strategies for encouraging patients to preschedule treatment and hygiene appointments
- Describe different patient reminder methods
- List both internal and external methods of marketing the dental practice

KEY TERMS

- patient recare system
- reactivation letter
- patient retention marketing
- new patient marketing

Besides being a healthcare facility, the dental office is also a business. A financially successful practice depends on a regular flow of patients. A patient who is disappointed at the treatment and care received may decide to find another dental office to attend. Each time a patient decides to leave the practice, the result is a loss of revenue.

Thus, each member of the dental team has a role to play in the development of patient relationships. The role of the dental administrator in maintaining and acquiring new patients in the dental office is an important one. In particular, the dental administrator is expected to develop patient loyalty by making a good first impression, making the patient needs a priority, communicating effectively with patients, and maintaining up-to-date contact information. Furthermore, the dental administrator must effectively manage a recare and reminder system and contribute to the marketing of the dental office.

DEVELOPING PATIENT LOYALTY

Developing patient loyalty to the dental office is an ongoing process that takes time and efforts on the part of every team member of the dental office. For instance, a patient who contacts the dental office for the first time may have many questions about his or her specific dental needs, and the office administrator must be able to answer those questions with confidence and clarity. Building positive patient relationships affects all staff members in that patients will begin to trust other staff members once they develop trust with one. The same holds true in situations where a patient loses trust in one staff member; that is, the loss of trust with one team member impacts the relationship with the whole team. The following are guidelines for the dental office administrator for developing trust and long-lasting patient relationships to build and maintain the patient base of the dental office.

Make a Good First Impression

You have only one opportunity to make a good first impression on a patient. The impression the dental administrator makes on patients, or anyone entering the dental office, strongly influences their perception of the dental office. Each person who comes into the dental office should be given immediate attention. If a patient enters the office for a scheduled appointment, consult the schedule and greet the patient by name. If the patient is a child, greet the child by name as well as the parent. Communicate any delays in the schedule immediately and offer the patient some form of comfort or distraction, such as a glass of water or magazines. For children, provide books or coloring materials that are age appropriate. Addressing patients on their arrival is an important part of building the patient relationship since it communicates to patients that they are important to the dental practice and it is a recognition that the patient time is valuable.

The goal of the dental administrator is to create a positive perception of the office for the patient, which will facilitate an enjoyable dental experience and lasting relationship. Moreover, a patient who feels a positive relationship with the dental office will be more likely to accept and follow through with treatment prescribed.

You can accomplish this goal by applying many of the professional guidelines discussed in earlier chapters, which are summarized below:

- **Dress professionally.** Your outward appearance is an indication of how you feel about yourself, your environment, and the business you work for. As a front office staff member, you are a frontline representative of the whole dental team. A clean, neat outward appearance communicates pride in the work you do and the people you work with.
- **Smile when speaking with the patient.** Being approachable is an essential element for relationship building. Smiling when greeting or speaking with patients portrays an approachable attitude that facilitates communication with others.
- **Greet the patient promptly.** Addressing patients and their reason for attending the office is a professional way to acknowledge patients' presence and communicate to them that they are important to the dental team. Patients who are left waiting at the front office quickly develop a negative impression of staff members and the quality of service. Furthermore, paying attention to people who enter the dental office avoids situations in which a front desk that is not attended to can become a situation for crime to occur.

checkPOINT

1. What are six techniques you can use to make a good first impression?

legal TIP

- Avoid leaving patient information where others can read the content—whether on paper or electronic.
- Charts should not be left out in public areas. Confidential information should be marked as such and protected from the view of others. Try to keep computers reflecting patients' information out of view, or use screen savers or other methods to protect the information as reasonably as possible.
- Avoid asking patients sensitive questions where other patients can hear the conversation.
- Avoid discussing confidential patient information with other dental team members where other people can hear the conversation

- **Do not carry on personal phone calls while working.** A patient who is in the reception area can overhear any telephone or face-to-face conversation you have with others. If you must make or receive a personal phone call, find an area where patients will not overhear your conversation. Personal conversations are unprofessional in an environment where patients are present.
- **If you are busy with another patient, give the patient who is waiting a verbal or nonverbal cue of acknowledgment.** If you are on the telephone, glancing up and nodding your head and smiling is a nonverbal way to give a patient a cue that you are aware they have come into the office, and will be with them as soon as you can. If you are speaking to another patient face to face, interrupt your conversation briefly to acknowledge the other person and inform them that you are currently with a patient and let them know when you will be with them. If you see the patient and you do not acknowledge his or her presence, the patient will perceive this as being ignored.
- **Keep the front desk and reception area clean and well-organized.** Patient charts and other paperwork are considered confidential in the dental office. Leaving information on the front desk where it can be viewed by others violates patient confidentiality. Keep paperwork on the front desk in a neat, organized manner to avoid visual access by other patients.

In addition to adopting these practices, be prepared to respond intelligently to any questions a prospective patient may pose to you regarding the dental practice. A list of questions you may have to field is provided in Box 9-1.

Focus on the Patient First

Creating a patient-centered dental practice means that the focus of the practice is on providing services that the patient wants. The patient-centered practice places the needs of the patient first and takes the emphasis off of the patient as someone for the dentist to treat. For example, the patient-centered practice will have appointment hours that are accommodating for patients, such as in the evening or on weekends, an after-hours emergency contact will be available for patients and has

BOX 9-1
Fielding Questions From Prospective Patients

Below are questions that potential new patients may ask the dental office administrator when they call or come into the dental office. Consult with the office manager or dentist to gain answers to these questions so that you are prepared to discuss them with a potential or new patient.

- Is the dentist a member of the appropriate dental association?
- Do you practice current infection control procedures at the office?
- Will the office accept insurance assignment of my dental benefits?
- Will I be offered different options for treatment?
- Is the dentist available for after-hours emergencies?
- Are the facilities neat and clean?
- Does the dentist do various procedures, or will I be referred out for many procedures?
- What hours are you open?
- Do you treat children?
- Does the dentist involve the patient in the treatment planning phase?
- Do you have a facility that provides special assistance or care, such as wheelchair access, nitrous oxide, and premedication?
- Do you offer payment plans for treatment?

what IF ?

Imagine you are entering a dental office as a new patient for your first appointment with the dentist. As you approach the front desk, the dental administrator turns to you and says, "I'll be just a sec; I have to finish this call." She then proceeds to continue a conversation on the phone, which appears to be a personal call, as it revolves around upcoming weekend activities. Five minutes later, the dental administrator hangs up the phone and turns to you and says, "OK, so, how can I help you?" If you were the patient in this scenario, what would your first impression be? How could the dental administrator have behaved more professionally in this situation?

With this scenario in mind, the first impression given is that the patient is not important to the dental practice, and the dental administrator representing the practice is not a caring, concerned individual. Acknowledging a patient when he or she enters the dental office is important for sending the nonverbal message that the patient is important to the practice and his or her time is valuable. In this situation the patient was acknowledged; however, the manner which the administrator used gave the patient the impression that the dental administrator was hurried. The choice of unprofessional language used in the communication "just a sec" should be replaced with "I'll be a few minutes." Always tell the patient approximately how long you will be. If you are going to be "just a sec," you are telling them you will be "one second," which is unrealistic. Always give a close approximation such as "I will be about 5 minutes, I am just finishing a call." The dental office administrator in this situation should have completed her phone call out of listening range to the patient. Moving to another area of the practice would have been more effective. Her personal call was unprofessional in the presence of a patient. What made matters worse was that she made the patient feel unimportant by making the patient wait until she finished making her weekend plans. Keep in mind that the dental office is a place of business and your personal affairs should be kept to a minimum and designated to specific areas. If you can, avoid conducting personal business at work.

systems in place that educate patients on all aspects of their dental treatment. Ultimately, the team of a patient-centered practice listens to the patients and provides solutions for their concerns. Exceptional customer care for each and every patient in the office is the focus and assists in successful relationship building.

Treat each patient as if he or she is the most important person in the dental clinic. This means, give patients your full attention when they are in the office, return phone calls in a timely manner as promised, and always thank them when they call or come into the office. When ending a telephone call, say "Thank you for calling" and when a patient is about to leave the office, say "Thank you for coming in today," acknowledging that the patient has chosen to attend the dental office can be a welcome compliment. Remembering details about patients when they are in the office goes a long way toward building relationships and practice loyalty. Mention birthdays, vacations, and other special events that you are aware of regarding the patient.

Keep Information Up-to-Date

Each time the patient comes in to the practice, confirm that there are no changes in address, phone number, work number, or insurance coverage. Patients often forget to let their dentist know that they have a new work number or cellphone number where they can be reached. A quick check by asking, "Have there been any changes to your phone number, address, or insurance information that we have on file?" should elicit the information you need. Keeping the demographic information up-to-date is just as important as keeping a patient's health history current in the chart. Your responsibility is to ensure that the patient chart is current. To contact the patient, you must have the correct mailing address and telephone number. Sending time-sensitive mail such as account statements to incorrect addresses creates frustration for you and the current occupant of the address. In Chapter 8, we discussed the importance of updating patients' health history on a regular basis. In addition, as children grow older and become adults, maintaining the health history information in the chart is important and can be easily overlooked; therefore, it is important to consider the child the same way you would an adult patient in this regard.

checkPOINT

2. What is the goal of the dental office administrator in creating a positive first impression?

Follow Up and Follow Through

Each patient in the dental practice must be contacted, by a phone call, letter, or postcard, at some point during the 12-month period after his or her last appointment. Always follow up with patients regarding treatment that has been done or needs to be done, and follow through by contacting them in the method and timeframe

> **Administrative TIP**
>
> You may find that there are patients attending the dental office who have a first language other than English. Part of providing good customer service in developing the patient-centered practice includes accommodating patients to make as much information as understandable and accessible as possible. A diverse patient population can be accommodated by providing new patient, health history, and health history update forms in multiple languages. Health insurance companies provide forms in multiple languages for their clients that can be accessed via the Internet by you or the client. The American Dental Association also provides links for dental office personnel to Web sites that can provide information. Translating any form into another language used in the dental office you are working in can be done by a member of the staff who is fluent in the language.

promised. Not staying in touch with patients could mean a loss of a patient and revenue for the practice. This chapter highlights some of the marketing strategies commonly used in the dental office for patient relationship development.

Inform Patients of All Treatment Details and Costs

Another way to foster goodwill with the patient is to clearly disclose all relevant treatment details, especially related to cost and financial arrangements. Use a detailed treatment outline form and financial responsibility form to outline patient responsibility. Being upfront about the costs and length of treatment avoids unpleasant surprises when treatment is complete. Chapter 15 covers the particular elements involved in treatment planning and how to effectively present a treatment plan to a patient.

RECALL/RECARE SYSTEMS

A **patient recare system,** also known as a recall system, is a proactive method of scheduling future appointments with patients and reminding the patients of these appointments. Note that in this text, the term *recare* is preferred, as the term *recall* can have negative associations and can make the patients feel that their appointment is not important. The dentist is not "recalling" the patient back to check whether the dentistry needs to be replaced, much like how a car company recalls a car for a defective part. Thus, avoid the use of the word *recall* when informing patients of their need to return to the hygienist. Other terms used to describe this type of appointment include continued care and preventive care.

The reminder and recare system can be paper-based (letters, cards), electronic (computer database), or by telephone. The critical component in the recare system is that patients are receiving their notification of a recare appointment and that the office administrator documents all communications with patients. The patient recare and reminder system is an integral part of maintaining patient relationships in the dental office.

Regardless of the type of system in place in the dental office, they all have the same goal: maintaining patient flow through relationship maintenance. It is important for the patient to feel the need and the importance of returning to the dental office on a regular basis. Creating the patient's perception of the practice begins with the dental administrator and continues as the staff members place importance on and emphasize the value of the recare appointment. Without the perception of value, patients will be more hesitant to schedule or maintain a recare appointment. Good verbal skills, team communication, and patient education are an important combination for a successful recare system.

The main types of recare systems used in dental offices are as follows:

- Prescheduled recare appointments
- Written correspondence and telephone recare systems

One of the many concerns in a dental practice today is having an effective recare system. Any recare system is only as good as the person responsible for its success, and that person must monitor it constantly in order for the system to be effective. The dental office administrator is largely responsible for the success of this system.

BOX 9-2
Appointment Prescheduling

Avoid this scenario:

Administrator: Do you want to schedule your appointment now?

Patient: No. I'll have to call you.

Use these alternatives:

Administrator: Mr. Jones, our hygienist, Jane, would like to see you in 3 months. She has an opening on Monday July 14 or Tuesday July 15. Which day is better for you?

Or

Administrator: If you schedule your appointment now, I will mail you a reminder card 3 to 4 weeks prior to the appointment, and if you need to reschedule it, there will be no problem at all.

These suggested scripts focus on getting around patient concerns regarding scheduling appointments too far in advance. Scheduling an appointment too far in the future may make patients feel locked in. Maintain control of the appointment schedule by reminding patients well advance of their appointment.

Prescheduling Recare Appointments

Prescheduling recare appointments means scheduling a patient's next appointment before he or she exits the practice after a completed appointment. This can be a very effective recare system for several reasons:

- Patients have an appointment in the schedule, and the patient has requested to be contacted if an appointment earlier than the one already scheduled becomes available.
- The goal of effectively maintaining the daily schedule and the level of production is much more easily achieved since patients do not have to be encouraged to set appointments after they have left the practice.

A general rule of thumb when prescheduling recare appointments is never to ask a closed-ended question. A closed-ended question solicits a "yes" or "no" answer, and often the answer is "no." Box 9-2 provides some scripts that can be used for navigating through objections when prescheduling patients. Encouraging the patient to schedule the next appointment before leaving the dental office begins with the clinical team while the patient is in the operatory. For example, a patient who has come in for an annual examination with the dentist is told that she needs to return for an appointment for a filling. The dentist explains to the patient the risks involved in waiting too long before getting the treatment and the advantages to having the tooth treated early. When the patient arrives at the front desk, she informs you that she did not bring her schedule and will have to call you. Your role is to make appointment scheduling for the patient hassle free. In this situation, you can do the following:

- Offer the patient an appointment that is at the same time on the same week day in the future; oftentimes, patients will schedule appointments on specific days where free time is more likely, such as the patient who schedules appointments every second Friday because that is a regular day off for him.
- Inform the patient that you will call her later on in that day or early the next day. Some people lead very busy lives, and it is often more convenient for the patient to be contacted about scheduling the appointment rather than expecting the patient to contact the office.
- Offer to e-mail the patient. Electronic forms of communication such as cellphones and e-mail are common in the workplace. Many people prefer the freedom of answering e-mail letters at a time that is convenient for them, for example, when they are at home in the evening.

checkPOINT

3. What are two advantages of prescheduling the patient appointment?

In fulfilling your responsibility of ensuring that the daily schedule is filled appropriately, your skill of encouraging patients to and assisting them in scheduling their appointments will become proficient. As your relationship develops with the patient, the trust the patient has for you will facilitate the appointment scheduling process as he or she will come to expect your ability to anticipate what appointment day and time is most favorable to him or her. Chapter 10 focuses on appointment scheduling and provides tips on how to create a productive schedule.

Written Correspondence and Telephone Recare Systems

Written correspondence recare systems involve sending letters to patients to remind them of future needed treatment. These letters can also be used to introduce an exciting new method for treatment. Letting patients know what treatment is available to them can encourage them to make an appointment and often serves as a personalized reminder.

Such correspondence is a gentle and effective way of maintaining contact with patients, particularly if it has been some time since they have been in to the dental office. Sending a letter to the patient who has not been in the dental practice for quite some time is often referred to as a **reactivation letter**. Figure 9-1 provides a sample of a letter aimed at reactivating the patient to the dental office. A telephone call is always made approximately 2 weeks to 1 month after the letter is sent out as a way to follow-up on receipt of the letter and attempt to schedule an appointment for the patient.

Recare cards are also used to correspond with patients and are mailed out monthly. Each patient in the practice has a particular time frame in which the dentist or hygienist recommends he or she return to the practice, or that the patient requests he or she be notified. Most patients are asked to return for an examination and cleaning every 6 or 12 months. This means that on the 6 or 12 month time period from when the patient was last in the dental office, he or she will get a notification to return to the office for his or her examination and cleaning.

Augustine Dental Clinic
2596 Calvin Street
Luther, MA
30210

January 19, 2010

Dear Mr. Knox:

According to our records, it has been 18 months since your last visit to our clinic.

Our goal is to help as many people as possible to achieve oral optimum health. We are committed to this goal and want you to know that we are concerned about your oral health.

At this time, we recommend that you visit our office for a periodic checkup. This includes a review of your oral health, oral cancer screening, and dental hygiene education session.

Please call 363-0001 to schedule your visit.

Sincerely,

Jane Keller
Office Administrator

FIGURE 9-1 **Patient reactivation letter.**

A telephone recare system is a system used where each patient is called 1 month prior to his or her appointment. The office administrator is usually responsible for completing this task. It is an effective system for many reasons:

- It provides a personal touch for the patient by using a direct contact method.
- It allows enough time in advance of the appointment to reschedule if the patient requires.
- It provides enough notice for the patient to make the necessary arrangements to attend the appointment.
- It provides an opportunity for the office administrator to confirm patient information such as demographics, insurance coverage, and patient concerns, before coming into the dental office.

When using a telephone recare system, it is more productive if you use an area where you will not have any interruptions, such as a private office, and dedicate a set amount of time each time to make the phone calls. Planning to telephone patients at a time when they are more likely to be accessible, such as after supper, or in the morning will result in a more productive session. Limit the number of staff members who call the patients to 1 or 2. Patients will often call back and leave a message to speak with the staff member who called them, not realizing that any person who answers the phone is able to assist them. Always let patients know that they can speak to anyone when they call to confirm or reschedule their appointment.

checkPOINT

4. What is the purpose of a reactivation letter?

Once the telephone call has been made to the patient and the appointment is rescheduled or confirmed, a recare card indicating the appointment date and time is then mailed to the patient.

Patient Reminders

Reminding patients of scheduled appointments is a large responsibility of the dental office administrator. Different types of patient reminders used in the dental office and methods of effective scheduling are discussed next. The patient reminder cards are very important marketing materials used in the dental office.

Telephone Reminders

Each patient who has an appointment in the dental office must receive a phone call one business day prior to the appointment. Make the reminder phone call simple and direct. Use terminology that the patient understands. The following are examples of effective telephone reminders:

- Use the following if you speak directly to the patient:
  "Good morning Mrs. Brown. This is Sandy from Saddlelake Dental Clinic calling. How are you this morning? (Wait for response.) I am calling to confirm your appointment with Dr. Jones at 9:00 AM tomorrow morning. (Patient will confirm attendance.) We're looking forward to seeing you then. Have a good day."
- Use the following if you get voice mail or an answering machine:
  "Good morning Mrs. Brown. This is Sandy from Saddlelake Dental Clinic calling to conform your appointment with Dr. Jones at 9:00 AM on Tuesday morning. Could you please call our office to confirm this appointment at (999) 555-1234? Thank you and have a good day."

Notice that the word *confirm* is used in these reminder phone calls instead of *remind*. Avoid using the word *remind* when confirming an appointment with a patient, as it can come across as condescending. "Confirming" the appointment sounds much more professional.

When a patient informs you that they are unable to make their appointment time, the appointment should be rescheduled immediately. Chapter 10 focuses on rescheduling appointments and effective terminology to use in this task. Having a short-call list, which is a list of patients who wish to come in and see the dentist on short notice,

Administrative TIP

The best time to make reminder phone calls is between 9:30 AM and noon the day prior to the appointments. If a patient is unable to make the appointment and needs to reschedule, having this information earlier in the day will make it easier to fill the opening in the schedule. If you wait until later in the day to make the reminder phone calls and a patient reschedules an appointment, you will have less time to fill the opening and the chances of being left with an opening in the schedule are greater.

will be helpful in situations in which patients reschedule the day before their appointment, as these newly vacant time slots can then be filled. When all of the patients on the schedule have been called, a notation as to the status of the call—such as "confirmed," "no answer," or "left message"—should be made on the schedule.

Mailed Reminder Cards

Although calling patients is often seen as the most effective way to remind them of appointments, some dental offices may choose to mail a reminder post card in place of, or in addition to, a phone call. Reminder cards are usually mailed out approximately 1 to 2 weeks prior to the appointment day to patients who have scheduled their appointments weeks or months in advance. The reminder card includes the date and time of the upcoming appointment and may be used for annual dental examinations, oral cancer screenings with the dentist, or scheduled dental cleanings with the hygienist. Figure 9-2 provides some examples of such a card.

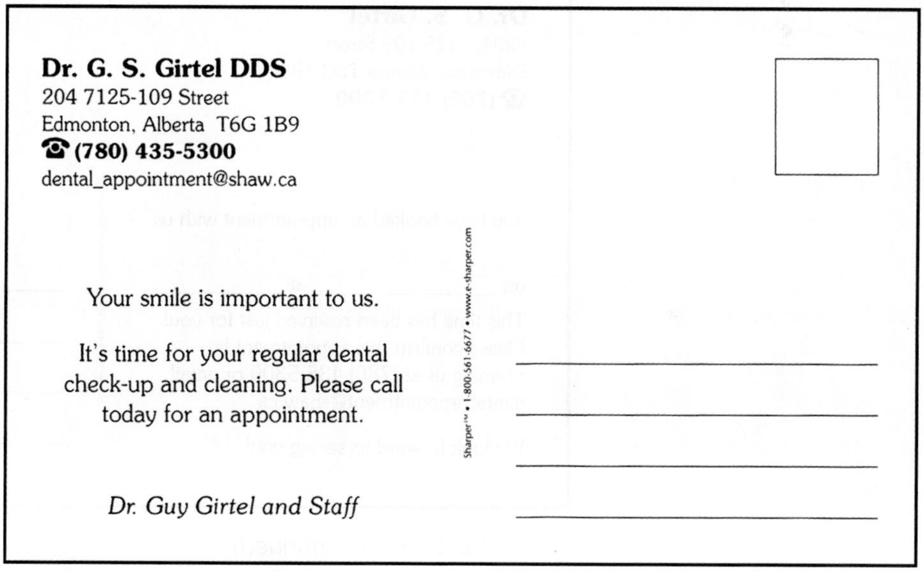

Dr. G. S. Girtel DDS
204 7125-109 Street
Edmonton, Alberta T6G 1B9
(780) 435-5300
dental_appointment@shaw.ca
Your smile is important to us.
It's time for your regular dental check-up and cleaning. Please call today for an appointment.
Dr. Guy Girtel and Staff
Sharper™ • 1 800-561-6677 • www.e-sharper.com

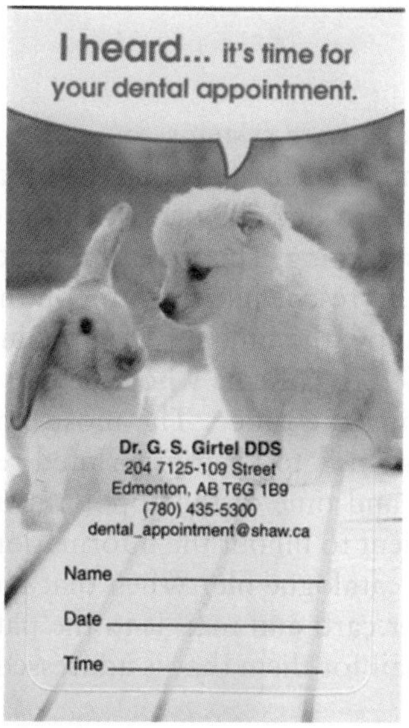

FIGURE 9-2 **Reminder postcards and appointment cards.**

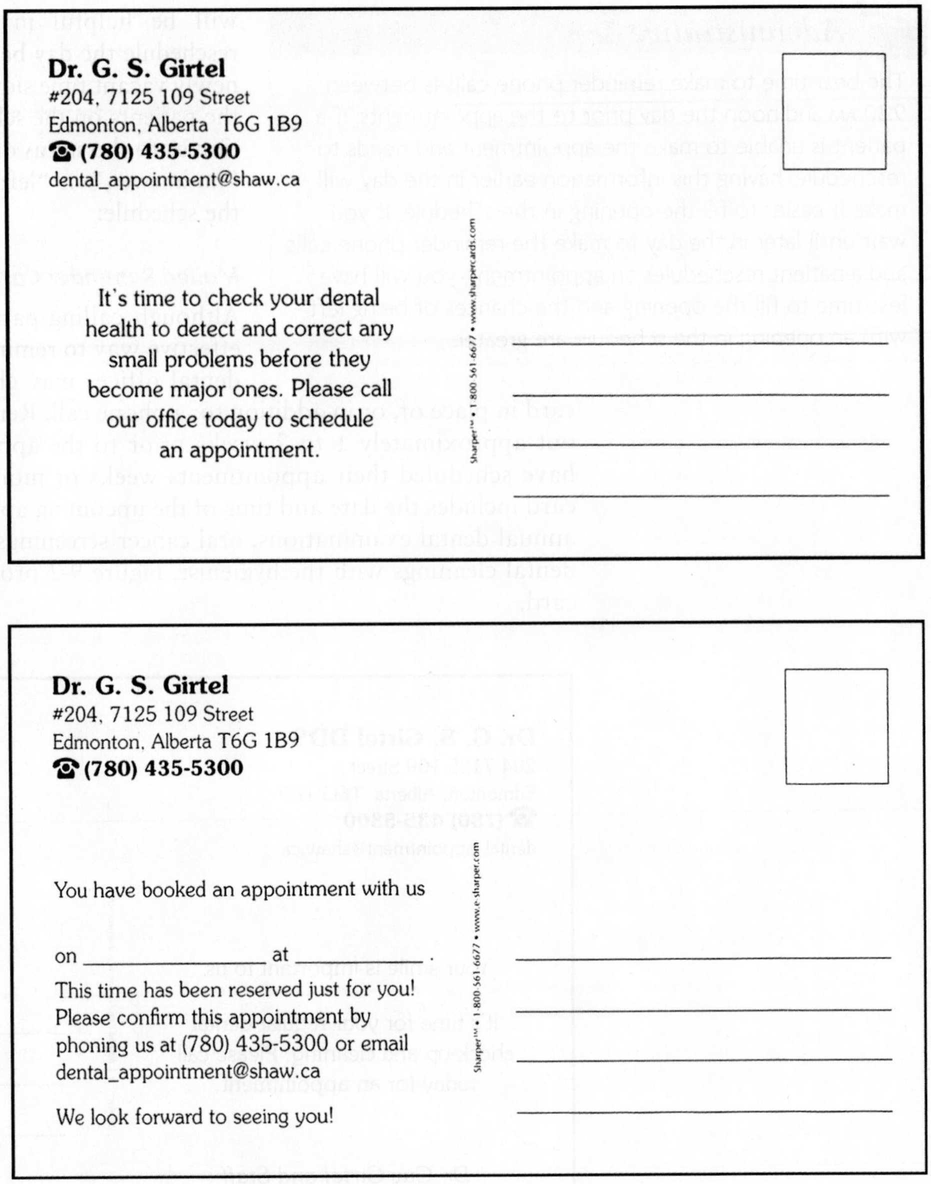
Dr. G. S. Girtel
#204, 7125 109 Street
Edmonton, Alberta T6G 1B9
(780) 435-5300
dental_appointment@shaw.ca
It's time to check your dental health to detect and correct any small problems before they become major ones. Please call our office today to schedule an appointment.
Sharper™ • 1 800 561 6677 • www.sharpercards.com
Dr. G. S. Girtel
#204, 7125 109 Street
Edmonton, Alberta T6G 1B9
(780) 435-5300
You have booked an appointment with us
on ______________ at ___________ .
This time has been reserved just for you!
Please confirm this appointment by phoning us at (780) 435-5300 or email dental_appointment@shaw.ca
We look forward to seeing you!
Sharper™ • 1 800 561 6677 • www.e-sharper.com

FIGURE 9-2 *(Continued)*

Computerized dental recare systems can create a personalized letter to the patient reconfirming the importance of visiting the office so the hygienist can check for any special areas of concern and the dentist can proceed with the periodic examination and oral cancer screening. This type of reminder provides patients with a reasonable amount of time to reschedule their appointment if required, or enough time to arrange in order to allow the time for the appointment.

Such cards are mailed to patients who schedule their next appointment months in advance before leaving the office. The most effective way to maintain an appointment reminder system is to keep preprinted reminder cards on hand with an area to record the date and time of the appointment and the name and address of the patient. Ask the patient to fill out the information on the card and then place the card in a monthly card catalogue file. When that month comes around, simply put a stamp on the reminder card and mail it to the patient. Patients are always pleasantly surprised to see mail for them that is addressed in their own handwriting! Fol-

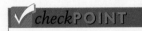

> **✓ checkPOINT**
>
> 5. What are two examples of patient reminders?

> ### *Administrative* TIP
>
> If a patient is scheduling a series of appointments, try to book them on the same day and time each week. If the appointment card does not allow for a list of appointments to be written on the card, give the patient a card that covers the first 2 weeks of appointments. When the patient returns for the last appointment written on the card, provide him or her with a new card for the upcoming appointment dates. Providing the patient with one card for each appointment may leave the patient feeling overwhelmed. The chance of an appointment card being lost or misplaced would also be greater.

low up with a phone call to confirm the appointment at least 2 days prior to the appointment. Confirmation of an appointment is important in maintaining a productive daily schedule. Providing patients with enough time to reschedule allows time for you to fill the vacant appointment time.

Appointment Reminder Cards

Patients who schedule an appointment for some time in the upcoming weeks are often given an appointment reminder card before leaving the dental office. An appointment card always includes the name of the patient, the date and time of the appointment, and the name and address of the dentist. Appointment cards with a removable sticker with the date and time are very popular, as patients can easily place the sticker on their calendar as a reminder (bottom of Fig. 9-2A).

MARKETING

To be successful in today's economy, businesses, including dental offices, must compete for market share. One way that dental offices compete for market share is by incorporating marketing strategies into business practices. All businesses have a marketing program that is made up of many strategies that complement each other. In the dental office, there are strategies put into place that the office administrator is responsible for integrating into everyday tasks. The reminder calls and cards we discussed earlier are one way of advertising the dental office and maintaining the patient flow in the practice.

All team members are responsible for contributing to the marketing of the dental practice. Each staff member should promote the practice by educating patients about the importance of maintaining good oral health and telling their friends and family about the dental clinic they work in. If the staff members in the dental office cannot speak positively about the practice and the philosophy it stands for, the chances are good that many patients will feel the same way and will seek out another dental office. In the dental office, there are two main types of marketing: marketing aimed at retaining patients and marketing aimed at attracting new patients.

Patient Retention Marketing

Patient retention marketing refers to the marketing that is done within the dental practice to retain patients. It starts with the first impression that the dental office administrator gives to patients when they call the office to make an appointment or come into the office. The perception that the patients have of the dental office is partially created through the internal marketing. The biggest influence on successful internal marketing comes from the dental team members. For example, the dental office administrator sets the tone for the patient by being cheerful and professional at all times. The dental assistant shows empathy and competence by ensuring that the patient is comfortable. The dentist provides quality dental treatment for the patient, and the dental hygienist educates the patient on the importance of good oral health. This brief example shows how each staff member contributes to the positive dental experience for the patient with a view to having the patient return to the clinic in the future.

The following suggestions are used in dental offices and aimed at patient retention. These suggestions can also double as tactics used to obtain new patients.

Clean and tidy dental office. Keeping the front office area clean and presentable includes dusting, tidying books, straightening chairs in the reception area, and maintaining a neat and organized looking front desk. Incorporating standard precautions into the clinical areas and making patients aware of this fact is also a way to impress upon, and let patients know that the utmost care and attention to detail are valued in the dental office.

Cheerful voice and friendly face at the front desk. Keeping an upbeat attitude encourages patients to come into the office. A friendly and sincere attitude is contagious and the office administrator who reflects this attitude often has a positive influence on the rest of the staff and the tone of the appointment. Patients will enjoy attending the office and an upbeat attitude can often decrease the effects of anxiety on a patient.

Staff enthusiasm. Staff members who are enthusiastic about where they work, the job they do, and the people they work with can create an atmosphere that is enjoyable for patients. An enthusiastic attitude promotes the dental office and reinforces to patients that they have made the right choice by being patients at the practice.

Staff identification tags. Once you have introduced yourself to the patients the first time you meet, you have the advantage of seeing their names on the schedule and reading the chart in preparation for their next appointment. This helps staff to remember patients and makes it easier to learn the patient names. However, patients may not always remember all of the staff members' names, which is the reason why each staff member should wear a name tag for identification. This allows patients to learn your name as they get to know you a little more at each visit. By getting to know staff members by their names, patients can much more easily develop loyalty to the practice.

Professional appearance. Dressing appropriately for your position and remaining aware of maintaining a professional appearance communicate to patients that you care about the image of the practice and are concerned that patients think positively about the office and the staff members.

Practice newsletter. A newsletter that is printed up and mailed out to all current patients of the dental office is an effective tool for keeping patients informed about the dental clinic. A newsletter usually includes information on topics such as new products, staff announcements, office closures, and educational information. Additional methods of patient retention marketing are listed in Box 9-3.

BOX 9-3
Marketing the Dental Practice

Patient Retention	Attracting New Patients
• Correspondence such as cards and letters to patients	• Office sign
• Relaxed environment	• Newspaper advertising
• Patient referrals from existing patients	• Yellow pages advertising
• Giveaways such as magnets and pens	• Tours of the office
	• Presentations at schools on oral hygiene
	• New patient incentives provided via a neighborhood welcome committee

Ultimately, patients are more inclined to return to a dental office where the staff enjoys each other and the patients and where they do not feel as if they are just another number. Being polite and respectful at all times and addressing the patient by name are helpful in achieving the goal of patient retention. When patients trust the healthcare professionals they use, they often encourage friends and family to become patients of the dental clinic. The greatest compliment any patient can pay to a dental team is to refer his or her friends and family!

Marketing to Attract New Patients

Any type of marketing done outside of the dental office has a goal of attracting new patients to the clinic. A sign displayed outside the building indicating where the dental office is located, a practice name and phone number listed in the phone book, and an advertisement in a newspaper are all examples of **new patient marketing.**

The following are some strategies that can be used to attract new patients to the dental office.

Staff business cards. All staff members should have a business card that tells who they are and the position they hold in the dental practice. When you are in a business situation such as a dental conference, you can very easily give out your business card so that your contact information is available to the individual who requires it. Patients also appreciate receiving a business card. As a dental office assistant, you will have many opportunities to provide a business card to patients, family, and friends as you assist in the recruitment and retention of patients to the dental practice.

New patient incentives. New patient incentives are used to attract new patients to the office and are often offered in the form of a service. For example, new patient incentives may include complimentary bite-wing x-rays with a new patient examination or a complimentary whitening product with a new patient examination. Other new patient incentives also include providing the person who refers a new patient with a gift certificate as a way to say thank you.

Web site accessibility. A very effective marketing strategy used by dental offices is the use of a Web site. Every day patients are searching the Internet for a dentist in their area. With the increase of computers in households and the number of people who have access to the Internet, part of the dental office marketing strategy should include attracting online consumers. The first impression of a dental office, for some patients, is made by a great-looking Web site. Additional ideas for new patient marketing for the dental office are provided in Box 9-3.

*check*POINT

6. Explain the difference between marketing the dental clinic to new patients and marketing the clinic to retain patients.

Remember, however, that all the new patient marketing that is done can be undone very quickly if there is no recognition of the barriers that can occur when new patients call the practice to make an appointment. Chapter 10 looks at some of those barriers and how to avoid them.

Chapter Summary

The dental office relies on the office administrator to represent the practice in a professional and positive manner. As the relationship between the patient and dental team builds, the tasks and duties of the office administrator can help maintain and grow the relationship. Effectively using reminder and recare systems develops patient loyalty. Patient reminders and other types of marketing, both internal and external, can create a positive image of the dental practice for the patient.

Review Questions

Multiple Choice

1. **The critical component in a recall system is**
   a. that it is computer- or written correspondence-based.
   b. that patients receive notification and the office administrator documents it.
   c. that patients feel recalled to the practice.
   d. that patients are in the schedule and accessible.

2. **Sending information to a patient who has not been to the dental office for some time is called a**
   a. recare card.
   b. reactivation letter.
   c. newsletter.
   d. hygiene update.

3. **Effectively using reminder and recard systems**
   a. develops patient loyalty.
   b. guarantees to increase revenue.
   c. creates more work.
   d. involves all staff members.

4. **An effective marketing strategy used in the dental office is**
   a. the use of a road sign.
   b. the use of a Web site.
   c. a mascot.
   d. monthly telephone calls.

5. **One of the many concerns of a dental practice today is**
   a. staff retention.
   b. having an effective recare system.
   c. production revenue.
   d. patient relationship development.

6. **Scheduling a patient's next appointment before leaving the completed appointment is termed**
   a. recare scheduling.
   b. prescheduling.
   c. auto booking.
   d. recalling.

7. **Acknowledging a patient when he or she enters the dental office is important because**
   a. it lets the patient know that you are busy and will get to them when you can
   b. sends a non-verbal message that the patient is important to the practice
   c. is a way of letting the patient know you are aware of their presence
   d. makes everyone feel better because you are nice to them

8. **It is important to keep patient demographic information up to date in order to**
   a. maintain accurate contact and financial information about the patient
   b. keep an up to date mailing address for time sensitive statements
   c. carry out the office administrator responsibilities
   d. all of the above

9. **Dressing professionally is an example of**
   a. focusing on the patient first
   b. making a good first impression
   c. keeping information up to date
   d. following up with the patient

10. **An example of fostering goodwill with patients is**
    a. disclose all relevant treatment and costs associated
    b. not staying in touch with patients through recall cards
    c. keeping the front desk neat and clean
    d. not acknowledging patients while you are on the phone

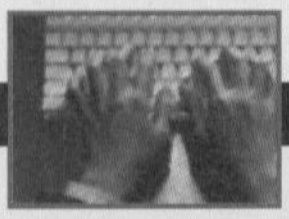

Hands-On Activity

1. Create a script with a classmate regarding a patient who must preschedule an appointment to see the hygienist in 3 months. How are you going to encourage the patient to schedule the appointment without sounding pushy?

2. Create a Web site home page for the dental office you work in. What will you include on the home page and how will you make it appealing to new patients?

chapter TEN

Appointment *Management*

OBJECTIVES

After completing this chapter, you should be able to do the following:

- Spell and define key terms
- Discuss the role of the dental office administrator in appointment scheduling
- Identify the differences between manual and computerized appointment scheduling
- Explain how Health Insurance Portability and Accountability Act (HIPAA) pertains to the daily schedule
- List common abbreviations used on the daily schedule and explain why they are used
- Explain the purpose of buffers and when it may be necessary for double booking
- Describe scheduling considerations for meeting patient needs and staff preferences
- Demonstrate how to schedule an appointment for a new patient, returning patient, emergency patient, and walk-in patient
- Demonstrate how to schedule a referral appointment for a patient

KEY TERMS

- manual appointment scheduling system
- computerized appointment management system
- units of time
- buffer times
- double booking
- dovetailing
- emergency patients
- walk-in patients

A priority of the dental office administrator is to ensure that the daily schedule is filled and that patients are scheduled efficiently. Managing the daily flow of patients in the dental office is the most important duty of the dental office administrator. The effective management of the schedule affects every staff member in the dental office and can make the difference between a day that runs smoothly and one that is full of frustration. The dental office administrator is responsible for the schedule and the effect that it has on the other team members. Keeping this in mind as you schedule patients will help you to understand why this is such an important duty in the dental office.

OUTLINE

In previous chapters, we discussed the importance of having a professional and positive attitude at all times while in the dental office. As you schedule patients and prioritize the appointments in a way that is manageable for all team members, your attitude must remain positive. With time and practice, this will become second nature. As you embark on your career, you will need to focus on developing these skills.

To assist you in acquiring these skills, this chapter presents both manual and computerized appointment management systems. Also presented are guidelines on maintaining the schedule, scheduling considerations, and scheduling appointments for various types of patients, along with how to provide patients with referrals to dental specialists and other providers.

APPOINTMENT SCHEDULE

Each dental office has a scheduling system that is preferred by the dentist. Both manual and computerized scheduling systems are used in dental offices, with varying designs. Whether a manual or a computerized system is used in the practice, the basic guidelines for scheduling are the same. The type of scheduling system used depends on the number of dentists in the practice, the office hours available for scheduling, the number of hygienists, and the number of patients in the clinic.

Manual Appointment Scheduling

Still used by many dental offices, the **manual appointment scheduling system** consists of an appointment book that displays either 1 day or 1 week of appointments per two-page spread, typically for a full year. Appointment books come in many shapes, sizes, and colors and have varying numbers of appointment columns for each day, to fit the needs of different sizes of dental offices. For example, a dental office with only one dentist and one hygienist may use a manual appointment book that has two or three columns. A dental practice that has two or three dentists may use an appointment book that has four or more columns. Some dental offices use appointment schedules that have as many columns as they do operatories, whereas others correlate columns to practitioners.

Located at the top of the column is the name of the practitioner or operatory. Located vertically down the left-hand side of the page are the times available for booking appointments. The first appointment time available is at the top, and the last appointment time available is at the bottom. The appointment times are usually divided into intervals of 10, 15, or 20 minutes. Each appointment booked must include the following information:

- Name of patient (first and last)
- Phone number
- Reason for visit

Some areas of the schedule are blocked off, or unavailable, for scheduling patient appointments. These times are set aside for the dentist for many reasons: lunch, a break, a meeting, or phone calls. On a manual schedule, this time is blocked off by crossing out the space with an X or drawing lines through the time block. Each dental office has a specific way of blocking out time. Be sure to write the reason for the time being blocked out. For example, if the time is being blocked out for a staff meeting, write "staff meeting" at the beginning of the time block. In the manual appointment system, the time blocked out for various reasons must be written into each day in the book.

Some dental offices like to reserve one time block each day for emergency patients, either at the beginning of the day or in the middle of the day. Some dentists also prefer to have their personal obligations placed on the daily schedule as a reminder to themselves of the obligation and to remind staff not to schedule any patient immediately before, during, or immediately after the obligation.

Before you book patients into the schedule, make sure that you are scheduling the patient in for the correct amount of time. Section "Units of Time" discusses how to determine the amount of time needed for different types of treatment. The daily appointment schedule is copied and posted in certain areas in the dental office every day.

> **checkPOINT**
>
> 1. Describe manual appointment scheduling.

Computerized Practice Management Programs and Appointment Scheduling

> **legal TIP**
>
> The schedule should be posted in areas that are not accessible by patients or where patients cannot read the schedule, as per the HIPAA guidelines. The daily schedule is a record of all patients who attended the dental office on a particular day. For this reason, the schedule is a legal document, and changes such as cancellations and emergencies should be written into the schedule as they happen and should not be deleted permanently. At the end of the day, the schedules should be removed and shredded, not thrown in the garbage since they contain personal information about patients.

Using the computer to manage scheduling, as well as other such tasks as maintaining patient and financial files, is common in the dental office. In a dental practice that maintains a busy flow of patients on a daily basis, the use of computers to manage the patient flow can cut down on the amount of time needed to schedule patient appointments, process transactions in patient accounts, and manage patients' dental health information. Many types of software packages are available specifically for the dental environment, and new ones are being developed continually.

Generally, the dentists and the office manager together select a software package based on its features. Many dentists and employees require a software package that can manage the many different preferences of the practitioners and the schedules they keep. The number of employees that can access the software at once is an important factor in the selection process, since a busy dental environment requires that many clinicians and administrative employees can access different patients' information all at once.

Commonly, computer software programs must be upgraded on a periodic basis. Typically, the manufacturer of the software program sends a disc of information that needs to be installed on the computer to upgrade components of the software program. One person is usually responsible for maintaining upgrades to the software program. Unless it is specified that it is your responsibility to install the upgrades, the office manager or dentist will likely maintain this area.

Dental practice management programs are generally made up of two components: administrative components and clinical components. As a dental office administrator, you need to be familiar with both the components, to understand how one area affects the other. The administrative components of the software assist in maintaining the patient flow in the practice and is made of the demographic and financial information, whereas the clinical components assist in the diagnosis, treatment, and education of patients and includes the clinical chart and radiographs, as well as educational material used for treatment planning. Figure 10-1A and B provides examples of both the administrative and clinical components of the patient's chart. Regardless of the differences among dental practice management programs, there are common elements between all of them that are covered in this chapter and others. Specifically, the appointment management component of the dental practice management program is presented later. The program components for financial transactions, inventory, in-office communication, referrals, and patient records are presented in other chapters, where appropriate. Box 10-1 is a list of some of the many dental practice management programs available in Canada and the United States.

Electronic scheduling is the most common feature in a computerized dental practice. Setting up and tracking appointments is performed most efficiently with a **computerized appointment management system.** Figure 10-2 shows an example of a daily appointment schedule in a computerized scheduling system. Many different types of computerized appointment systems are available, but all have the same goal, which is to manage the patient flow of the dental office. However, just as with the manual system, the system used is only as effective as the individual operating the system.

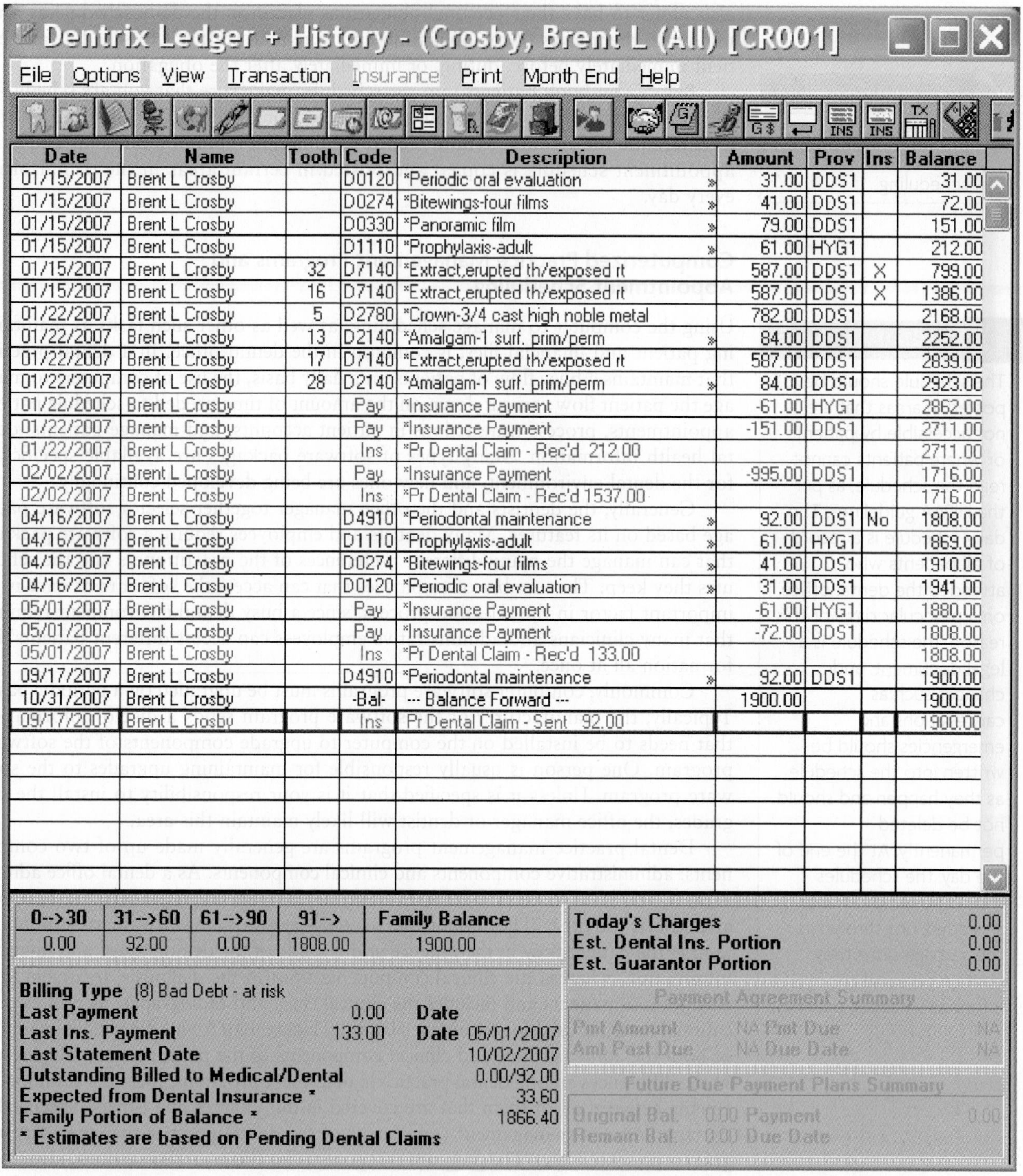

Date	Name	Tooth	Code	Description	Amount	Prov	Ins	Balance
01/15/2007	Brent L Crosby		D0120	*Periodic oral evaluation »	31.00	DDS1		31.00
01/15/2007	Brent L Crosby		D0274	*Bitewings-four films »	41.00	DDS1		72.00
01/15/2007	Brent L Crosby		D0330	*Panoramic film »	79.00	DDS1		151.00
01/15/2007	Brent L Crosby		D1110	*Prophylaxis-adult »	61.00	HYG1		212.00
01/15/2007	Brent L Crosby	32	D7140	*Extract,erupted th/exposed rt	587.00	DDS1	X	799.00
01/15/2007	Brent L Crosby	16	D7140	*Extract,erupted th/exposed rt	587.00	DDS1	X	1386.00
01/22/2007	Brent L Crosby	5	D2780	*Crown-3/4 cast high noble metal	782.00	DDS1		2168.00
01/22/2007	Brent L Crosby	13	D2140	*Amalgam-1 surf. prim/perm »	84.00	DDS1		2252.00
01/22/2007	Brent L Crosby	17	D7140	*Extract,erupted th/exposed rt	587.00	DDS1		2839.00
01/22/2007	Brent L Crosby	28	D2140	*Amalgam-1 surf. prim/perm »	84.00	DDS1		2923.00
01/22/2007	Brent L Crosby		Pay	*Insurance Payment	-61.00	HYG1		2862.00
01/22/2007	Brent L Crosby		Pay	*Insurance Payment	-151.00	DDS1		2711.00
01/22/2007	Brent L Crosby		Ins	*Pr Dental Claim - Rec'd 212.00				2711.00
02/02/2007	Brent L Crosby		Pay	*Insurance Payment	-995.00	DDS1		1716.00
02/02/2007	Brent L Crosby		Ins	*Pr Dental Claim - Rec'd 1537.00				1716.00
04/16/2007	Brent L Crosby		D4910	*Periodontal maintenance »	92.00	DDS1	No	1808.00
04/16/2007	Brent L Crosby		D1110	*Prophylaxis-adult »	61.00	HYG1		1869.00
04/16/2007	Brent L Crosby		D0274	*Bitewings-four films »	41.00	DDS1		1910.00
04/16/2007	Brent L Crosby		D0120	*Periodic oral evaluation »	31.00	DDS1		1941.00
05/01/2007	Brent L Crosby		Pay	*Insurance Payment	-61.00	HYG1		1880.00
05/01/2007	Brent L Crosby		Pay	*Insurance Payment	-72.00	DDS1		1808.00
05/01/2007	Brent L Crosby		Ins	*Pr Dental Claim - Rec'd 133.00				1808.00
09/17/2007	Brent L Crosby		D4910	*Periodontal maintenance »	92.00	DDS1		1900.00
10/31/2007	Brent L Crosby		-Bal-	--- Balance Forward ---	1900.00			1900.00
09/17/2007	Brent L Crosby		Ins	Pr Dental Claim - Sent 92.00				1900.00

0-->30	31-->60	61-->90	91-->	Family Balance
0.00	92.00	0.00	1808.00	1900.00

Today's Charges		0.00
Est. Dental Ins. Portion		0.00
Est. Guarantor Portion		0.00

Billing Type (8) Bad Debt - at risk
Last Payment 0.00 **Date**
Last Ins. Payment 133.00 **Date** 05/01/2007
Last Statement Date 10/02/2007
Outstanding Billed to Medical/Dental 0.00/92.00
Expected from Dental Insurance * 33.60
Family Portion of Balance * 1866.40
*** Estimates are based on Pending Dental Claims**

Payment Agreement Summary
Pmt Amount NA Pmt Due NA
Amt Past Due NA Due Date NA

Future Due Payment Plans Summary
Original Bal. 0.00 Payment 0.00
Remain Bal. 0.00 Due Date

A

FIGURE 10-1 Computerized patient chart. (A) Administrative component. **(B)** Clinical component. DENTRIX images courtesy of Henry Schein Practice Solutions, American Fork, UT.

Advantages

If used effectively, however, the computerized practice management system offers many advantages over the manual system and can save time and make the office administrator's job much easier. For instance, entering information into the daily schedule such as lunch, employee breaks, and office hours only has to be performed once in the computerized system during the initial setup, whereas the manual system

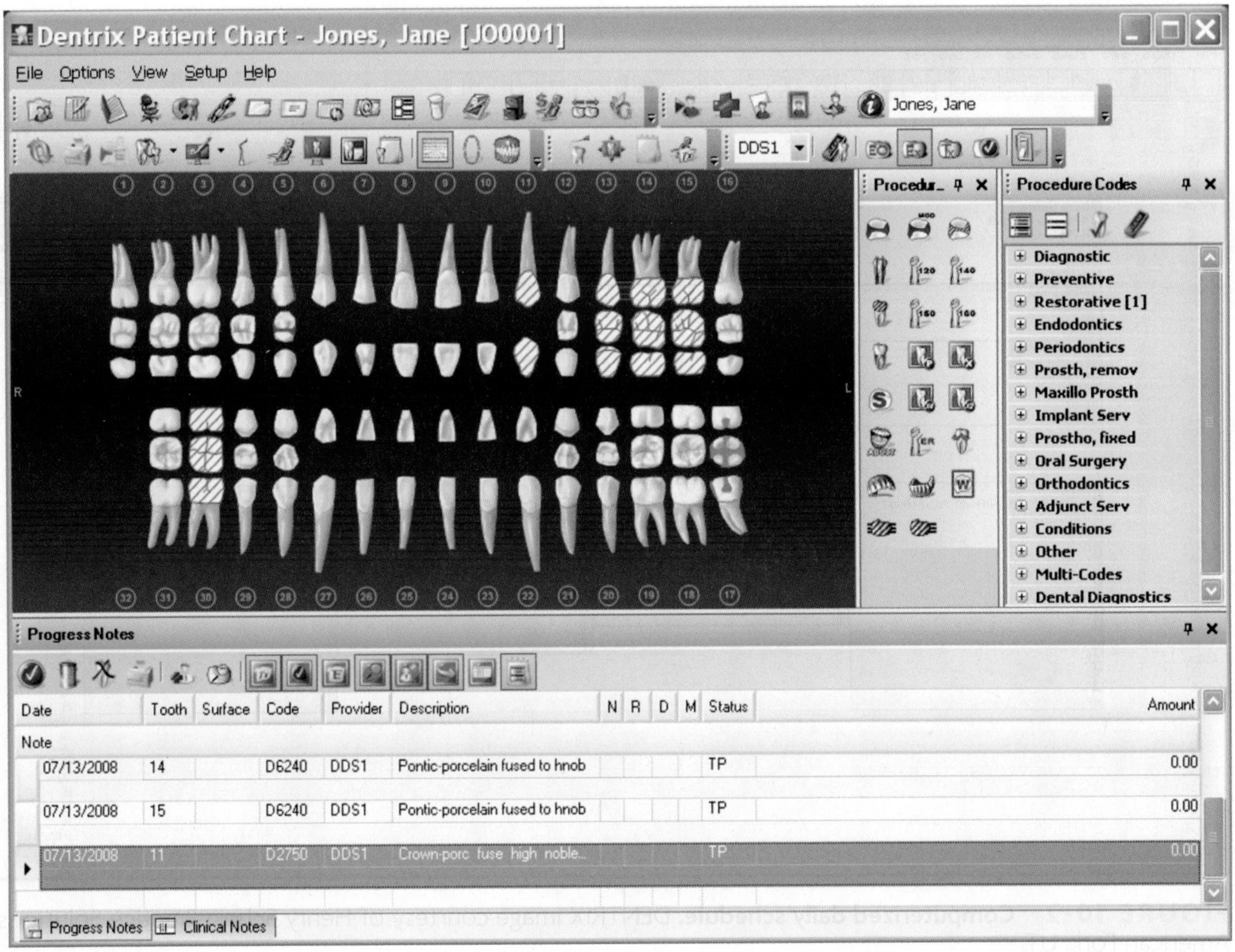

B

FIGURE 10-1 *(Continued)*

requires daily manual entry of this information. The integration of the patient's chart and all its components, appointment schedule and letters, insurance claim filing into one program enables you to perform many functions at once. One component of computerized dental management software that is particularly advantageous is the ability to send insurance claims electronically to insurance carriers and receive a response regarding the amount of payment toward treatment. Sending the claim and receiving the response takes less than 1 minute and is performed in the presence of the patient with the goal of collecting the difference owing from the patient prior to them leaving the office. The response from the insurance carrier can be printed

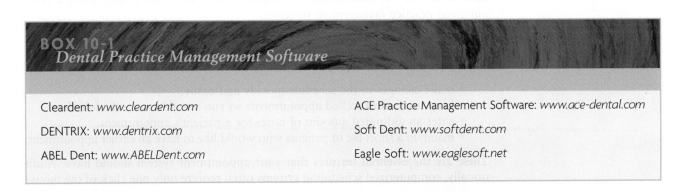

BOX 10-1
Dental Practice Management Software

Cleardent: *www.cleardent.com*

DENTRIX: *www.dentrix.com*

ABEL Dent: *www.ABELDent.com*

ACE Practice Management Software: *www.ace-dental.com*

Soft Dent: *www.softdent.com*

Eagle Soft: *www.eaglesoft.net*

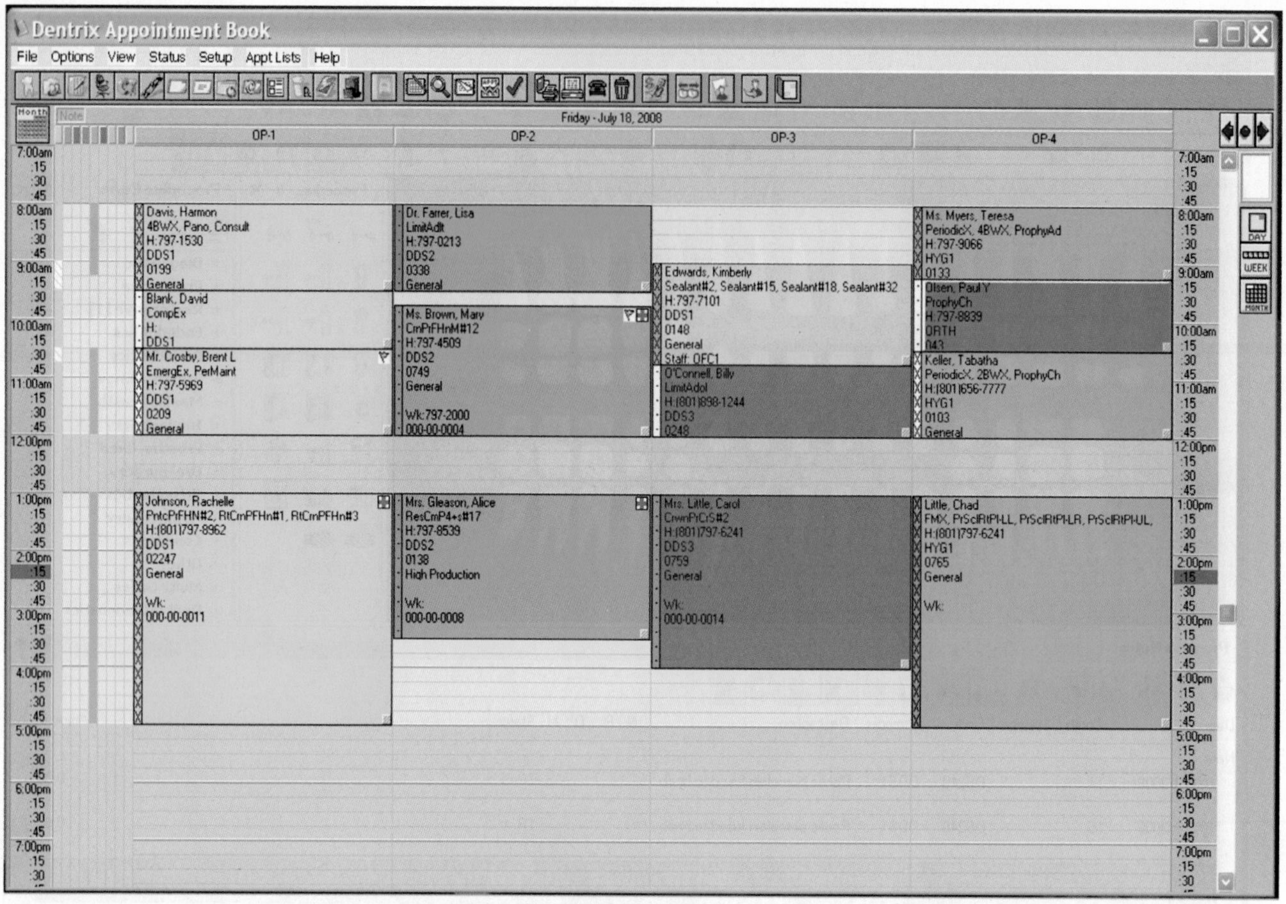

FIGURE 10-2 Computerized daily schedule. DENTRIX image courtesy of Henry Schein Practice Solutions, American Fork, UT.

out and a copy can be given to the patient. This method of electronic claims submission reduces the overall accounts receivable outstanding and provides immediate information from the insurance carrier regarding the patients' coverage. Chapter 15 provides a more in-depth look at electronic insurance claims submission.

The use of a computerized system provides a way for the office administrator to access patient charts quickly to determine which patients are due for recare appointments and which patients have missed appointments and require rescheduling (Figs. 10-3 and 10-4). This system also allows the staff to easily view patients' digital radiographs, moments after they have been taken in the operatory. This is advantageous to you as a way of maintaining an accurate recare system and ensuring that patients are maintaining their recommended recare schedule. Box 10-2 provides an overview of the features and transactions that can be performed using a computerized practice management program.

Features

A good patient scheduling application will allow you to

- make changes to the schedule quickly and easily;
- keep track of cancelled appointments so you are able to reschedule them;
- enter an unlimited amount of notes for a patient's appointment;
- maintain a short list of patients who would like to have an earlier appointment.

These are the essential features that your appointment system should have. Additionally, computerized scheduling systems often require only one click of the mouse

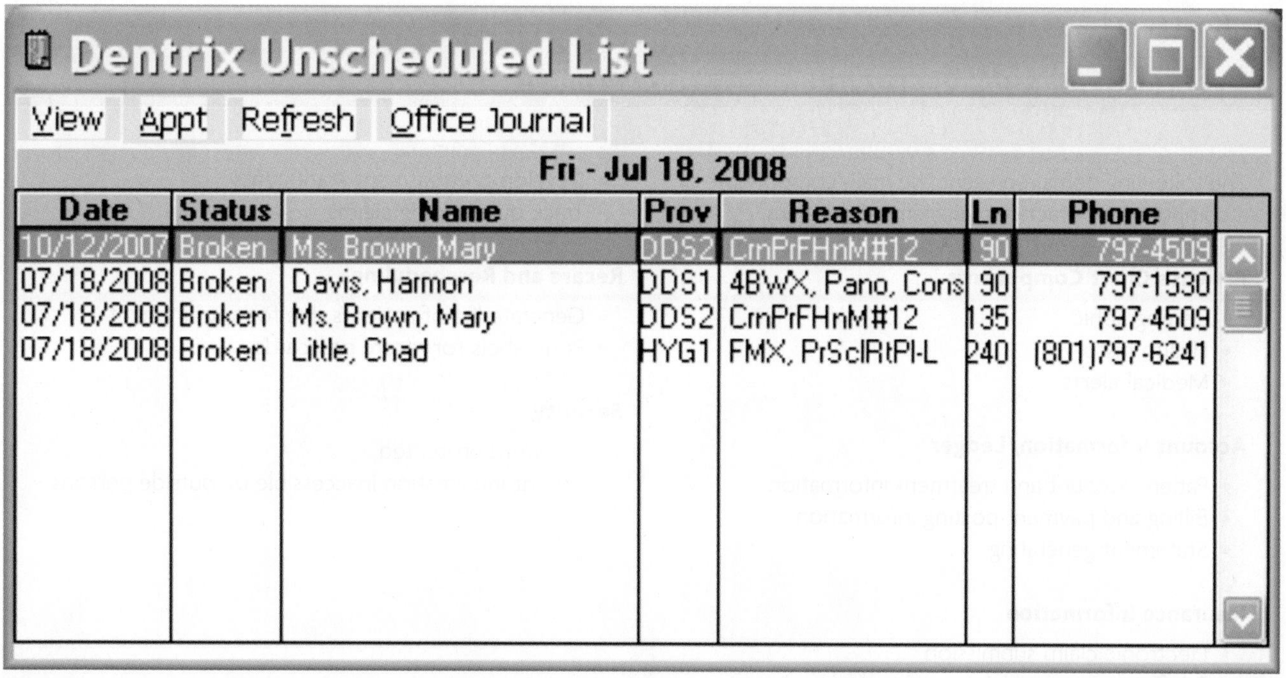

Date	Status	Name	Prov	Reason	Ln	Phone
10/12/2007	Broken	Ms. Brown, Mary	DDS2	CrnPrFHnM#12	90	797-4509
07/18/2008	Broken	Davis, Harmon	DDS1	4BWX, Pano, Cons	90	797-1530
07/18/2008	Broken	Ms. Brown, Mary	DDS2	CrnPrFHnM#12	135	797-4509
07/18/2008	Broken	Little, Chad	HYG1	FMX, PrSclRtPl-L	240	(801)797-6241

FIGURE 10-3 Reschedule patient list. DENTRIX image courtesy of Henry Schein Practice Solutions, American Fork, UT.

to add an appointment, reschedule an appointment, and view the day, the week, or the month of appointments booked. They allow you to access a patient's account and quickly go to the next appointment and vice versa. When a patient calls to schedule an appointment, his or her account can be easily accessed and, if there is a balance owing, the patient can be informed and asked to pay the balance at the time of the appointment.

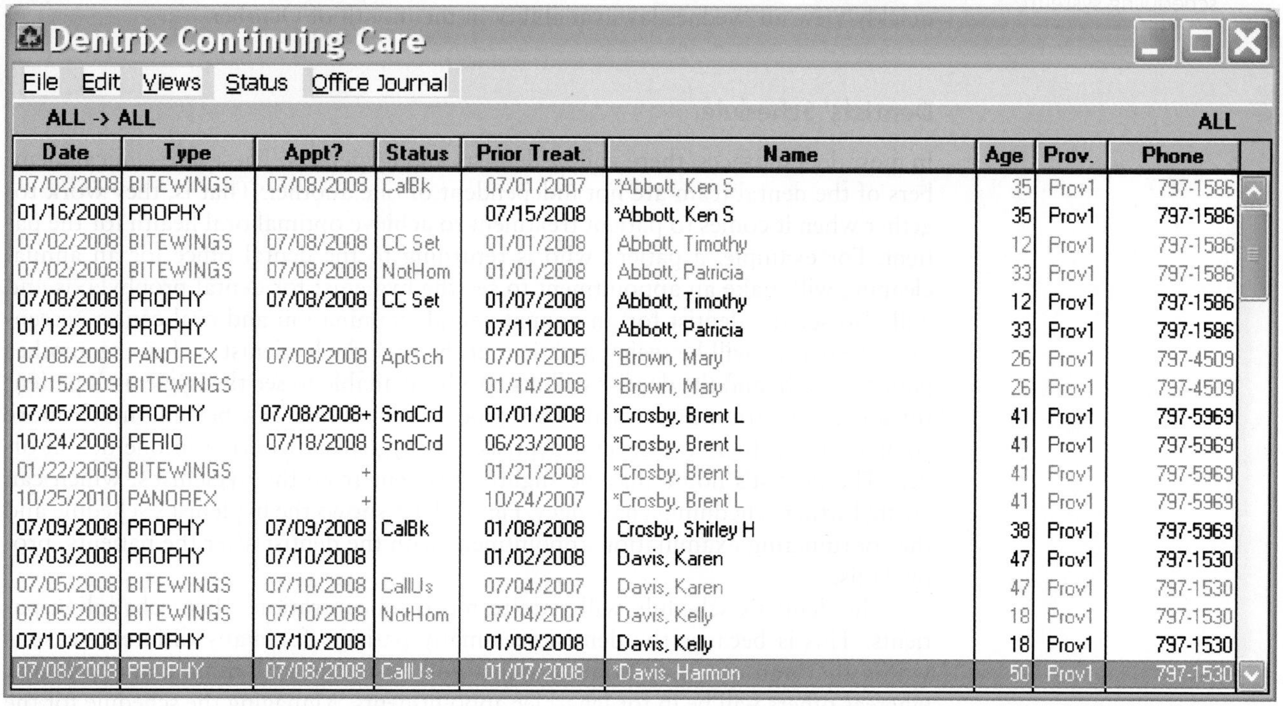

Date	Type	Appt?	Status	Prior Treat.	Name	Age	Prov.	Phone
07/02/2008	BITEWINGS	07/08/2008	CalBk	07/01/2007	*Abbott, Ken S	35	Prov1	797-1586
01/16/2009	PROPHY			07/15/2008	*Abbott, Ken S	35	Prov1	797-1586
07/02/2008	BITEWINGS	07/08/2008	CC Set	01/01/2008	Abbott, Timothy	12	Prov1	797-1586
07/02/2008	BITEWINGS	07/08/2008	NotHom	01/01/2008	Abbott, Patricia	33	Prov1	797-1586
07/08/2008	PROPHY	07/08/2008	CC Set	01/07/2008	Abbott, Timothy	12	Prov1	797-1586
01/12/2009	PROPHY			07/11/2008	Abbott, Patricia	33	Prov1	797-1586
07/08/2008	PANOREX	07/08/2008	AptSch	07/07/2005	*Brown, Mary	26	Prov1	797-4509
01/15/2009	BITEWINGS			01/14/2008	*Brown, Mary	26	Prov1	797-4509
07/05/2008	PROPHY	07/08/2008+	SndCrd	01/01/2008	*Crosby, Brent L	41	Prov1	797-5969
10/24/2008	PERIO	07/18/2008	SndCrd	06/23/2008	*Crosby, Brent L	41	Prov1	797-5969
01/22/2009	BITEWINGS	+		01/21/2008	*Crosby, Brent L	41	Prov1	797-5969
10/25/2010	PANOREX	+		10/24/2007	*Crosby, Brent L	41	Prov1	797-5969
07/09/2008	PROPHY	07/09/2008	CalBk	01/08/2008	Crosby, Shirley H	38	Prov1	797-5969
07/03/2008	PROPHY	07/10/2008		01/02/2008	Davis, Karen	47	Prov1	797-1530
07/05/2008	BITEWINGS	07/10/2008	CallUs	07/04/2007	Davis, Karen	47	Prov1	797-1530
07/05/2008	BITEWINGS	07/10/2008	NotHom	07/04/2007	Davis, Kelly	18	Prov1	797-1530
07/10/2008	PROPHY	07/10/2008		01/09/2008	Davis, Kelly	18	Prov1	797-1530
07/08/2008	PROPHY	07/08/2008	CallUs	01/07/2008	*Davis, Harmon	50	Prov1	797-1530

FIGURE 10-4 Recare appointment list. DENTRIX image courtesy of Henry Schein Practice Solutions, American Fork, UT.

BOX 10-2
Features of a Computerized Practice Management Program

The following items represent the main components of a computerized practice management program

Patient's Chart Components

- Demographic
- Health history
- Medical alerts

Account Information/Ledger

- Patient account and treatment information
- Billing and payment posting information
- Statement generating

Insurance Information

- Electronic claim submission
- Printing insurance claims
- Develop pretreatment statements
- Track outstanding claims

Recare and Rescheduling

- Generate list of patients due for appointment
- Print labels for recare postcards

Security

- Password protected
- Patient information inaccessible by outside persons

checkPOINT

2. What is one advantage of a computerized scheduling system?

Advanced practice management programs provide features such as color-coded appointment types, daily to-do lists, patient arrival alerts, and time slot finders, which allow the user to locate specific day or time availability at a glance. For example, if a patient is returning to see the hygienist in 6 months and asks to schedule an appointment on any Wednesday morning in the month of October, you can quickly view all Wednesday availability in the month of October.

Dentists' Schedule

In most dental offices, there will be dentists and hygienists. These two clinical members of the dental team are not independent of one another. That is, they work together when it comes to patient treatment to achieve optimal oral health for the patient. For example, a patient who is returning to the dental office for an annual cleaning will make an appointment to see the hygienist for dental prophylaxis and will also see the dentist for an annual dental examination and oral cancer screening. The dentist will be seeing a patient at the time the hygienist is cleaning another patient's teeth, and the dentist will need to be available to see the hygienist's patient for an examination afterward. This type of scheduling can become much more complex when there are several dentists and hygienists working in one dental office. The dentist's hours may be slightly different from the hygienist's, which can create further scheduling challenges. Figure 10-5 shows the hygienist's schedule and the coordinating examination appointment with the dentist after the patients' prophylaxis.

The dentist's schedule will require more concentration when scheduling patients. This is because the dentist sees many patients for many different reasons within the span of a day. Some patients will be in for a 30-minute appointment, whereas others will be in for lengthier appointments. Managing the schedule for the dentist is much like a puzzle where you need to find the right size piece, or appointment, to fit in certain openings.

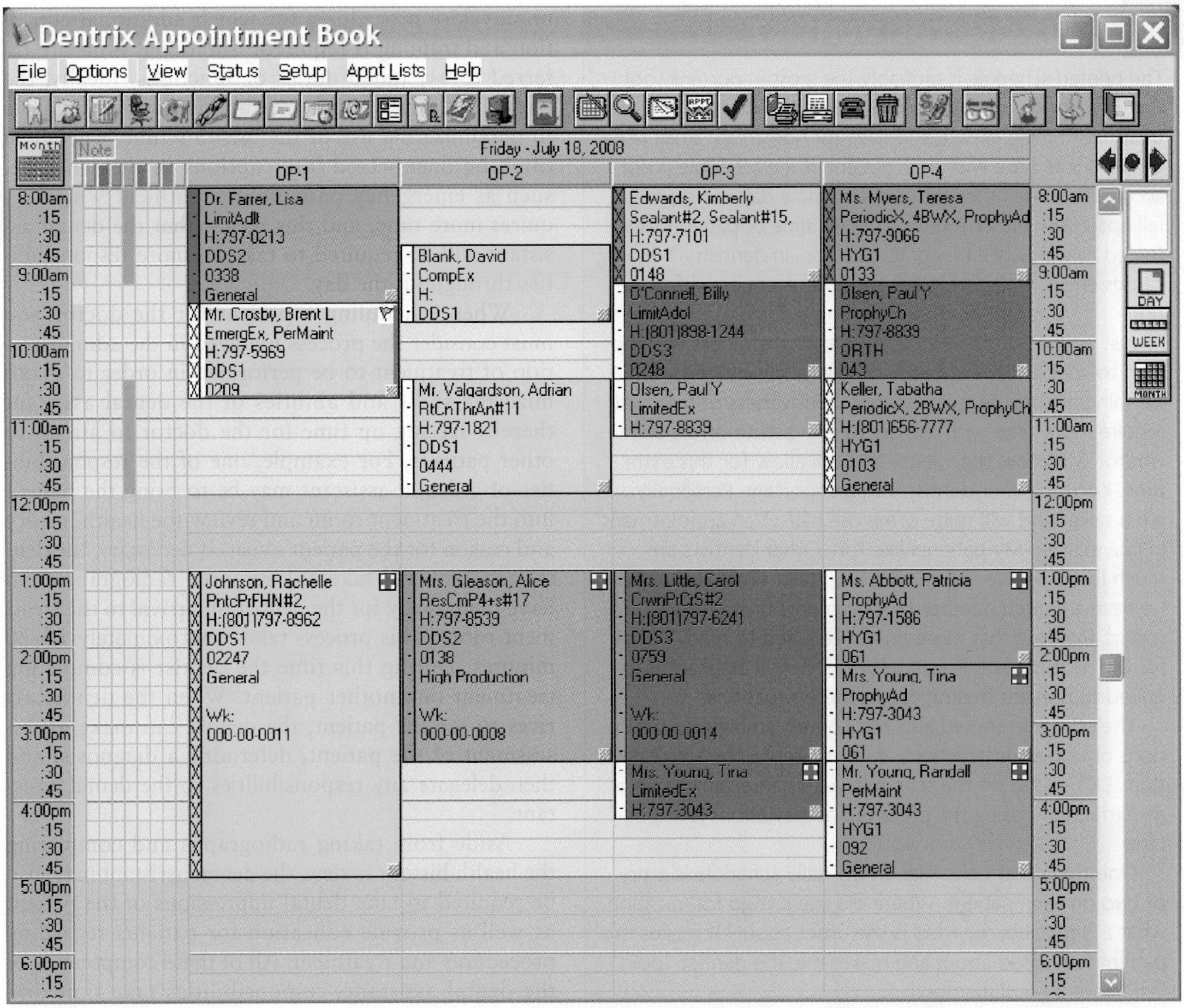

FIGURE 10-5 Hygienists' schedule. DENTRIX image courtesy of Henry Schein Practice Solutions, American Fork, UT.

Hygienists' Schedule

Hygienists, unlike dentists, provide specialized treatment to patients, including dental prophylaxis, treatment follow-up, and periodontal treatment. Every effort must be made for the hygienist's schedule to not conflict with the doctor's schedule. That is, if a patient is seeing the hygienist for a dental prophylaxis and expecting an examination afterward, you must make sure the dentist has time in the schedule to complete the examination. Most appointments with the hygienist will be for a set time period, such as a standard 45 minutes or 1-hour time schedule per patient. If the hygienist is seeing a patient on a treatment plan, the patient may require more than one appointment to be scheduled and a time slot of more than 1 hour to be scheduled. Later in this chapter, we will focus on the nuances of successfully scheduling a dentist and hygienist in the same time frame.

checkPOINT

3. For what reasons do patients come in to see the hygienist?

Dental Assistants' Schedule

The dental assistant is an integral part of the clinical team. It is quite unlikely that the dentist will be able to fully perform his or her job without the assistance of a dental assistant. Dental assistants have clinical responsibilities that can include

Tip FROM THE DENTIST

The printed schedule is probably the most important tool that I use in the execution of my day. I depend on it for treatment timing, breaks, and even for how much small talk I can afford to have with each patient. If the schedule is not accurate and well thought out, the whole day will quickly fall apart with either too much down time or patients being forced to wait while I hurry to catch up. In dentistry, hurrying causes errors, which translate into lost revenue and frustration.

Just as important as accuracy is thoughtfulness with regard to special patient needs or special clinic needs. Certain patients, because of apprehensiveness or fear, will require more time with the dentist. An astute office administrator will know the clients and will allow for this extra time. Knowing your dentist is also important. Personally, I am a talker and will quite often use half of an appointment in idle chatter. My patients like this. Other dentists are much less talkative and require less "talk" time. Some clinics have a limited number of instruments or treatment rooms, meaning that more time is required to ready things for the next patient. Respect for the dental assistant is required to prevent frustrations in these situations.

The schedule should also not contain ambiguous definitions or unclear instructions. If, for example, the abbreviation "EX" is used on the schedule, is this an examination or an extraction? Using the preferred abbreviations is important!

One thing that I also like on my daily schedule is a tip or two on each patient. Where did she just go for vacation, what is her hobby, or what is she upset about? It makes the patient feel cared about and makes me, the dentist, look like I have a good memory!

noninvasive procedures for which additional education and training is required. Additional skills are referred to expanded duties or functions. Ideally, the goal of creating a productive appointment schedule is to maximize the use of the doctor's time. There can often be unexpected interruptions in the schedule, such as emergency patients or treatment which requires more time, and this means that the dental assistant will be required to take on more responsibilities throughout the day.

When scheduling a patient for the doctor you must consider the process involved in the administration of treatment to be performed in order to maximize the skills and abilities of the dental assistant thereby freeing up time for the doctor to attend to other patients. For example, one of the responsibilities of a dental assistant may be to bring the patient into the treatment room and review the health history and reason for the patient's visit. If necessary, the dental assistant will take any required radiographs and have them ready for the dentist on arrival to the treatment room. This process takes approximately 15–20 minutes. During this time the dentist is completing treatment on another patient. When the dentist arrives to see the patient, the dentist can make an assessment of the patient, determine a diagnosis, and then delegate any responsibilities to the dental assistant.

Aside from taking radiographs and completing the health history review, the dental assistant may also be required to take dental impressions of the patient as well as provide education for patients regarding procedures and treatment. All of these components of the dental assistants responsibilities take time and thus, should be considered in the appointment schedule. Figure 10-6 shows how a dental assistant's time is integrated into the daily schedule. Later in the chapter when we discuss double booking and dovetailing, the role of the dental assistant in that area will again come into focus.

MAINTAINING THE SCHEDULE

One of the most important responsibilities of the dental office administrator is maintaining the daily schedule. This means that the schedule must not only be booked, but the patients must be scheduled in a way that maximizes the time of every member of the clinical team. For example, the dental hygienist will often see a patient for dental prophylaxis prior to the dentist seeing the patient for an oral examination. If you schedule the patient to see the dental hygienist and not enough time is provided for treatment, the dental hygienist may not finish treatment and the patient will have to reschedule or, the dentist will not be able to see the patient for an oral examination and will have unexpected free time. Your responsibility is to ensure that the patient is scheduled for the appropriate amount of time needed to have a productive appointment schedule. To effectively maintain the schedule in a dental office, you must understand the units of time used in such a schedule, as well as the use of abbreviations, buffers, double booking, and dovetailing. Understanding these concepts

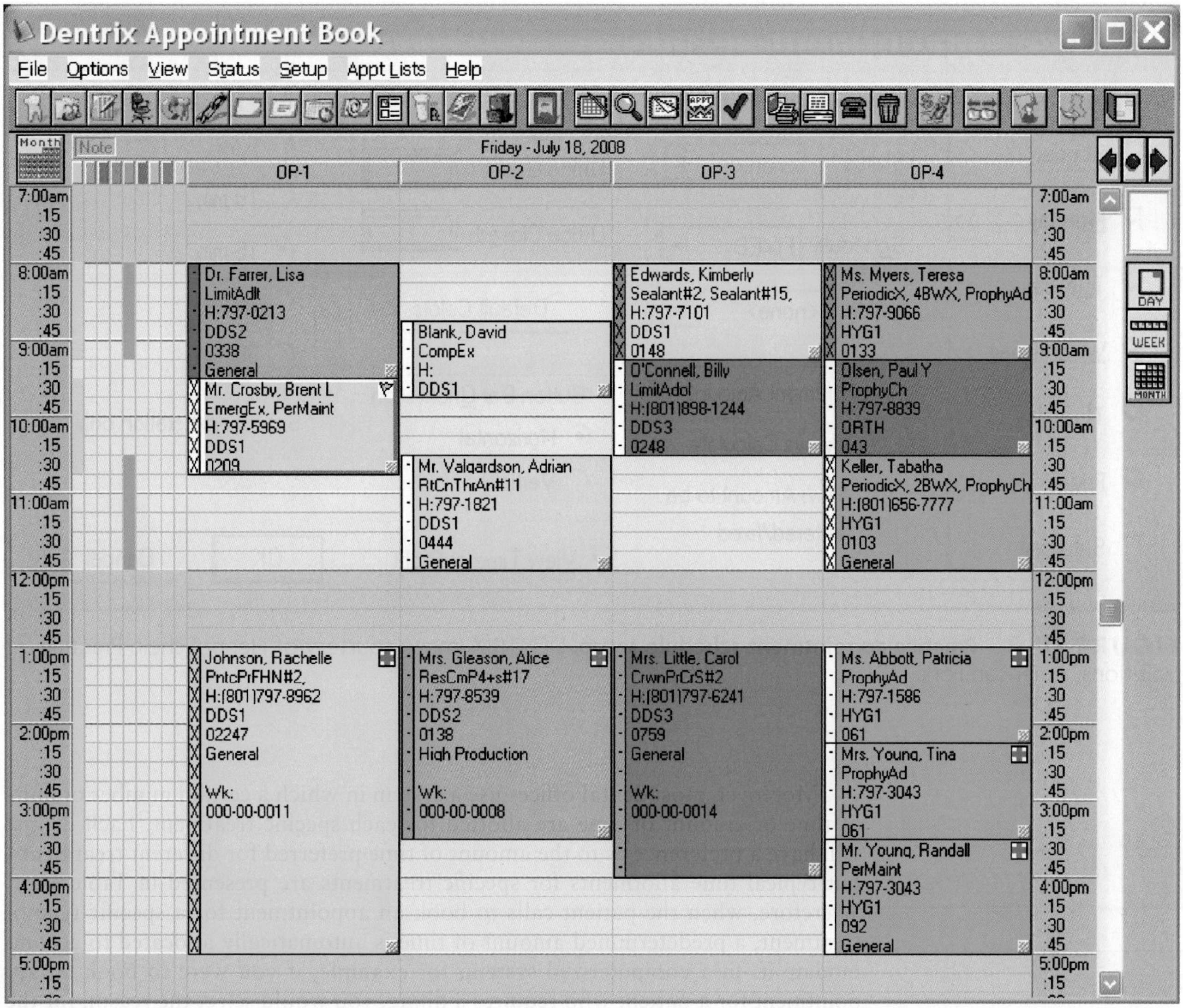

FIGURE 10-6 Dental assistants' schedule. DENTRIX image courtesy of Henry Schein Practice Solutions, American Fork, UT.

and the responsibilities of the clinical staff members will assist you in creating a productive schedule. These concepts are discussed later. Note, too, that the Tip From the Dentist information box provides some valuable insight into how the dental office administrator can create a schedule that helps make the day run more smoothly in the dental office.

Units of Time

In the dental office, the amount of time required or allotted for treatment is often described as a certain number of **units of time**. For example, in many dental offices, one unit of time is equal to 15 minutes and the daily schedule is thus divided into 15-minute increments. This approach makes scheduling relatively straightforward. For instance, in this case, if the dentist requests 3 units of time for the procedure, 45 minutes of time should be scheduled for the appointment. In Chapter 15, when we discuss patient billing and insurance, we will look more closely at how units of time translate into dollars billed and at the uniform coding system required by insurance companies. Figure 10-7 shows the appointment schedule setup options in the computerized practice management program.

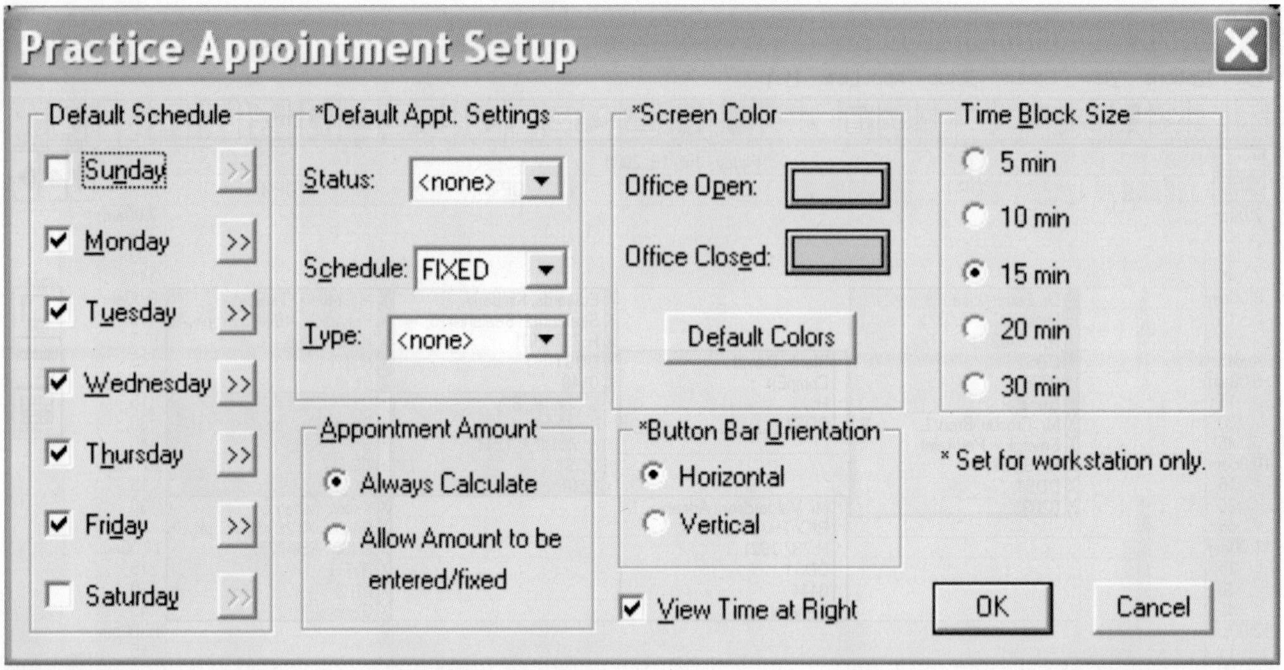

FIGURE 10-7 Practice appointment schedule setup. DENTRIX image courtesy of Henry Schein Practice Solutions, American Fork, UT.

Moreover, most dental offices use a system in which a certain number of units of time or amount of time are allotted for each specific treatment. Each dentist will have a preference as to the amount of time preferred for different treatments, but typical time allotments for specific treatments are presented in Table 10-1. Therefore, when the patient calls to book an appointment for a specific type of treatment, a predetermined amount of time is automatically allocated to accommodate it. In a computerized system, for example, if you were to book an appointment for a patient who requires a filling, you would select the reason for the appointment and the computer would automatically set the amount of time the doctor prefers. The amount of time is adjustable, however, as the doctor may ask for more or less time.

Such use of structured appointment times allows for efficient management of the schedule and of the time of the practitioners while they are in the office. In addition to this, the creation of the daily schedule is much more easily achieved and planning the day or week in advance is possible.

Scheduling Abbreviations

It is very important that the abbreviations used in the dental office are adhered to when scheduling appointments. If you are unsure of an abbreviation used, ask! Guessing or creating your own abbreviation and using an abbreviation that could have multiple meanings will only lead to confusion for the medical staff. For example, if you are scheduling Mrs. Jones to see the doctor because she requires an adjustment to her crown and you are unsure of what the abbreviation may be, choosing to put CA to symbolize crown adjustment could be read as many things by staff members who are not familiar with the abbreviation, such as cancer, cancellation, and so on. Be mindful of what information you put on the schedule. Table 10-2 provides examples of some abbreviations used for procedures in the daily schedule.

TABLE 10-1 Appointment Time Allotment

Treatment	Time Allotment (minutes)	Units of Time (1 unit = 15 minutes)
Recall, emergency, or specific examination	30	2
Root canal therapy	45 (× 2 appointments)	3
Crown preparation	60	4
Cement crown or bridge	30	2
Restoration—anterior tooth	45	3
Hygiene (dental prophylaxis)—adult	60	4
Hygiene—child under 10 years	45	3
Denture adjustment	30	2
Consultation examination	45	3
Root planing	60	4
Restoration—posterior tooth	60	4
Restoration—primary tooth	30	2
TMJ examination	75	5
New patient examination	45	3

Each dentist will have preferences as to the amount of time preferred for scheduling appointments, as will each hygienist. The above are guidelines designed to provide you with an overview of the types of appointments scheduled and time requirements for treatment.

TABLE 10-2 Scheduling Abbreviations

Treatment	Abbreviation
Root canal therapy	RCT
New patient examination	NPExam
Emergency examination	Emerg
Recall examination	Recall or Rc
Denture adjustment	Dent Adj
Crown preparation	Cr Prep (tooth number)
Bridge preparation	Br Prep (teeth numbers)
Filling	Flg (tooth number)
Oral surgery	Ext (tooth number)
Bone grafting	Bone Gft (quadrant)
Dental prophylaxis	Hyg or Scale/Prophy
Root planing	Root Planing

The above is a list of abbreviations that can be used on the daily schedule. Each dental office will have its own preferred abbreviations, and this list is meant to provide a guideline only.

Buffers

Buffer times are times that are blocked off on the schedule as if they were patient bookings but that are used for emergency appointments and various office activities. The number of emergency appointments in a given day or week is impossible to predict but emergency appointments are likely to happen, and the only way to accommodate such appointments in the schedule is to use buffer times. Buffer times can also be added to the schedule to accommodate certain administrative tasks that the dentist must accomplish, such as making phone calls or writing up notes for a letter. The first appointment of the day or last appointment of the day is usually a desirable time for buffer times.

Double Booking

Double booking refers to when two patients are intentionally scheduled at the same time to see the dentist. This is not a regular occurrence but does happen. Often, double bookings are made when the treatment planned for one or both of the scheduled patients necessitates what would otherwise be significant downtime on the part of the dentist. Such bookings occur in the following instances:

- When scheduling a patient who requires a procedure such as a denture reline, in which the patient must wait in the operatory for a certain period of time.
- When scheduling an emergency procedure, in which the patient is asked to wait for radiographs to be developed.
- When scheduling a patient who is having an in-office whitening procedure performed, in which the patient must remain in the operatory for a period of time.

Often, there is a dental assistant who is available to supervise and manage patients who are in situations in which they are receiving treatment that does not require the dentist to be in the operatory, such as the whitening procedure.

checkPOINT

4. What are the two reasons when patients may be double booked?

Dovetailing

To dovetail an appointment means that either the first or last 15–30 minutes of the patient's appointment involves duties or procedures that can be managed by the dental assistant. **Dovetailing** the appointment schedule is crucial to maintaining the appointment schedule because it maximizes the time for all the clinical staff and allows the dentist to delegate responsibilities where necessary. First of all, it is important to recognize when the dentist is needed most during the procedure. Second, being familiar with the duties that a dental assistant can perform, that is, knowing what the dentist can delegate, is important for effective dovetailing. Figure 10-6 demonstrates what dovetailing looks like in the appointment schedule. Once the duties are delegated to the dental assistant, the dentist can attend to a patient in another treatment room with another dental assistant.

SCHEDULING CONSIDERATIONS

Throughout the appointment scheduling process, being aware of the dentists' preferences concerning scheduling is important for effective maintenance. For example, being familiar with the amount of time a dentist prefers for certain procedures, or knowing the office policies regarding emergency patient scheduling, as well as considering how the type of patient appointment required will affect the appointment bookings, all determine how you maintain the appointment schedule. The next section outlines some of the elements you must consider when scheduling patient appointments.

Patient's Scheduling Needs

Before you schedule an appointment for a patient with the dentist, you should ask yourself the following questions regarding the patient:

- What is the reason for the appointment?
- How long has the patient been experiencing symptoms of pain? (Sudden or for a period of time.)
- What day and time is the patient looking to make an appointment for?
- Does the patient depend on transportation assistance?
- Does the patient need to see more than one staff member (dentist and hygienist)?
- If the patient has dental insurance, will this visit be covered by the insurance?
- If involved in a work-related accident, does the patient have the appropriate documentation or contact information for the dentist to complete?

Not every patient you speak with will have the same insurance coverage, needs, or requests. Knowing this information will help you to schedule appointments for patients much more effectively.

The management of the daily schedule is the responsibility of the office administrator, and for this reason it is important that the control of the schedule remains with the dental administrator and not with the patient. Allowing patients to pick and choose when they would like to come in will send a message that patients can rearrange their appointments to suit their schedule. For example, a patient who calls and says he is in pain and would like to get in to see the dentist as soon as possible will probably take the appointment time you provide. If the patient tells you that he cannot come in today and the only available time he has is 2 days from now, the patient is likely not in severe pain. Try to accommodate patients, but do not let them dictate when the doctor will see them. If a patient calls and requests an appointment for Friday morning at 10 AM, but you have a patient scheduled at that time, politely let the patient know the doctor will be seeing a patient at that time and offer the following suggestions:

1. The next available appointment time on the Friday.
2. The next available appointment at 10 AM.
3. Encourage patients to schedule an appointment at a time that might not be preferred and place their name on the short call list to get them in earlier to see the dentist.

Staff Members' Scheduling Preferences

Managing the schedule not only means learning how to schedule patients and accommodate their needs and requests, but also accommodating the needs and requests of the dentist or hygienist and how they prefer to schedule appointments. Some dentists prefer to remain punctual and receive their patients on time throughout the day and, therefore, will request that you schedule adequate time for treatment as per their request. Other dentists will not be as concerned with being on time to see patients. You will need to take this into consideration when booking patients.

Consideration must also be given to the dentists' preferences regarding the time of day certain types of treatments are scheduled. Some dentists may prefer to perform longer treatments first thing in the day or only on certain days. Moreover, dentists may be more naturally productive at certain times during the day, and therefore may wish to schedule certain types of appointments at certain times to maximize their productivity. The dentist or dental assistant will inform you of these preferences.

The dentist may also have preferences regarding how unscheduled visitors are handled during the day. Dental supply companies often have representatives who visit dental offices and request to speak with the dentist regarding new products or equipment available. The dentist may or may not be keen to speak with these representatives. You will need to check with the dentist as to his or her preference in these matters. Some dentists may prefer that the office manager speak with sales representatives and schedule time in the schedule at a later date for the dentist to meet with them if necessary. Another type of unscheduled visitor is the dentist's friends, colleagues, or family members. Some dentists would like to be notified immediately if a family member phones or comes into the practice or if other dentists are requesting to speak to them. Always determine in advance how the dentist would like these situations handled.

Understanding the needs of the dental assistant is also important when scheduling appointments. If the dental office has only one crown preparation kit available, you will need to consider that the kit will have to be sterilized after use before using it again. Or, if there are only four operatories available, scheduling too many short treatments close together may not give the dental assistant enough time to prepare rooms. For this reason, it is beneficial for the dental administrator to understand how a treatment is performed from start to finish in order to effectively schedule treatments. Observing the dentist from time to time in the operatory will help in this understanding, and help you to gain confidence in educating patients on the importance of good oral health.

checkPOINT

5. What are the three questions to keep in mind when evaluating a patient's scheduling needs?

HOW TO SCHEDULE APPOINTMENTS?

There are four main types of appointments you will schedule in the dental office:

- new patients
- returning patients
- emergency patients
- walk-in patients

Each of these types of patients requires that different questions be answered at the time of the booking to schedule the appointment.

New Patients

When a patient who has never seen the dentist before calls the dental office to make an appointment, this person is considered a new patient. The initial conversation you have with a new patient can make or break the patient's desire to see the dentist.

The most important thing to remember is to accurately record the information the patient provides; this means repeating back to the patient the phone number and address he or she provides you with. Have him or her spell his or her name for you; do not assume that you are correctly spelling it.

Another consideration when scheduling new patients is that a new patient examination requires more appointment time for the dentist than a returning patient examination. At a new patient appointment, the dentist must review the patient's dental history and health history, perform a complete oral examination and oral cancer screening, and diagnose any radiographs taken. This can take up to 45 minutes, and any other treatment the patient requests will require additional time to complete. Follow the guidelines for new patient appointment scheduling in Procedure 10-1 when booking a new patient.

Returning Patients

Besides new patients, you will also be scheduling appointments for returning patients, those who have had appointments at the dental office before. Procedure 10-2 presents the method for scheduling appointments for patients who are returning to the dental office.

PROCEDURE 10-1 *Scheduling New Patient Appointments*

1. Establish that the patient is a new patient and assess the amount of time required for the appointment. Ask the following questions when the patient calls to schedule an appointment:
   - Have you seen Dr. Jones before?
   - Is there a specific reason you wish to see the dentist?
2. Collect the following information from the patient:
   - Name (ensure correct spelling)
   - Address
3. Explain the policy of the dental office regarding payment and cancellations and explain what information the patient is required to bring. Preparing the patient for any out-of-pocket expenses he is responsible for will avoid any frustrations that may be experienced by unexpected costs. Always be upfront about the office policies with patients if you expect them to follow it.
4. Provide the patient with the address and location of your office. Provide directions to the office, if needed, pointing out any relevant landmarks. This will help the patient be on time and will keep an efficient schedule.
5. Confirm the patient's contact preference: home, work, or on their cell phone. Let the patient know that you will call her at the requested number and the approximate time to expect your call. For example, "I will be confirming your Wednesday appointment on Tuesday morning around 10 AM."
6. Always thank the patient for calling the dental office and confirm the appointment date and time. Thanking patients for calling is a polite way of letting them know that not only do you appreciate the call, but you appreciate that they have chosen your dental office to be a patient in. Confirming the date and time lets patients know that their appointment has been scheduled and confirms that you have scheduled the patient on the correct date and time as agreed.
7. If the patient is coming to the dental office from a referral, call the other dental office and obtain any available radiographs or information regarding the patient. Having any information regarding the patient's health or dental history ready for the dentist to review before seeing the patient will help prepare the dentist and other staff members for a smooth appointment.

Administrative TIP

Keep a handy desk calendar at the front desk. If patients are without their own calendars or planners, loan them yours. This will make it easier for them to remember what days they will be available for the appointment. This is particularly helpful if the appointment is being scheduled in another month.

Emergency Patients

Patients who call the dental office because they are experiencing oral pain or have broken a tooth are considered **emergency patients** and must be given priority in scheduling. Sometimes it is difficult to determine whether a patient is indeed an emergency patient. Use the questions below as a guideline to determining emergency patient status and as a way to gather information for the dentist prior to the appointment. Use the patient's chart to record the information. In any case, if a patient is experiencing oral pain, swelling, or bleeding, consider him or her an emergency patient.

- Are you experiencing any discomfort?
- What tooth do you think it is (upper/lower, right/left)?
- Can you describe the discomfort for me (throbbing/shooting pain)?
- Is there any swelling?
- When did the discomfort start?
- Are you taking any pain relievers? How often?
- Do they seem to be working?
- Can you come in today?

*check*POINT

6. What are four questions you might ask a patient who is in pain and wanting to make an appointment?

The dental office you work in may have a specific policy regarding emergency patients. Be sure to consult your policy manual to deal effectively with patients who are experiencing discomfort. Use the time slots set aside for emergency patients to schedule the appointment. If the time slots are unavailable, check with the dental assistant or dentist to find an appointment time for the appointment.

PROCEDURE 10-2 *Scheduling the Returning Patient*

1. Provide the patient with the next available appointment time for the procedure he or she needs. If the patient has a specific date and time request, see if you can accommodate him or her or find a similar date and time.
2. Offer the patient one specific time and date. An example would be, "Dr. Smith is available to see you on Wednesday, June 5th at 9:30 AM." Avoid saying, "I have Wednesday, Thursday, or Friday afternoon openings—which would you like?" If the specific date and time are not appropriate for the patient, offer another specific date and time.
3. Schedule the patient into the daily schedule. Always do this while the patient is in front of you or on the phone to you to avoid forgetting.
4. For patients making an appointment in person, write the appointment information onto an appointment card and give this to them. Having the information written on a card will allow patients to write the appointment into their schedule at home or place the card where they will be able to see it as a reminder.
5. Thank the patient for scheduling the appointment. Always smile and let the patient know that her loyalty is appreciated. Politeness and manners often portray this gratitude.

Walk-In Patients

Walk-in patients are those who show up at the dental office without a scheduled appointment. Each dental office will have its own policy regarding walk-in patients. Some dental offices invite walk-in patients by putting the phrase, "Walk-in appointments available," on their office sign. The relevant office policy will dictate how these patients are handled. If a patient walks in to the clinic and wants to see the dentist that day because of some emergency reason, he or she is considered a walk-in patient, and it will be up to you to inform the dentist that the patient is waiting, if the office policy allows for walk-in patients. If there are emergency time slots available, you can inform the patient of the times and provide him or her with the option of returning during one of the times. Alternatively, you can ask the patient to wait until the dentist is available. If the patient is not in any pain and there are no openings on that day, encourage the patient to schedule an appointment to see the dentist on another day. Keep in mind that the office policy and the dentist's preference should govern this decision.

SCHEDULE INTERRUPTIONS

From time to time, the schedule will have to be adapted for different reasons. Patients may arrive late for their appointment, cancel shortly prior to their appointment, or miss their appointment. Sometimes the dental office may have to reschedule appointments due to illness or tragedy. Interruptions in the daily schedule are common in the dental office, and an effective office administrator will handle them with professionalism and tact.

Patient Cancellations

When patients call to cancel their appointment, you should first ask if they would like to reschedule the appointment. The information should be written on the daily appointment schedule and then in the patient's chart. The reason for writing this information on the daily schedule is to let the dentist know the reason the patient is canceling and that the appointment has been rebooked. If the patient is rescheduling an appointment that is midtreatment, emphasize the importance of keeping the follow-up appointment. If the patient does not want to reschedule, offer to call him back in 2 days. Let the patient know that you will inform the doctor of his

BOX 10-3
Documenting Cancellation in a Patient's Chart

June 30, 2006—Jane called and cancelled her appointment 1 hour prior to appointment time. Her son was ill, and she was unable to get a babysitter. She rebooked for July 13, 2006. [your initials here]

cancellation and rebooking status. Make a note to call the patient to rebook the appointment in 2 days and to call again 2 weeks later, if he does not respond. To fill the cancellation, access the short call list you have available and calling patients who would like to come in earlier. Box 10-3 is an example of how to document a cancellation in the patient's chart.

check POINT

7. What steps should you take when a patient cancels an appointment?

A patient who cancels appointments may be displaying a fear or anxiety reaction to the dental treatment. If the patient cancels more than one appointment, ask him or her if he or she is concerned about the treatment he or she is scheduled to receive. Encourage the patient to come in and start with a more relaxed or less comprehensive form of treatment and to speak to the dentist about any concerns he or she has at that time.

Late Patients

When a patient arrives for an appointment later than scheduled, it can cause a delay in the schedule for the rest of the day. Depending on the office policy, you may have to ask a late-arriving patient to reschedule the appointment. If a patient calls to inform you that he or she is on his or her way but will be a certain amount of time late, you should check with the dental assistant or dentist to confirm that there will still be enough time to complete treatment. Inform the patient of the decision and thank him or her for calling. Most patients who are going to be 10–15 minutes late can still be seen, and, if they are calling to let you know, they are still willing to keep what they can of the appointment. Patients who are late on a regular basis should be informed that their being late is putting a delay in the schedule for the rest of the day. The office policy will dictate how to handle these patients, whether it means rescheduling the patient or booking the patient at the end of the day only.

Missed Appointments

Patients who do not make their appointments and do not call to inform the dental office that they will not be coming, often referred to as a no-show, can create a lot of frustration in the dental office. Some dental offices have a policy of calling patients when they do not show, finding out the reason, and then rescheduling the appointments. If a patient no-shows more than once, an office policy may be that the patient must place a U.S.$50 booking deposit on their account prior to the appointment. If the patient makes the appointment, the U.S.$50 is used as a credit toward the treatment; otherwise, it is used as a charge for scheduling time to see the dentist and not showing up. Always document this information in the patient's chart. Patients who have a tendency to forget their appointments or show up late should be contacted 1 or 2 days prior to the appointment to get confirmation from them that they will attend.

Dental Office Cancellations

Dentists and hygienists may from time to time have to deal with personal matters that prevent them from seeing their scheduled patients, such as illness, family emergencies, or unforeseeable events. Rescheduling patients is often the result. The patients being

PROCEDURE 10-3 *Making a Referral Appointment*

1. Have the patient's chart in front of you, along with the referral slip of the dental office you are calling. There will be specific information the dental office you are referring to needs to have in order to schedule an appointment. Complete the referral form before making the call, and the information you will need to provide will be on the form in front of you. The following information is necessary:
   - Name, address, phone number, and birth date of the patient
   - Parent or guardian's name (if a minor)
   - Reason for the appointment (consultation or treatment?)
   - Dental insurance information
   - Emergency?
   - Radiographs provided?
2. Record the name of the person you spoke with and the date and time of the call on the referral slip and in the patient's chart. If you need to access this information at a later date, you will need to have it in one location.
3. Photocopy the referral slip and give the original to the patient. A copy should be placed in the patient's chart. If radiographs are being sent to the specialist's office, make an additional photocopy of the referral slip and attach the radiographs to it for their use.
4. Make sure the information is documented in the chart. By completing the chart with the information, the chart then shows proof that the dentist's request for treatment was followed through with.
5. Inform the patient of any office policies you were advised of from the dental office referred to.

rescheduled do not need to be told the specific reason for the change. If patients ask for a reason, provide a general explanation. Give the patient as much notice as possible. Call the patient and say, "Dr. Jones has been called away from the office unexpectedly. Would it be convenient for you to come in next week to see the doctor for your appointment?" Most patients will be very understanding of the situation. If the dentist is away for more than a few days unexpectedly, another dentist could be suggested for treatment. Provide patients with the name, address, and phone number of the other dentist. Your office policy should provide this information.

checkPOINT

8. What should you do if you need to reschedule patients?

REFERRALS TO DENTAL SPECIALISTS OR OTHER PROVIDERS

Part of the duties of the dental office administrator involves the scheduling of referral appointments to dental specialists or other doctors. Chapter 1 provides a list of all the types of dental specialists available. It is not unusual for the patient to have to wait 1–4 months for an appointment with a specialist. Procedure 10-3 presents guidelines to follow when making a referral appointment for a patient.

Chapter Summary

The effective management of the daily schedule can provide a smoothly run day for all staff members in the dental office. The dental office administrator is responsible for the scheduling of patients. Whether the schedule is produced manually or through the use of a computerized system, the basic guidelines involved in scheduling patients remain the same. The dental administrator should adhere to office preferences and policies regarding abbreviations used, amount of time to schedule for certain procedures, and when time is to be set aside. Scheduling challenges such as emergency patients and cancellations must be handled professionally and effectively to preserve the relationship with the patient and uphold the standards of the practice. Knowing the office policies regarding new patient scheduling, late patients, and patients who cancel or miss their appointments can assist in the proper handling of these delicate situations.

Review Questions

Multiple Choice

1. **Buffers, in the daily schedule, are**
   a. times set aside for lunch breaks.
   b. time periods in the schedule not used.
   c. time periods used for office activities.
   d. used in case a staff member is late.

2. **In most dental offices, the basic unit of time in the schedule is**
   a. 11 minutes.
   b. 15 minutes.
   c. 30 minutes.
   d. 1 hour.

3. **Dovetailing**
   a. occurs when a scheduling error has been made.
   b. maximizes the dentists' time.
   c. creates a chaotic schedule.
   d. allows the dental assistant to try new things.

4. **A computerized practice management system allows you to**
   a. access the Internet more easily.
   b. manage the recare system.
   c. organize your day.
   d. manage the dentist easily.

5. **Walk-in patients**
   a. call and schedule appointments.
   b. may not always be seen for an appointment.
   c. walk in to the dental office and ask to see the dentist.
   d. depend on buffers in the schedule.

6. **Which of the following is not an advantage of a computerized patient schedule?**
   a. Make changes to the schedule easily.
   b. Enter a limited amount of notes for an appointment.
   c. Track cancelled appointments.
   d. Maintain a list of patients who would like an earlier appointment.

7. **An important tool for the dentist is**
   a. the staff's vacation list.
   b. the daily schedule.
   c. the recare list.
   d. the names of patients who cancelled.

8. **Double booking is**
   a. patients booked on the same day and time for 2 weeks.
   b. family members scheduled one after the other.
   c. two patients scheduled at the same time.
   d. one patient scheduled twice.

9. **When a patient calls to cancel his or her appointment, you should**
   a. ask the patient the reason why he or she is canceling.
   b. explain the office policy regarding cancellations.
   c. ask the patient when he or she would like to reschedule it for.
   d. sympathize with the patient and cancel the appointment.

10. **Which of the following procedures could a double booking be scheduled for?**
    a. A patient who requires root canal therapy.
    b. A patient who requires radiographs and must wait for them to be developed.
    c. A child who is anxious about dental treatment and requires a restoration.
    d. An elderly woman who is seeing the hygienist for scaling.

Critical Thinking

1. The dental assistants are complaining to you that you are scheduling too many emergency patients into the schedule in 1 day. The office policy states that if a patient is in pain, you must find a place in the daily schedule to place them. What would you say to the dental assistants? Who would you ask for assistance, if any?

2. Mrs. Jones has called the clinic three times this week and asked if she could get in sooner to see the dentist. She is not in any pain and insists her situation is not an emergency since she is taking tylenol for any discomfort. You are concerned because of the frequency of calls. What do you say to Mrs. Jones? Use a classmate to role play with.

3. Dr. Johnson has arrived 30 minutes late this morning. The first patient of the day, Jane Smith, is upset about the delay and has just gotten up out of her seat and is coming toward the front desk. What are you going to say to Jane?

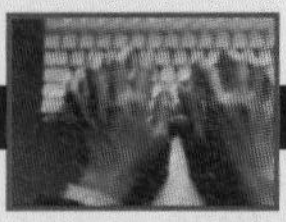

HANDS-ON ACTIVITY

1. Create a one-page script regarding how to effectively handle patients who have cancelled their appointments at the last minute. You need to provide the patient with some options in your script.
2. Create a schedule for the dental office for 1 day, showing the lunch, break time, and a staff meeting at 3 o'clock. There is one hygienist and one dentist in the office working today. Have a classmate simulate making a call to you and wanting to schedule an appointment for her and two family members to see the hygienist and the dentist today.
3. Develop a brochure that outlines the office policy for treating emergency patients in the dental office. Include what you will require for financial, demographic, and health history information.

chapter ELEVEN

Staff Management

OBJECTIVES

After completing this chapter, you should be able to do the following:

- Spell and define key terms
- List the contents of the policy and procedure manual in the dental office
- Explain how to develop a policy and procedure manual
- Discuss the importance of monthly staff meetings and morning meetings and their purpose in the management of the dental office
- Explain guidelines for the office manager in hiring, evaluating, and terminating staff
- Describe how to develop and maintain a continuing education policy in the dental office

KEY TERMS

- office policy and procedure manual
- policy
- procedure
- mission statement
- organizational chart
- job description
- morning meetings
- working interview
- employee evaluation

OUTLINE

- **Office Policy and Procedure Manual**
  - Contents of a Policy and Procedure Manual
    - Practice Description and Organization
    - Office Procedures
    - Personnel Policies
    - Task Descriptions
    - Emergency Procedures
  - Development of the Policy and Procedure Manual
- **Staff Meetings and Communication**
  - Monthly Staff Meetings
  - Morning Staff Meetings
  - Open Door Policy
- **Hiring, Evaluating, and Terminating Staff**
  - Hiring
  - Evaluating
    - Preparation
    - Agenda
    - Feedback
  - Taking Disciplinary Action and Terminating
- **Continuing Education**
  - *Chapter Summary*

The most valuable assets in the dental office are the staff. Working together, as a team, is crucial for a dental practice to operate successfully. A team that works together well not only has a common goal but also agrees with the philosophy of the practice used in meeting the goal and incorporates shared communication techniques and flexibility in doing so. Providing guidelines for dental team members to follow is critical for effective management. This chapter provides insight into the management of staff personnel in the dental practice and the specific responsibilities delegated to office managers and, in some situations, dental office administrators. In particular, this chapter presents the contents and development of a policy and procedure manual, conducting staff meetings, hiring, evaluating, and terminating staff, and managing continuing education opportunities.

OFFICE POLICY AND PROCEDURE MANUAL

Like any business, a dental office requires clear policies and procedures that are followed by all employees to run efficiently. Thus, each employee in the dental office must be familiar with the guidelines in the policy and procedure manual. These written policies and procedures ensure consistency in business practices. Moreover, some policies and procedures in the dental office must be followed to remain within legal and ethical guidelines prescribed by its regulating and accrediting agencies.

An **office policy and procedure manual** is a document that is written by an owner or a manager of the dental office and provides the office policies and recommended procedures to be followed. A **policy** in the dental office refers to the recommended guidelines concerning a specific area of practice, for example, financial policies or employee vacation policies. A financial policy may outline the methods of payment that are accepted in the dental practice. A vacation policy may stipulate a required amount of time in which an employee must be employed with the company before vacation time is awarded. Be careful not to confuse a policy with a rule. Rules are not meant to be broken; policies imply flexibility, unless otherwise stated. For example, a vacation policy in the dental office states that all employees must work a minimum of 3 months before requesting vacation time. A dental assistant who has worked slightly less than the required time period may request vacation time and discuss with the office manager a special circumstance that requires him or her to be away from his or her position. The office manager can make the decision to either uphold or deny the request, using the vacation policy as a guideline. In addition to policies, the office manual outlines procedures. A **procedure** is an outline of a step-by-step process that must be followed for the accurate performance of a particular task. For example, including the daily office opening and closing procedures in the manual are useful as a reference for those who are unfamiliar with this area of the dental office. An office policy and procedure manual combines both policies and procedures in one document to provide a central resource for all employees.

New employees in the dental office are often introduced to the office policy and procedure manual as part of their orientation to the office, as answers to common questions regarding employment are often provided in the policy manual. The policy and procedure manual is a source of information for all employees regarding task procedures and employee expectations. Each office will have a manual devised by the dentist or dentists in accordance with their preferences for the dental clinic. As the dental practice grows, or changes and new policies develop, or policies are replaced, the policy and procedure manual is updated. Each employee in the dental office is asked to read the policy and procedure manual and confirm that he or she has read and understood its contents by signing a confirmation form. The purpose of this form is to impress upon the employee the importance of the manual and the necessity for understanding its contents. Each employee should be familiar with the policy and procedure manual because it provides the guidelines used in the office by all members of the dental team and is a frame of reference for employees for carrying out procedures as well as effectively communicating with patients, which contributes to a functional dental team. Figure 11-1 is an example of a dental office policy and procedures manual.

checkPOINT

1. What is the difference between a policy and a procedure?
2. Why should each employee be familiar with the policy and procedure manual?

Contents of a Policy and Procedure Manual

The contents of a policy and procedure manual in the dental office depend greatly on the size and type of dental environment. For example, a dental office that is a group practice, that is, one in which there are more than two dentists, may have policies outlining the dentists' specific hours of work and preferences as to when they require their office administrator or dental assistant to be available for work. That is, each dentist may have specifications that will be outlined in the manual. A dental office where only one dentist practices may not include as much detail and

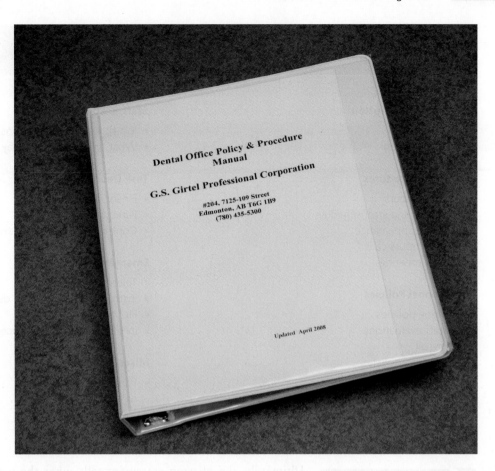

FIGURE 11-1 Policy and procedure manual.

variation in the office manual. However, dental office manuals may include topics that are relevant regardless of the size of the practice. The following topics are typically covered in an office policy and procedures manual:

1. Practice description
2. Office procedures
3. Personnel policies
4. Task descriptions
5. Emergency procedures

Box 11-1 provides a breakdown of the items that may be included under these general headings.

Practice Description and Organization

The first section of the policy and procedure manual includes a description of the dental practice, which includes an organizational chart and outlines the philosophy of the dental office. The organizational structure and office responsibilities of the dental team can vary from office to office and over time, depending on the number of employees in the dental office. The structure of any organization can be presented in diagrammatic form as an **organizational chart**. By depicting the chain of command and the interrelationships between staff members, this chart can promote effective communication among departments and employees.

The philosophy of the dental practice can also be referred to as a mission statement. The **mission statement** of any business is a statement of the goals and philosophy of the business (Box 11-2). A mission statement is designed to illustrate the purpose of the company. Often it will include a description of how the company is unique through the service it provides and the methods used to provide the service.

BOX 11-1
Office Policy Manual Index

Practice Description
- Philosophy
- Organization

Office Procedures
- Office hours
- Doctor and staff schedule
- Office appearance
- After hours calls
- Staff meetings

Personnel Policies
- Hiring policies
- Staff evaluations
- Payroll
- Vacation policies
- Sick leave
- Dress code
- Termination policies

Staff Responsibilities
- Job titles and descriptions
- What to do on a slow day

Task Descriptions
- Financial policies
- Patient policies
- Control of accounts receivable

Emergency Procedures
- Telephone numbers
- Instructions in case of a dentist's absence
- Fire procedure
- In-office emergency procedure

Miscellaneous
- Various items

checkPOINT

3. What is the purpose of an organizational chart?
4. Why is a mission statement important to the organization?

Ultimately, the mission statement tells what the main goal of the company is, that is, what it intends to accomplish and it does so by summarizing how the actions used to meet the intended goal will be guided. The mission statement further illustrates the character of a company and is motivational to staff and clients.

Office Procedures

The office procedures section of the policy manual includes items such as the following:

- *Office hours:* The regular operating hours of the dental office are outlined in this section of the manual. This section also includes statutory holidays recognized by the office.
- *Opening and closing procedures:* This section outlines specific procedures for staff to follow regarding the preparation of the office prior to patient arrival

BOX 11-2
Office Philosophy and Mission Statement

Our dental practice is a team-oriented, patient-centered practice. We believe in the best possible care for our patients and will do our best to give them that care. We will provide this care to our patients by being honest, in our daily work and in society. We treat each patient the same—in a friendly, caring manner—and will never prejudge his or her ability to pay for services. We offer many choices and alternatives for complete comprehensive care for our patients. We create a workplace that is safe and productive through teamwork, openness, and with employees who take responsibility for their actions, and our skills are continually updated for the benefit of our patients' care and our professional growth.

in the dental office as well as tasks to perform at the end of the work day, before leaving the office.

- *Personal appearance:* This includes the recommended dress code for staff in the clinical and administrative areas of the dental office. This section may also include policies regarding a uniform allowance for staff members.
- *Emergency and after-hours calls:* The office policy regarding patient emergencies and contacting the dentist would be addressed in this area of the manual. The procedure to follow for making alternate arrangements for patients when the dentist is not available is also outlined here.
- *Staff meetings*: The frequency and duration of staff meetings, as well as any expected contribution from staff members, are outlined.

Personnel Policies

The personnel policies focus on the specific concerns of staff members by addressing areas such as the following:

- Hiring policies
- Staff evaluations
- Payroll
- Vacation policies
- Sick leave
- Dress code
- Termination policies

Figure 11-2 provides information that may be considered under each of the areas concerned with personnel policies. The types of personnel policies listed in this area will be specific to the dental office in which you are employed.

Task Descriptions

This section includes procedures regarding financial policies, patient policies, and maintaining control of accounts receivable. For example, one such procedure included in this section might be the updating of patient medical history forms. The procedure should outline the frequency that the forms must be updated, which can vary in length from 6 months to 1 year, and the purpose of the update. An updated health history form allows the dental practitioner to consider how a specific health condition may influence treatment outcomes. The purpose for collecting updated health information should be outlined in the policy manual since this allows each staff member to explain the reason to the patient based on the policy outlined.

The task description section of the office manual also includes specific information regarding scheduling preferences and an outline of how much time is recommended for specific procedures and how many appointments are necessary to complete treatment. For example, major restorative treatment such as crown and bridge preparation may require two separate appointments. As the dental office administrator, you must be aware of the length and duration of appointments to facilitate a patient's treatment. Furthermore, this section of the office manual provides information regarding how to communicate effectively with different types of patients, such as a script for managing the care of emergency patients. An example of such policies is provided in Box 11-3.

Emergency Procedures

A section regarding the correct steps to take during an emergency situation is necessary in the policy and procedures manual. All dental team members must be aware of and understand their role in an emergency situation. That is, they must know where they must be and what task they must perform should an emergency

Hiring Policies

The following procedure is followed when hiring new employees in this office:

- All potential employees are interviewed by the Office Manager
- A 2nd interview is scheduled with potential employees with the Office Manager and one other staff member. The Dentist will meet with the interviewee at this time, either briefly or at length, as per his request.
- Before hiring, a minimum of 2 work references must be checked.
- The Office Manager is responsible for the contact and set-up of all new hires.
- All new employees are on probation for a period of 3 months.

Staff Evaluations

Each year, all team members will have an evaluation, or performance review. These meetings are set-up to discuss strengths and weaknesses and how any necessary improvements can be made. Job expectations are also reviewed at this time. Employees are expected to rate their own progress in preparation for the meeting.

Payroll

All employees in this office are paid on an hourly basis. It is the responsibility of each staff member to submit their individual hours a minimum of one working day before their last working day on each month.

Hours paid does not include the time of arrival ,15 minutes prior to clinic opening, nor staying after hours to do work.

Employees are paid on a monthly pay schedule, the last day of each month, with an advance on the 15th of each month. Cheques are issued on these dates.

Holidays and Vacation Times

As per Employment Standards, the following outlines the general holidays that are recognized by this office.

Employee eligibility for pay on these holidays will depend on their individual situation.

New Year's Day (January 1)
Family Day (3rd Monday in February)
Good Friday (Friday before Easter)
Victoria Day (Monday before May 25)
Canada Day (July 1 or 2)
Labour Day (1st Monday in Sept)
Thanksgiving Day (2nd Monday in October)
Remembrance Day (November 11)
Christmas Day (December 25)

Staff are allowed the following number of weeks for vacation according to the number of weeks they are employed.

- 2 weeks after 1 year of employment
- 3 weeks after 5 years of employment

Vacation pay at the rate of 4% of wages earned is paid to the employee during these times.
Vacation times are to be discussed with the Dentist at least two months in advance and a written request must be submitted.

Sick Leave

Employees who are unable to attend work due to illness must contact the Office Manager directly as soon as they are aware they will not attend. Providing as much time as possible to ensure a replacement is essential to the practice. Time off due to illness is time off without pay.

Dress Code

In order to ensure the safety of employees and assist them in performing in a safe manner, the following dress code must be adhered to in this office:

Dental Assistants: Uniform and White soft soled shoes
Dental Hygienists: Uniform and White soft soled shoes
Business Staff: Uniform,Lab coat over their attire or a business suit.

Make-up, perfume and jewelry are fine, as long as it is not overdone.
All staff members must wear their name/title badge while working in the clinic.

Termination of Employment

Our office follows the guidelines of the Alberta Employment Standards. For every year of employment, 1 week notice will be provided, to a maximum of 8 weeks notice. Permanent employees are expected to provide two weeks notice.

Staff members will receive written warnings should they not perform their expected duties and responsibilities to the specifications and expectations of the Dentist. If after 3 written warnings, an improvement is not noticeable, employment will be terminated with the appropriate amount of weeks notice provided.

FIGURE 11-2 Personnel policies.

BOX 11-3 *Patient Policies*

Emergency Patient Procedures

Patients who are experiencing tooth pain, swelling, or bleeding should be seen as soon as possible on the day they telephone. Collect as much information as you can from the patient regarding the signs and symptoms the patient is experiencing, the tooth affected, and how the patient has been managing the discomfort. Consult with the dentist or the dental assistant to select a time in the schedule if an appointment time or buffer time is not available. If you are unable to accommodate an emergency patient in the dental office, be prepared to provide the patient with alternate care arrangements, specifically, contact information for another dental clinic, or emergency facility. If you are able to accommodate the patient, it is preferable that you inform the patient that there may be a wait, as you are putting them in on an emergency basis without a scheduled appointment. Notify the patient that at this appointment the dentist will make a diagnosis and relieve any discomfort, however, it is possible that the treatment required may occur at a subsequent appointment, if necessary. The patient should be given the next available appointment to complete treatment, before leaving the dental office.

Pediatric Patients

It is our policy that pediatric patients must be accompanied by a parent or guardian. Remember that the child is the patient, NOT the parent. Greet children as they come in to make them feel more at ease. Our operatories are an open concept design, and children are welcome to watch while their parents receive dental treatment, provided it is not too gruesome.

Geriatric/Special Needs Patients

Some patients may require assistance to get into the building. There is an elevator they can use. Some may require a staff member to meet them at the main door and escort them. Treat elderly patients with respect; address them as Mr. or Mrs., unless they state otherwise.

Late Patients

If a patient is late by 15 minutes or less of their appointment time, whatever treatment can be provided in the time remaining will be performed, and, if required, unfinished treatment will be rescheduled. If a patient is later than 15 minutes, he or she will need to reschedule, in all fairness to others. It is preferable to consult with the treatment provider (dentist or hygienist) in these circumstances, and he or she will make the final decision.

Patients who Fail to Show for the Appointment

Call patients who do not show up for a scheduled appointment immediately—within 15 minutes of the start of the appointment. Reschedule them or put them on the reschedule list. After two no-shows, refer the patient file to the office manager.

Difficult Patients

Difficult patients should be dealt with in a calm, friendly manner. If the patient becomes verbally abusive, ask him to stop and tell him you will only continue this conversation when he stops the abuse. If you need assistance, have the office manager deal with him.

occur in the dental office. An emergency situation in the dental office could be any of the following:

- A patient losing consciousness
- Fire occurring in any area of the office
- A patient having trouble breathing
- A person in the office choking
- Allergic reactions

Each dental office has emergency procedures that must be followed by each member of the dental office. It is important for you to know exactly what your role is in the emergency procedure. If you are responsible for making the phone call to the emergency center and you are unaware that this is your responsibility, it could mean the difference between life and death. Emergency telephone numbers and a step-by-step process for fire and other emergency situations must be available to all

BOX 11-4 *Emergency Procedures*

Telephone Numbers

- Police/fire/ambulance: 9-1-1
- Dentist's cell: (512) 222-5555
- Dentist's home: (512) 123-4567

Fire Procedure

In case of fire, follow the steps below:

1. The office administrator should call 9-1-1.
2. The office manager should ask all patients to leave the clinic.
3. The dentist should instruct all staff members to leave.
4. Exit through the back door of the office, turn right, go down the stairs and out the back door of the building.
5. The dentist should be last person to leave the office: check to make sure no patients or staff remain and that all doors are closed, not locked.

Office Medical Emergency Procedure

1. The office administrator should call 9-1-1.
2. The dentist should stay with the patient.
3. The hygienist or office manager should assist the dentist.
4. The hygienist or office manager should meet the ambulance at the main door.

employees. Box 11-4 provides sample emergency procedures in the dental office, as they may appear in this section of the policy and procedure manual.

checkPOINT

5. What are examples of an emergency in a dental office?

Development of the Policy and Procedure Manual

Developing an office policy and procedure manual can be a time-consuming task. Computer software programs are available that provide an outline and template for office policy manuals. As a member of the dental team, you may be required to develop all or part of the office policy manual, at some point in your career. Whether you are using a computerized template or developing the manual from scratch, keep the following guidelines in mind to assist you in its creation:

- Consult with the dentist regarding his or her preferences in any of the specific sections of the manual, before starting.
- Solicit the opinions of team members in the development of sections of the manual such as patient communication scripts. Senior staff members may provide insight into effectively communicating with patients based on past experience.
- Use the guidelines of dental regulatory bodies and licensing agencies in developing policies. Include policies that ensure compliance with Health Insurance Portability and Accountability Act (HIPAA) and Occupational Safety and Health Administration (OSHA) guidelines.
- Create scripts and forms for employees to use in order to accurately complete tasks as required.
- Keep the manual in a central area where all staff members will have access to it and it will be kept secure.

checkPOINT

6. What points should you consider when developing an office policy and procedure manual?

STAFF MEETINGS AND COMMUNICATION

Maintaining regular communication with staff members is important to prevent miscommunication among staff members and management. Ensuring that communication remains positive and effective between staff members is carried out in various ways in the dental office. The three most effective ways to communicate with staff and promote a positive team environment are as follows:

- Monthly staff meetings
- Morning meetings
- Open door policy

Monthly Staff Meetings

Monthly staff meetings have a purpose of regenerating the team's commitment to the office and refocusing on the goals of the practice and how the individual team members can help achieve them. Such meetings should be held on a monthly basis and should be viewed as an opportunity for team members to communicate with each other. Some dental offices assign each staff member an opportunity to manage the monthly staff meeting. The following tips can help you direct a staff meeting successfully:

- Try to select a time during office hours in order to hold a staff meeting. There may be a prearranged policy regarding staff meetings and when they will be held, for example, the first Monday of every month. The meeting may be held during the day to include the lunch break and the lunch is catered to accommodate all staff members. The meeting should be approximately 1–2 hours in length.
- The meeting should be held in an area that is free from distractions and where all staff members feel comfortable in speaking freely. A staff room or meeting room in the office is most suitable. An area where patients cannot overhear what is being discussed is most preferable.
- Create, distribute to all staff, and adhere to an agenda, or list of topics to discuss in the meeting. This will ensure that everyone is aware of the process of the meeting and where their contribution is expected. Furthermore, an agenda allows the person chairing the meeting to refocus the group if necessary and provides an opportunity for all items on the agenda to be addressed. Box 11-5 provides an agenda outline to be used in facilitating a staff meeting.
- Include every member of the team in the meeting. Do not ask one person to answer the phone or receive deliveries; use an answering service. Leave an informative message on the answering machine for callers, which provide information about when the call will be returned. In the event that a delivery occurs or a patient comes into the office, staff members should alternate in attending to these responsibilities. Prior to the start of the meeting, ask for volunteers to take on these responsibilities should they occur.
- Every member of the dental team should contribute to the meeting by providing suggestions for improvement or areas of concern they require assistance with. This can be encouraged by asking each member of the dental team to bring one item of discussion to the meeting that they feel either requires attention or is working well.
- Encourage team members to bring a possible solution if they have a complaint to voice at the meeting. A staff member who feels that a task or procedure

BOX 11-5
Monthly Staff Meeting Agenda

1. Review previous meeting agenda and minutes.
2. Focus on upcoming month or 3 months.
3. Review goals and attainments of previous month.
4. Discuss patient feedback/concerns.
5. Have individual staff members discuss relevant department issues.
6. Discussion solutions to any issues.

should be changed in the dental office should be encouraged to provide a solution for discussion at the meeting. Encouraging all staff members to involve themselves in the discussion toward change can bring about a solution quickly, and one which the most agrees with.

- Consider providing food or an educational presentation to encourage attendance at meetings. A lunchtime meeting is desirable when lunch can be provided for staff members. Dental product and supply companies often provide "lunch and learn" sessions for staff in the dental office. The dental supply representative attends the dental office, lunch is provided for the staff members, and an educational seminar is given to staff regarding a specific product. The seminar usually is 1 hour in length. An added benefit is that most staff members can receive continuing education points as required by the professional licensing body.

If conducted properly, employees will look forward to staff meetings because they provide an opportunity for dialogue with coworkers regarding topics of concern and solutions are often discovered. A sense of camaraderie is also fostered as all staff members are apprised of the latest improvements and changes in the dental office, and their suggestions are integrated into the modifications.

Morning Staff Meetings

Morning meetings are typically held before seeing the first patient of the day. With the entire dental team in attendance, the intention of the meeting is to review the daily schedule and discuss areas where team members can assist one another in managing the flow of patients. Once the office has been prepared for the arrival of patients, time should be set aside prior to the office opening for the meeting. The morning meeting is short, usually 10 minutes, and should be held at a time when all staff members can attend. It is designed to improve the overall efficiency and consistency of communication among staff members regarding the patient flow in the dental office for the day ahead. The daily schedule and the patients who are attending the clinic that day are the focus of the morning meeting. The dental practitioners are informed of patient concerns, which can range from financial, medical, or personal. As the dental office administrator, your responsibility regarding the morning meeting consists of informing the dentist or dental hygienist of any information or issues the patient has raised when the appointment was scheduled. For example, if a patient coming in to see the dentist has just returned from a vacation in Europe, remind the dentist of this since it is a good conversation starting point when the patient arrives. Another example may be to inform the hygienist that a patient they are seeing has requested that radiographs not be taken at the appointment. Although each patient should give permission prior to any treatment performed, providing the hygienist with this information allows for preparation regarding an explanation for the purpose of radiographs. Ensuring that all staff members have the same information about each patient from the start of the day will create positive attitudes and the cohesiveness required to create a productive day. Box 11-6 provides an agenda

BOX 11-6
Morning Meeting Agenda

1. Open the meeting with an invitation for staff to identify personal concerns (phone call expected, leave early).
2. Discuss the number of patients being seen that day.
3. Point out any concerns for the dentist or hygienist to note regarding patients.
4. Address acceptable times to schedule emergency patients.
5. End with a positive/thoughtful quote.

checkPOINT

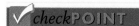

7. What is the purpose of the morning meeting?

that can be used to facilitate the morning meeting. Guidelines for facilitating a morning meeting are as follows:

- Have the person most informed about the schedule for the day facilitate the morning meeting, typically the office administrator or scheduling coordinator.
- Ensure that the entire team is present at the meeting to have the greatest communication success.
- Make sure there is at least 10 minutes to have the meeting.
- Keep staff members on track by focusing discussion on the daily schedule.

Open Door Policy

Facilitating effective and positive staff communication can be performed by maintaining an open door policy by the office manager. This means that all members of the dental team are welcome and encouraged to approach the office manager regarding questions or concerns that may arise. Being available to team members at any time sends a message that team member concerns are valid and important. The office manager should inform each member of the team of the open door policy and maintain an approachable demeanor toward staff to follow through with this.

Often, when it gets busy in the dental office, there may not be time to communicate personally with staff members. In such situations, using the office e-mail system can provide an avenue for communication from the office manager. Information and messages can be sent to employees regularly and quickly, and responses can be received just as easily. In other situations, however, direct personal communication is required, for example, when recognizing employees for outstanding work and on special occasions, such as birthdays. Such recognition adds to the cohesiveness in the dental team.

HIRING, EVALUATING, AND TERMINATING STAFF

The office manager in the dental office serves as the liaison between the dentist and the staff. Often the dental office administrator will assist the office manager in carrying out duties related to staff management and development. If you become an office manager, a large amount of your time will be spent on issues related to staff management, specifically, hiring, evaluating, and terminating staff. This responsibility can be a challenging one and for this reason requires a fair amount of preparation in carrying out the tasks involved. In a small dental practice, the dental office administrator may be required to assist the dentist in carrying out these duties. In a practice with more than one dentist, an office manager will likely handle all staff-related responsibilities. Your understanding of the process involved with hiring, evaluating, and terminating employees will prepare you for the opportunity to assist with, or take on, the responsibility of staff management and help you to gain a better understanding of the staff management process. The section that follows focuses on staff management and the components relating to effective management in this area.

Hiring

One of the responsibilities of an office manager in the dental office involves the management of employees. Hiring, one component of the staff management process, is the first step to building a winning dental team and requires a unique set of analytical and interpersonal skills, including crafting a job description for the open position and interviewing and assessing prospective employees.

Before beginning the search for candidates for a position, you must first develop a **job description**, or written outline of the specific duties and responsibilities related to that position. Figure 11-3 provides a sample job description for a clinical

JOB DESCRIPTION: DENTAL ASSISTANT

Job Summary
The Dental Assistant is a professional employee, trained to provide direct assistance to the Dentist. The Dental Assistant functions under the direction, instruction and supervision of the Dentist.

Qualifications
- Must be 18 years of age or older and able to read and write consistent with job requirements
- Has at least one year of experience as a Dental Assistant
- Holds registration from an accredited school of Dental Assisting and is registered to practice in Alberta
- Shows evidence of fulfilling health requirements of the clinic
- Has a reliable means of transportation

Responsibilities
- Assists the Dentist chairside
- Seats the patients and does a preliminary evaluation of their health history and chief complaint
- Reports all findings to the Dentist in a professional manner
- Sets up and breaks down rooms for each procedure using proper infection control and barrier techniques
- Sterilizes all instruments and equipment as required by the clinic standards
- Practices honesty, dependability and confidentiality regarding all patient matters
- Correctly documents treatment notes and dental charting as required
- Assists with front office duties as needed and as available

FIGURE 11-3 Job description: clinical staff member.

employee in the dental office, and Chapter 1 provides a job description for a dental office administrator. The job description serves several purposes. First, it can be used in advertisements aimed at prospective employees to give them an idea of what the position entails. Second, it can be used by the office manager to evaluate the suitability of a potential employee for a position. Finally, it can be used after a person is hired to evaluate his or her performance, relative to established expectations.

*check*POINT

8. What is the purpose of a job description?

Ensuring that the job description is written correctly and accurately is the responsibility of the office manager. When duties and responsibilities change, the job description must be updated to reflect these changes. Asking employees to assist in updating their job descriptions is beneficial for the team, since it includes staff members in the cooperation of changes in the practice.

Writing job descriptions can be performed using a computer software program, if required. Job descriptions and their format vary between dental offices. The job description example in Figure 11-3 uses three main categories. More detailed job descriptions may use the following categories:

- Job title
- Supervisor
- Position summary
- Hours
- Location
- Employment requirements
- Duties
- Evaluation process
- Salary or pay scale range

Any revisions made on the job description should be included on the form.

Employees hired in the dental office can be recruited by advertising in the classified section of the local newspaper, through word of mouth, or through an educational institution. Regardless of the type of advertising, always request that each applicant for the position submit a resume with the application. In Chapter 20, we will discuss the recruitment process in more depth.

Interviewing applicants may be the sole responsibility of the office manager. When the list of applicants has been shortened to two or three, other staff members may become involved in the interviewing process. The goal of including staff members in the decision-making process is to garner as many opinions as possible about the potential employee from all staff and better assess whether the person will fit with the present team.

The interview process in the dental office is arranged by the office manager or office administrator. The people involved in the interview process make the decision as to how the interview will be carried out. That is, whether it will be a formal interview that involves a structured question-and-answer format or a more relaxed conversational style interview, is at the discretion of the manager or dentist. Regardless of the preferred interview format, it is necessary to set aside time at some point in the day in order to have a face-to-face interview with the applicant.

If an advertisement has been placed in the classified section of the newspaper, it is likely that there are resumes that have been submitted or applicants have attended the dental office to complete a job application form (Fig. 11-4). Once you have compiled all resumes and applications, you will need to review them and select the most suitable candidates for an interview. A suitable candidate will have either previous job experience or an academic background that prepares the person for working in a dental office, such as a dental administration or clinical certification. The advertisement for the position should include the following components:

- Title of the position and a brief description of the main duties. Providing all of the detailed information of the position is costly to include in the job advertisement and should be discussed at the job interview. Keep the description brief.
- Describe the type of personality required for the position. Words such as friendly, enthusiastic, or hard working should be used to describe the personality best suited for the position.
- Hourly wage or salary information. If the remuneration is dependent on the applicant's experience, this should be indicated in the job advertisement. You could also request that the applicant indicate his or her expectations regarding salary when the application is submitted.
- Contact information for the position, such as the name and address of the dental office and how the applicant should apply, that is, should the person fax or mail his or her resume, or come to the office in person to apply.

Interviewing candidates requires a certain amount of time throughout the work day be set aside. Each suitable applicant should be contacted and a day and time for an interview should be offered. The amount of time set aside for one interview should be approximately 1 hour. Conducting an effective and productive job interview depends on asking the right questions. Make sure the questions you ask are relevant to the position in question. Prepare a list of questions to ask the applicant and stick to the questions to conduct the interview within the time allotted. The object of the interview is to assess the ability of the applicant to perform the duties of the position in a way that complements the dentists' style of managing the dental practice. Box 11-7 provides a list of some of the questions asked of potential employees at a job interview. Try to avoid asking closed-end questions, since this type of question is not likely to provide the insight needed in making a hiring decision. Another method of questioning used in job interviews involves the use of a hypothetical situation posed to the applicant. The applicant is presented with a hypothetical scenario and asked to describe how the situation should be managed. The response of the applicant provides an indication of how the situation would be handled in real life and can influence the hiring decision.

Throughout the interview process, the applicant will provide information about his or her work habits, skill proficiency, and overall attitude concerning the position. Sometimes information can be provided to the interviewer in the form of red flag; that is, the candidate will provide information that can signal an attitude that could pose as a potential problem if the candidate were to be hired. For example, if during the interview the candidate was highly critical of a previous employer or supervisor,

APPLICATION FOR EMPLOYMENT

PERSONAL INFORMATION **DATE OF APPLICATION:** ______

Name: ______
Last First Middle

Address: ______
Street (Apt) City, State Zip

Contact Information: ( ) ( ) ______
Home Telephone Mobile Email

How did you learn about our company? ______

POSITION SOUGHT: ______ **Available Start Date:** ______

Desired Pay Range: ______ **Are you currently employed?** ______

EDUCATION

	Name and Location	Diploma Received	Area of Study
High School			
College or University			
Specialized Training, Trade School, etc...			
Other Education			

Please list your areas of highest proficiency, special skills or other items that may contribute to your abilities in performing the above mentioned position.

FIGURE 11-4 **Job application form.**

PREVIOUS EXPERIENCE

Please list beginning from most recent

Dates Employed	Company Name	Location	Role/Title

Job notes, tasks performed and reason for leaving:

Dates Employed	Company Name	Location	Role/Title

Job notes, tasks performed and reason for leaving:

Dates Employed	Company Name	Location	Role/Title

Job notes, tasks performed and reason for leaving:

REFERENCES

Please provide the names of three references who can provide information concerning your skills for the position applied for. Do not include names of friends or family members.

Name ____________ Phone ____________ Position ____________

Name ____________ Phone ____________ Position ____________

Name ____________ Phone ____________ Position ____________

I agree to have my references contacted in regards to the position I have applied for.

Applicant Name (Print) Applicant Signature Date

FIGURE 11-4 *(Continued)*

BOX 11-7
Interview Questions

- How comfortable do you feel asking patients for money?
- What are your best qualities (strengths)?
- What areas of dental administration would you like to improve in?
- How do you react in stressful situations?
- What would your past employer say is your greatest strength?
- What area of this position will be most challenging for you?
- How would you manage an angry patient?
- What work experience have you had that will benefit you in this position?
- How do you intend to continue learning about advances in the administration of the dental office?
- Where do you see yourself in 5 years?
- Can you describe a situation where you dealt with a patient who was anxious about dental treatment?
- How would you manage a situation with a colleague who was upset with you–or with whom you were upset with?
- How would you respond to a patient who was dissatisfied with one of the staff members in the office?

it could indicate that the individual may have difficulties working with other people or taking direction from others. Asking the candidate additional questions relating to getting along with coworkers may provide further information about the individual's abilities in this area. Box 11-8 gives additional examples of red flags to be recognized at the interview.

The dentist usually has the final say in the hiring of new employees in the dental office. This is often the reason that a second interview is requested. Once the candidate selection has been narrowed down to one or two potential employees, a second interview is held with the dentist, and possibly one other staff member, in attendance. The dentist may have a more in-depth line of questioning for the candidate that focuses on the use of scenario-based, or behavioral questions. For example, the dentist may pose a scenario to the potential employee, such as "You have just received a call from Mr. Jones who is experiencing a lot of pain in a fourth

BOX 11-8
Red Flags in the Interview Process

- **Canceling the interview.** If the candidate cancels the interview for reasons other than an emergency, this could indicate that getting the job is not that important.
- **Asking about salary and time off right away.** A candidate who addresses concerns about salary and time-off eligibility at the start of the interview is likely more interested in what they can get, which means that loyalty and work ethic may be lacking.
- **No research about the industry or organization.** A candidate who has not taken the time to research the dental office by either searching the company Web site or asking about the company early in the interview, a lack of genuine interest in the company may be evident.
- **Silence.** A candidate who is quiet and responds minimally to questions may not be the ideal candidate for a dental office administration position. Pay attention to how the candidate communicates with you during the interview, this could indicative of communication will occur on the job.
- **Poor references.** Every employee hired in the dental office should provide the names of past employers who can provide information about past work performance. If the references who are contacted provide information regarding the applicant which is not favorable, or the candidate is unable to provide employment references, be wary, as this may be indicative of a candidate who has not shown positive work performance in the past.

quadrant molar. Mr. Jones insists that he would just like to have a pain reliever and he will be fine. He does not want to make an appointment to see the dentist. How are you going to respond to Mr. Jones?" In this scenario, your response should include the importance of the diagnosis made by the dentist to prescribe the correct medications. The second interview may also involve providing the candidate with a tour of the office, and meeting other members of the dental team. Alternatively, the second interview may be less structured and involve a more hands-on approach to the duties of the position. The second interview may include the candidate either observing or working in the dental office for a short period of time, such as a few hours or a full day. If the candidate returns to the dental office for a few hours of work or observation, this is referred to as a working interview. A **working interview** can be suggested to gain a more in-depth picture of the applicant and the working environment and the applicant works either voluntarily or with pay for the prospective employer. This type of interview allows both the employer and potential employee to ascertain if the position is suitable. The nature of the administrative duties in the dental office may require knowledge of a particular computer program, familiarity with the dental treatment philosophy, and knowledge of the treatment provided. If the potential employee does not have a firm grasp on these components, a training period is usually provided when hired and the working interview may be limited to certain tasks such as telephone answering, filing, and assisting with appointment scheduling. Throughout the working interview, the employee will have the opportunity to work with other members of the team, for this reason it is important to solicit information from other staff members about their experience with the candidate to assist you in your evaluation. The following questions could be used as guide:

- Did the candidate offer to help other staff members or patients?
- Was the candidate interested in learning about processes used in the office?
- Did the candidate take notes?
- Was the appearance of the candidate appropriate and professional?
- Did the candidate perform the tasks assigned in an acceptable manner?
- Does the candidate agree with the philosophy of the dental practice?

It is important to solicit the advice from other staff members who have worked directly with the candidate during the working interview. Often staff members observe work habits of other employees which may not have been seen by the dentist, office manager, or administrator. Once the working interview is complete, advise the potential employee that you will contact him or her by the end of the next working day. This time period allows the employer to discuss and evaluate the candidate's performance and also gives the candidate an opportunity to ponder the reality of working in the dental office.

Before hiring any employee, the office manager must be prepared to perform a **reference check.** Checking references means contacting past employers of the applicant to verify employment experience and work ethic displayed by the applicant. Just as with job interviews, there are questions that cannot be asked legally and preparation for reference checks is necessary. Figure 11-5 provides an example of reference check questions to ask. A minimum of three references should be contacted, and all of them should be past employers of the applicant. Contacting a personal friend of the applicant is not likely to provide you with an accurate picture of the candidate's work habits.

Once a decision has been made as to the hiring of the new employee, an employee agreement is usually presented for signature. Each employee is given his or her own individualized employee agreement. The information found on an employee agreement includes the following:

- Position
- Wages
- Period of employment

legal TIP

During the interview, it is important to stick to the list of prepared questions used for interviewing prospective employees in the dental office. Asking questions that may be construed as discriminatory should be avoided. This includes any questions that pertain to a person's age, religion, or marital status. In other words, if the question does not relate to the position applied for and the duties of the job, the question should be asked of the applicant. For example, asking the applicant if he or she is married is not a legally acceptable question to ask because the information gained by asking the question can be used to discriminate against the person. Other questions that should be avoided are any questions related to race, creed, color, sex, age, disability, or marital status.

REFERENCE CHECK

Dental Office Professional Corporation

CANDIDATE	DATE	CHECK CONDUCTED BY
POSITION	**DEPARTMENT**	**HIRING MANAGER**

INSTRUCTIONS

Please complete this form when you check a candidate's references.

BACKGROUND

How long have you known [Candidate's Name]?

JOB RESPONSIBILITIES

What position(s) did he/she hold? What were his/her primary responsibilities?

STRENGTHS AND WEAKNESSES

Describe are his/her strengths and weaknesses.

COMMUNICATION SKILLS

Does [candidate] have strong written communication skills? Presentation skills?

FIGURE 11-5 Reference check.

INTERPERSONAL SKILLS
How well did he/she get along with his/her manager? With teammates? With customers?

MANAGEMENT STYLE PREFERENCE
Under what management style does he/she perform well?

TIME MANAGEMENT
Does he/she manage his/her time well? Does he/she successfully prioritize and manage his/her workload effectively? Is he/she punctual and reliable?

ATTITUDE
How would you describe his/her attitude toward his/her job? During difficult or stressful situations?

REASON FOR LEAVING
Do you know why he/she left your company? –or– Do you know why he/she is interested in a position outside your company?

COMMENTS

FIGURE 11-5 *(Continued)*

- Tax withholding
- Working hours
- Vacation times
- Confidentiality agreement

Figure 11-6 is an example of an employee agreement that includes all of these categories and an explanation of each category.

Evaluating

All employees must be evaluated at some point during their employment. The frequency of evaluation is specific to each dental office. For example, some dental offices have a policy of an annual evaluation; others provide a biannual evaluation. It is important to evaluate employees on a regular basis. New employees are often evaluated 3 months after their start date, and then at their 1-year anniversary.

An **employee evaluation** is also known as a performance appraisal. It is designed to assess the on-the-job performance of employees and provide annual goals in the clinic that they can personally attain. All employees are required to sign and date their evaluations. Employee evaluations should be a positive experience.

Often, an employee's self-evaluation is part of the evaluation process. Typically, the employee is given a self-evaluation form 1 week prior to the evaluation date and asked to complete it. This practice provides the employee with a guide as to what areas will be evaluated and can make the process less anxiety provoking. Furthermore, it gives the employees the opportunity to acknowledge their weaknesses or areas that need improvement, which can make the office manager's job much easier during the evaluation.

Often, an employee's self-evaluation is part of the evaluation process. Typically, the employee is given a self-evaluation form 1 week prior to the evaluation date and asked to complete it. This practice provides the employee with a guide as to what areas will be evaluated and can make the process less anxiety provoking. Furthermore, it gives the employees the opportunity to acknowledge areas that require improvement and a chance to seek out direction as to how the challenges he or she is experiencing can be overcome. Some examples of general questions used in a self-evaluation are as follows:

- What skills have helped you achieve success in your current position?
- What area of your position is the most challenging for you?
- Do you feel you need further training or education in a specific area of your position?
- What have you achieved in the past year in your position that you are most proud of?
- Are there any other areas in the dental office you would like to consider working in?

The process of the employee evaluation can be a daunting task, and one that can be anxiety provoking for both the employee and employer. The following guidelines can be used for performing the employee evaluation. Providing the employee with a self-evaluation to prepare prior to the meeting assures the employee of the items that will be discussed at the review. Figure 11-7 is an example of an employee self-evaluation questionnaire. The questionnaire used can be tailored to the dental office specifically by adding questions and developing a preferred format.

Preparation

The employee evaluation should be conducted at a time and place where no distractions or interruptions will occur. Generally, the employee review is conducted on an annual basis, usually around the anniversary date that the employee began the position. The meeting should last approximately 1 hour. Schedule the review

EMPLOYEE AGREEMENT

Dated this _______________ day of _______________, 20 _____.

Between

Dental Office Professional Corporation (hereinafter referred to as the "Company")

AND

_____________________________ (hereinafter referred to as the "Employee")

1. **Position**

You will serve in a _______________ capacity as _______________ of the Company. Your supervisor will be _______________ and your duties will include, but not be limited to those attached (Attachment A), and may change over time.

2. **Wages**

You will be paid a salary at an hourly rate of $ _______________ per hour. Wages are paid on a monthly basis, on the last working day of every month, with an advance given on the 15th of the month. This hourly pay rate will be subject to adjustment pursuant to the Company's employee compensation policies in effect, from time to time.

3. **Period of Employment**

Your employment with the Company will be 'at will' meaning that either you or the Company will be entitled to terminate your employment at any time and for any reason, as per the regulations set out by the Province of Alberta, Employment Standards Act.

4. **Tax Withholding**

All forms of compensation referred to in this agreement are subject to reduction to reflect applicable withholding and payroll taxes.

5. **Working Hours**

Hours of work are dictated by the daily patient schedule, and includes the following hours, on the following days : Monday and Tuesday 11am until 8pm, Wednesday and Thursday 7:30am until 3:30pm and Friday 7:30 until 1pm.

6. **Vacations**

As per the Employment Standards Act, employees are entitled to the following vacation time:
After one year of employment : 2 weeks
After five years of employment : 3 weeks

Vacation pay is calculated at the rate of 4% of the employees' monthly gross wage. The employee has the option of having vacation pay paid on a monthly basis, or on a 'as need' basis.

7. **Confidentiality Agreement**

You agree that during your employment with the Company, you will not improperly use or disclose any confidential or proprietary information about the Company.

This agreement accepted on the ___________________________ day of ___________________________, 20_____.

____
EMPLOYEE

____
WITNESS

____
PROFESSIONAL CORPORATION REPRESENTATIVE

FIGURE 11-6 Employee agreement.

Employee Self-Evaluation of Performance

Name of Employee:
Job Title:
Date of Evaluation:

1. Please give a summary of job your responsibilities.
2. How do you feel about your performance as an employee over the last year? (Please discuss areas such as: attitude, motivation, initiative, quality of work, and productivity.)
3. What kinds of skills have you needed to fulfill your responsibilities over this past year? (For example: organizational, interpersonal, written & verbal communications, problem-solving skills.)
4. What have you accomplished over the last year? (For example: personal or company goals met, tasks accomplished, or anything you feel most proud of.)
5. What would you like to accomplish over the next year? (For example: performance improvements, tasks, goals, new skills.)
6. What other skills or experience do you have that you would like to be using in your job?
7. What would help you better perform your work responsibilities? (For example: communication skills, continuing education.)
8. How would you evaluate your overall performance over the last year?
9. Additional comments.

FIGURE 11-7 Employee self-evaluation.

approximately 2 weeks in advance and provide the employee with a self-evaluation form to complete for the meeting. The employee self-evaluation form will have questions that are similar in nature to the employee evaluation form completed by the employer (Fig. 11-8). In preparation for completing the employee evaluation form, gather the employees' file that should contain information such as the last performance review documents, a job description of the position the employee currently occupies, and any disciplinary or wage increase information. A past performance review in the employee file can provide information regarding areas requiring growth and areas of achievement and can assist in evaluating the employees' recent performance. A job description provides the objectives and competencies the employee should be meeting to perform the job effectively. The job description should be used as the basis of the evaluation.

Agenda

Developing an agenda of how the meeting will unfold is an effective way to keep the meeting on track, within the time allotted, and ensures you will address all areas of the performance review. Always begin the meeting in a friendly way, some employees may be anxious and putting them at ease right away will help in conducting a productive meeting. Make small talk with the employee about the weather or current events. If the employee seems overly anxious, address the issue by asking, "Are you nervous about this meeting?" Inform the employee of the agenda outline for the meeting; that is, what points will be discussed in the order of the agenda. Assure the employee that the goal of the meeting is to assist the development of the employee in his or her current position. You should then address the overall summary of the performance evaluation. Outline the strengths the employee has, and then address the challenges you see the employee experiencing in his or her role. Always use specific examples for both areas of strength and weakness. Allow the employee to explain the self-evaluation form he or she completed prior to the review. Ask the employee to cite examples if there are discrepancies between the employer and employee assessment. Discuss the final assessment of the evaluation, that is, the raise or promotion awarded, or why the employee will remain at the current pay scale or position. The

Employee Performance Appraisal

Name:	**Job Title:**
Department:	**Supervisor:**
Date of Review:	**Date of Last Review:**

Performance Ratings

1 _____ **Excellent:** Consistent performer who consistently exceeds expectations in all areas.

2 _____ **Good:** Frequently exceeds performance expectations for essential job duties.

3 _____ **Satisfactory:** Meets job requirements in accordance with established standards.

5 _____ **Improvement needed:** Overall performance acceptable, but improvement needed in one or more areas.

Performance Areas

1. Completes work on time and without sacrificing performance goals or standards.

RATING ____________
Comments/Examples:

2. Able to work on a team and willingly accepts assignments.

RATING ____________
Comments/Examples;

3. Initiates tasks without guidance.

RATING ____________
Comments/Examples:

4. Uses time and resources to accomplish work within appropriate deadlines.

RATING _____
Comments/Examples:

5. Accuracy and conciseness of written and verbal communication.

RATING ____________
Comments/Examples:

6. Works well with others in both informal and formal situations.

RATING ____________
Comments/Examples:

Improvements/Accomplishments:

Areas for further development and suggestions for achievement:

Overall Evaluation

Excellent
Good
Satisfactory
Improvement needed

Date of Next Review ______________________

Additional Comments:

This performance review has been explained to me and I understand the comments and overall evaluation.

______________________ ______________________

Employer Signature Employee Signature

____

Date

FIGURE 11-8 Employee performance evaluation.

rating system used should be outlined on the performance evaluation form. It should be clear to the employee what the achievement should be to gain an increase in pay or promotion. Each dental office is different in this regard. For example, developing a new skill through an educational program and used in a way that benefits the dental office may contribute to being awarded a raise in pay. Rating systems used will always address whether the employee is performing in the position at an unsatisfactory (below the minimum expected level), satisfactory (at the expected level), or excellent or exceptional level (performing more than the expected duties).

Feedback

Throughout the employee evaluation meeting, feedback is provided to the employee. It is important to provide honest feedback to the employee and provide examples to confirm the feedback you are providing. If the employee is having difficulty in achieving some of the objectives of the job description, provide some solutions for achieving the objectives. Giving the employee encouragement in situations of challenge can assist in helping the employee meet the objectives. As the meeting draws to a close, try not to end on a negative note. That is, if the employee needs to improve in certain areas, focus on how this improvement can occur. If the employee has made some major accomplishments over the past year, focus on those accomplishments. The employee should leave the meeting feeling hopeful that achievements are possible which further lessen the anxiety associated with future performance evaluation meetings.

Taking Disciplinary Action and Terminating

Employee termination is an inevitable event in the business of running a dental office. The reasons employees are terminated vary and are dependent on the policies regarding employee performance in the dental office. Reasons for termination can be a result of an employee wrongdoing such as the inability of the employee to do his or her job because he or she is unable to communicate effectively with patients, or despite repeated training with the computer program he or she is unable to properly use the computer. There are also reasons for terminating an employee that are out of the control of the employee, such as downsizing, or layoffs that occur because too many staff members are employed in the dental office and business has slowed down.

In the event that you must terminate an employee, always make sure that you are prepared to deliver the news to the employee and have followed the policies leading up to terminating an employee. In other words, do not fire an employee "on the spot" when you are angry about the situation. For example, an employee who arrives 30 minutes late for work for the fifth time in 1 month would anger most managers and the other employees who depend on them. In this situation, the employee should be asked to either leave the premises and return to the office the next day to discuss the situation or asked to wait in the manager's office. In the meantime, a period of time is provided for both employer and employee to prepare for what may be the inevitable result of termination.

Informing an employee that he or she will not be remaining as an employee in the dental office can be a difficult task for the office manager. There is a process that should be followed to come to the decision of termination. Before an employee is terminated, the following steps in the disciplinary process should be carried out:

- Having one-on-one meetings with the employee, including regular performance evaluations, in which any concerns with the employee's performance are discussed.
- Issuing a verbal warning to the employee regarding potential consequences of his or her failure to meet performance expectations.
- Recording in writing any concerns with the employee's performance.
- Issuing at least three written warnings prior to termination.

The first warning you give to an employee should be a verbal warning. This is often performed at the first instance of an employee not following office policy, for example, when an employee is late or does not complete a certain task. A record should be made and placed in the employee file that a verbal warning was given. Written, documented warnings are often used when a verbal warning has gone unheeded or a more serious concern arises, such as failure to show for work or breach of patient confidentiality. A written warning must be discussed with the employee and signed by the employee, and a copy provided to him or her. Generally, three written warnings are provided to an employee prior to termination. The written warning includes the date of warning, the area of concern, and points made during the discussion from both the manager and staff member. Providing the employee with a written warning to improve performance is documentation of failure to improve and, hence, grounds for termination. It also provides evidence should the employee decide to file a lawsuit against the employer.

During the meeting in which you are terminating the employee, the following guidelines are useful for ensuring the meeting is conducted as planned:

1. Review with the employee the steps followed regarding the number of verbal and written warnings and the days on which the warnings were issued.
2. Review the steps taken by both the employer and employee to ensure that progress was made regarding the area of concern, and ask the employee to describe what steps have been taken toward progress.
3. Discuss whether or not any progress has been made based on the steps required to make progress.
4. Specifically state to the employee that he or she is being terminated. It is important to be clear and direct to avoid misunderstanding. For example, for an employee who has been late six times in the last month you could say "Andrea, yesterday you were 30 minutes late, this was the sixth time this month that you have been at least 30 minutes late. You know this is a violation of the office policy. Everyone in the office must adhere to the same policies, so I must terminate your employment effective immediately."
5. Ask the employee if he or she understands the reasons for the termination. If he or she does not, provide an explanation.
6. Provide the employee with his or her final paycheck, including any vacation pay or unused sick time. Also include termination papers required to collect employment benefits.
7. Ask the employee to return any material that would be considered company property, such as keys, lab coats, or parking passes. Allow the employee approximately 30 minutes to gather personal belongings and return any company items to you.

checkPOINT

9. What steps are involved in the disciplinary process?
10. Why should an employee be given a warning in writing?

Administrative TIP

When addressing a performance concern with an employee, make sure that the first meeting you have with the employee is a positive one. Go over the issues involved in an exact manner to ensure a clear understanding of what must be improved upon. Using the job description, outline the expectations and pinpoint areas of concern. Make sure that you remind the employee of his or her value to the practice and your desire to help him or her be successful as a team member. Explain that consistent performance on his or her part creates success in his or her position. Outline the daily activities of the employee and the expectations for those activities. Ask the employee if there are any areas for improvement that he or she is unclear about. Provide a thorough explanation if required. Always end the meeting on a positive note; you want the employee to leave the meeting feeling hopeful, not dejected!

Once an employee is terminated, the other members of the staff may feel a sense of insecurity in their positions. The reasons for the termination are confidential and should not be discussed with the other staff members. It is important to reassure the other staff members that they can feel secure in their positions. A statement of verbal praise can be reassuring for staff members. The nature of the dental office allows employees to become familiar with patients and when an employee is terminated, patients may ask about the employee. Inform the patient that the employee no longer works in the office and assure them that the person who has replaced the employee will be providing the high quality of treatment they are used to receive. Maintain a professional attitude by not discussing any details regarding the situation, that is, whether or not the employee resigned or was terminated.

The disciplinary actions used in the dental office must be clear and outlined for all team members. Following the disciplinary process is important to avoid lawsuits from terminated employees. Providing a fair and equal disciplinary process is also important so that all team members are treated equally and know what to expect.

CONTINUING EDUCATION

The clinical employees in the dental office are responsible for acquiring a certain number of continuing education points each year to maintain their standing with their licensing body. Depending on the office policies, the office manager may have a role in helping to provide or facilitate opportunities for continuing education. Often the dental office administrator or the dental office manager will organize the lunch-and-learn educational seminars for the entire staff to attend. For example, dental supply and equipment companies often have a representative available to provide an educational seminar to dental office employees. The office manager is responsible for contacting the company representative and asking him or her to provide a seminar in the office. These seminars are often approximately 1-hour long, and continuing education points are awarded to all participants who attend. These educational seminars are referred to as a "lunch and learn" seminar. The company representative attends the office for 1 hour, usually during the lunch hour, and presents a product or procedure to the staff and provides lunch at the same time.

In addition to such formal educational programs, the office manager can provide staff with up-to-date information regarding the dental industry in other ways. Having dental magazines and journals available for staff members to read and encouraging staff to attend seminars offered outside of the dental office are options available for staff education.

Continuing education policies must be outlined in the office policy manual. Staff members must be made aware of their responsibility regarding educational obligations and what areas they can expect to receive assistance from the office manager.

Chapter Summary

The role of the office administrator can be expanded to include various staff management-related functions. As we discussed in this chapter, the contents and development of the office procedure manual as well as the maintenance of the manual help to maintain the rules to follow for the dental office to function effectively and provide a foundation to which all employees can refer. In conjunction with the policies outlined in the office manual, regular staff meetings also facilitate the regular communication required between management and staff members in the dental office. The office administrator has a role in the organization and management of the staff meeting, particularly in dental offices where the staff members are few and the office administrator takes on the responsibility of ensuring the staff meeting occurs.

The office manager or dentist takes on the responsibility of hiring, evaluating, and terminating staff in the dental office. Following the processes and policies established in this regard allows for a smooth transition in these areas to occur. The office manager or dentist may require the assistance of the office administrator throughout the hiring process, particularly when a second interview or working interview is required and feedback about the candidate's performance is requested.

Review Questions

Multiple Choice

1. **To provide effective management for employees, which of the following components are necessary?**
   a. Employment guidelines
   b. Regular hours
   c. Salary increases
   d. Morning meetings

2. **A working interview is beneficial to**
   a. give the applicant the chance to work in the office.
   b. gain a more in-depth picture of the applicant.
   c. assess if the applicant has skills.
   d. allow the applicant to accept the position.

3. **Staff meetings**
   a. should be held monthly.
   b. are an opportunity to air grievances.
   c. should be no longer than 45 minutes.
   d. are best held after office hours.

4. **Terminating an employee should be performed**
   a. after the first verbal warning.
   b. once a third verbal warning is given.
   c. after the third written warning is given.
   d. by the dentist.

5. **The hiring process can include all of the following except**
   a. working interview.
   b. reference check once the employee is hired.
   c. staff involvement with interview.
   d. review of office policies.

6. **Scripts and forms for employees to use to perform job tasks should be included in the**
   a. job description.
   b. employee handbook.
   c. policy and procedures manual.
   d. emergency procedures manual.

7. **Which of the following is a question that should not be asked by an employer during the candidate interview?**
   a. What would your past employer say regarding your work ethic?
   b. How many sick days have you taken this past year?
   c. Do you practice a particular religion?
   d. What day can you start work?

8. **Which of the following should be used as the basis of the employee evaluation?**
   a. Office policy and procedures manual
   b. Department of labor guidelines
   c. Outline of the job description
   d. Meeting agenda

9. **Which of the following statements best describes the employee evaluation process?**
   a. An on-the-job assessment of the employee.
   b. A process that involves the employee in job assessment and realistic goal attainment.
   c. An opportunity for the employee to admit weakness and fault.
   d. An evaluation of the dental practice and the employee based loosely on staff comments.

10. **Warnings regarding performance should be provided to the employee**
    a. only in writing.
    b. at a scheduled meeting.
    c. verbally.
    d. verbally first and then in writing.

Critical Thinking

1. If you were offered the position of office manager in a dental office, which areas do you think would be most challenging to you, and why?

2. Imagine that you are an office manager and that you are meeting with an employee to discuss his performance. There are a few aspects of the employee's performance that require improvement. Describe how you would discuss the issues with the employee and what steps would you take to ensure the employee could meet the goals set out?

HANDS-ON ACTIVITY

1. Develop a one-page outline for a policy and procedure manual for a dental office, with a description for each section.
2. An employee in the office has been wearing a lot of perfume and has been asked on two occasions to discontinue wearing perfume to the office. The employee arrived at work today wearing a lot of perfume. Write up a written warning for the employee regarding this infraction.
3. With a partner, conduct an interview for the position of office administrator. Draw up a list of questions to follow, and an agenda to keep the interview on track.

chapter TWELVE

Filing Procedures

OUTLINE

OBJECTIVES

After completing this chapter, you should be able to do the following:

- Spell and define key terms
- Identify the four basic steps followed to ensure accurate filing
- Describe the alphabetical and numerical filing systems
- Identify and describe other filing systems used in the dental office
- List the main types of filing cabinets and supplies
- Explain the impact Health Insurance Portability and Accountability Act (HIPAA) has on filing in the dental office
- Explain what active and inactive patient charts are and how they are stored in the dental office
- Describe the process used for transferring patient information
- List some guidelines for electronic filing

KEY TERMS

- conditioning
- indexing
- sorting
- storing
- alphabetical filing system
- numerical filing system
- geographical filing system
- subject filing system
- chronological filing system
- active patients
- inactive patients

Every time a patient comes into the dental office for an appointment or has a conversation with an employee of the office relating to his or her treatment, the patient's chart must be retrieved from the filing system, documentation must be made in the chart, and the chart must be replaced. In a busy dental practice, this can mean a large number of patient charts are handled throughout the day. Given this activity and the significance of the patient charts, paying attention to the filing system and correctly filing charts in their place is an important responsibility. Errors in filing charts can lead to frustration when the chart is required by a staff member to facilitate patient care. In addition to managing patient charts, the office administrator is typically responsible for filing financial documents, as well, which are filed separately from the patient charts. These include accounts payable and accounts receivable, payroll and monthly production, and income files.

Even though the maintenance of certain files in the dental office may be the responsibility of someone other than the dental administrator, such as the office manager, it is important for you to understand how all of the filing systems work. Many types of files will have to be accessed by other staff in the dental office, making it all the more important that filing procedures are followed consistently.

Therefore, this chapter provides you with essential information on how to establish and maintain an effective filing system. First, we will look at basic filing guidelines. Next, we will consider different types of filing systems used in dental offices. Then, we will cover storage equipment and supplies and the storage and transfer of files. Finally, we will discuss electronic filing.

BASIC FILING GUIDELINES

Before filing any kind of document, file, or chart in the dental office, some basic guidelines should be followed. The following four steps should be followed to ensure accurate and efficient filing: conditioning, indexing, sorting, and storing.

1. **Conditioning** refers to the preparation of the documents being filed. If a piece of paper is torn or has paperclips or staples attached, repair these documents by removing the paper clips and staples and taping any torn parts of the page. If the document being filed is for a patient's chart, make sure the document has the patient's name on it where it is visible. If there are two or more pages attached for the same patient, ensure that the patient's name can be found easily on each page.
2. **Indexing** refers to separating documents by type when filing. This means that patient documents to be filed into patient charts should be kept separate from other documents, such as invoices, which should be filed in accounts payable files.
3. **Sorting** means putting the group of records that you are going to file into some sort of order before filing them into the filing system. Patient charts should be put into alphabetical order (if an alphabetical system is used) or numerical order (if a numerical system is used). Financial documents should be put into alphabetical or monthly order in preparation for filing.
4. **Storing** refers to filing the records into the proper filing system. If the patient charts are being filed in alphabetical order by last name, follow this system for filing.

checkPOINT

1. What are the four steps involved in accurate filing?

COMMON FILING SYSTEMS

Even though computerized and paperless dental practices are on the increase, some documents still require the safe keeping and easy access afforded by hard copy files. An efficient filing system allows for access to information by any staff member who requires the document (Fig. 12-1).

Two main filing systems are used in dental offices: alphabetical and numeric filing systems. The filing system used in each dental office will be dictated by the preference of the dentist, the size of the office, the room available to store files, and the necessity for confidentiality of the files. Depending on the preference of the dentist, one may be used or both may be used for different purposes.

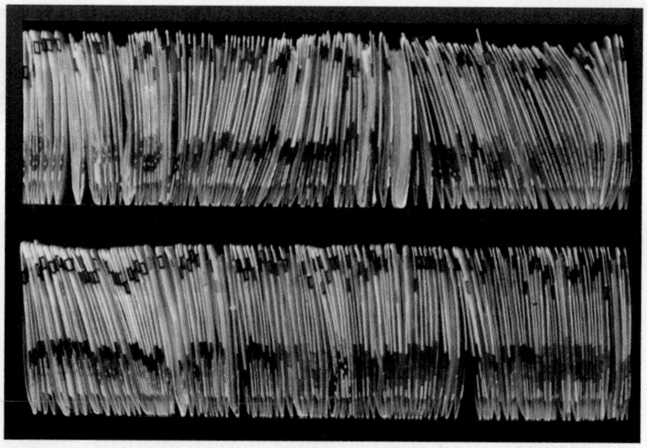

FIGURE 12-1 Filing system in a dental office.

Alphabetical Filing System

The **alphabetical filing system** uses the letters of some part of the name of the item to file. For example, in the dental office, patient charts may be filed in alphabetical order using the last names of patients. When filing alphabetically, rules must be followed to file charts in a logical manner. These rules refer to the indexing of the charts before filing them. When a patient chart is filed alphabetically, the name is filed by last name, first name, and middle initial. Each letter in the name should be treated as a separate unit. For example, two patient charts, one for Mr. David Christopher Jones and the other for Mrs. Elizabeth A. Smith must be filed. The charts would be filed in this order:

Jones, David Christopher
Smith, Elizabeth A.

In this example, J comes before S in the alphabet, so David Jones would be filed before Elizabeth Smith. Special attention must be paid to each letter in the name being a separate unit when the last names start with the same letter. For example, David C. Jones and Donald A. Janicks would be filed in this order:

Janicks, Donald A.
Jones, David C.

In this example, the first unit of the name, the letter J, is the same. Thus, the second unit in the name—in Janicks, the letter A and in Jones, the letter O—is used to index these two files. More details on alphabetical indexing are available in Box 12-1. Box 12-2 provides examples of alphabetical filing.

In preparation for filing alphabetically, place all the patient charts to be filed into groups alphabetically. Once you have performed this, take each letter group and work through the charts, placing them in alphabetical order using the second unit in the name, and then the third, and so on until they are in alphabetical order.

Use of color-coded labels on patient charts makes alphabetical filing easier. Figure 12-2 provides an example of such labels. When color-coded files in a letter category are filed together, they will all show the same colors. This feature makes it easy to identify whether a chart has been misfiled. For example, if the color of the letter A label is pink and the color of the letter G label is orange, it would be easy to spot a pink letter A file that has been misfiled among the orange letter G files. Figure 12-3 provides an example of a chart labeled for alphabetical filing. The use of an alphabetical file arrangement allows for easy browsing to find the patient chart in question. The alphabetical system is easy to use in the dental office because the alphabet is understood and used by all staff members. Furthermore, because there is no cross referencing required, that is, when searching for a patient chart which

BOX 12-1 Indexing Rules for Filing Alphabetically

- File by name according to last name, first name, middle initial, and treat each letter in the name as a separate unit. For example, Everett G. Formal should be filed as Formal, Everett G. and would be filed before Formal, Everitt G.
- Hyphenated names should be treated as one complete name. Lilian B. Howes-Smith would be filed as Howes-Smith, Lilian B. not as Smith, Lilian B. Howes.
- Last names beginning with Mac or Mc should be grouped together when filed; the preference will be that of the dentist or office administrator. Generally, Mac comes before Mc in keeping with alphabetical filing. It is important that consistency is maintained.
- File abbreviated names in order of how they are spelled out. For example, Wm. Applebee should be filed as Applebee, William, and John St. Johns should be filed as Saint Johns, John.
- File a married woman's chart by her name, not her husband's name. For example, Mrs. Angie Blackhart (Mrs. David Blackhart) would be filed as Blackhart, Angie not Blackhart, David Mrs.
- If a father and son are members of the clinic and have the same last name, use Jr. and Sr. in the indexing and on the name labels. Two patients with the same name who are not related should have patient name alert labels placed on their charts and their birth dates should be checked for verification when they do attend the clinic.
- Professional initials should be placed after a full name. Edward G. Robinson, J.D. should be filed as Robinson, Edward G., J.D.

begins with the letter "A" the individual can look directly under the "A" section of the filing to find the chart.

Numerical Filing System

The **numerical filing system** uses numbers to order files. Numbers used in this system generally consist of six digits. Using this type of filing system enables the person filing to organize the patient charts in numerical order and not have to be concerned with two patients having the same name, as each patient is assigned a unique number. A patient keeps the same chart number, even if his or her name changes, which helps avoid filing errors. However, using a numerical filing system requires a

BOX 12-2 Alphabetical Filing Examples

Sample Patient Names to be Filed in Alphabetical Order	Proper Alphabetical Order of These Names
Everett G. H. Forester	Artson, Artie A.
Eleanor Roosevelt	Evanson, Nicole L.
Artie S. Artson	Forester, Everett G. H.
Ms. Lili B. Millions	Grey, Cynthia E.
Mr. Duke A. Millions	Jackson, Karoline
Nicole L. Evanson	Millions, Duke A.
Maya Papaya	Millions, Lili B.
Bettyann E. Southward	Papaya, Maya
Cynthia E. Grey	Roosevelt, Eleanor
Mrs. Daniel Jackson (Karoline)	Simpson, Bart
Bart Simpson	Southward, Bettyann E.

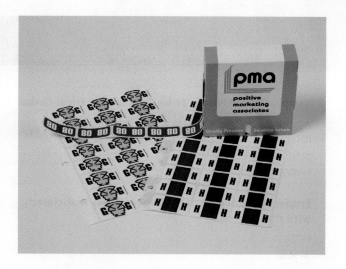

FIGURE 12-2 Dental chart labels.

cross-referencing chart to be available. Having a patient's chart filed by a number means that when the patient's chart has to be pulled from the files, one must first find the number that represents that patient.

A numerical filing system is a popular method for filing patient charts in medical offices. Larger group practice dental offices may file charts in this manner. The most significant advantage to using a numerical filing system is the degree of privacy that it allows. When patients have documentation filed into their charts, the chart is matched to the documentation by a number, which is found on the cross-reference list. The cross-reference list must be kept in an area away from the charts. Thus, if a patient's chart is inadvertently left on the front desk, on a counter, or in a place where other patients can view it, the patient's identity is protected. Of course, as has

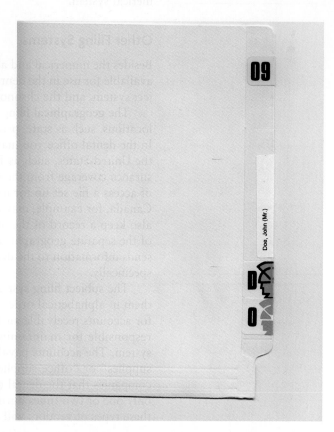

FIGURE 12-3 Chart labeled for alphabetical filing.

BOX 12-3
Numerical Filing Examples

Sample Patient Names to be Filed in Numerical Order

Anthony R. Scott 345690
Josephine T. Warble 197869
Stephanie M. Foods 345632
George Rudolph 762345

Proper Numerical Order of the Numbers Associated with these Names

197869
345632
345690
762345

Straight digit filing is similar to the method used for alphabetical filing in that when you have two initial digits that are the same, you keep moving to the next digit until you can determine which number comes first. For example, 345623 would be filed before 345690 because the numbers are the same until the last two digits, where 32 is filed before 90.

been discussed in earlier chapters, great care should be taken to avoid leaving patient charts where other patients can view them.

The correct way to file charts using a numerical filing system depends on the preference for use, as there are different ways of reading the numbers. Straight digit filing involves reading the number from left to right or top to bottom. Other dental offices may use a numerical filing system in which the number is read from right to left or bottom to top. Numbers can also be read in pairs for filing. For example, a numerical filing code such as 123456 can be read as 12, 34, 56. The filing method may involve using the last pair of numbers to file the chart. Whatever system is used, developing efficiency is the goal. Box 12-3 provides examples of filing using the numerical system.

*check*POINT

2. Describe the two main filing systems used in dental offices.

Other Filing Systems

Besides the numerical and alphabetical filing systems, several other filing systems are available for use in the dental office. These include the geographical system, the subject system, and the chronological system.

The **geographical filing system** involves the filing of items by their geographical locations, such as state, province, territory, or even location within a city or county. In the dental office you may have patients who work in other countries other than the United States, such as England or Canada. These patients may have dental insurance coverage from the country in which they are working, as a result. For ease of access a file set up for insurance companies that you must communicate with in Canada, for example, may assist in keeping records current and accessible. You can also keep a record of the insurance claim paid in the patients' chart. The necessity of the separate geographical file is useful particularly when the insurance company sends information to the dental office that may not necessarily pertain to the patient specifically.

The **subject filing system** involves categorizing items by subject file and placing them in alphabetical order of subject. Placing items in subject order is most useful for accounts receivable and accounts payable filing. In the dental office you will be responsible for maintaining the accounts receivable and accounts payable filing system. The accounts payable filing system may have a general file labeled "dental supplies" or "office supplies" these two files would hold receipts and invoices for companies that the dental office does not buy supplies from on a regular basis, but only one or two times during a period of year. Developing a general subject file for these types of vendors will allow for ease in purging files to keep them current.

A **chronological filing system** involves filing items by date. In a dental chart, for example, items in the patient's chart are filed in chronological order. The most recent or current item is filed on top, or first in the chart. To easily access information within a patient chart filing information based on the date, the patient received treatment at the dental office is the most efficient. When communicating with insurance companies, beginning with the date treatment was rendered is the preferred way to begin the discussion of a patient's information.

FILING EQUIPMENT

Open-Shelf

This type of file cabinet resembles a bookshelf in that it is open-faced and has approximately six to eight shelves (Fig. 12-1). This type of filing system can house the standard end-tab patient chart files used in the dental office because of the open concept it presents, and can house more files than a closed drawer file system.

Lateral File Shelves

This type of filing system can be two to eight drawers high and have retractable doors. This type of system can hold both legal and letter-sized files in the system. Shelves can be added easily to this system and therefore easily expand as the filing demands increase. The lateral filing shelves can also be locked for added security.

Vertical Filing System

This type of filing system resembles a filing cabinet where files are stored in a drawer. The cabinet is usually stacked two to four drawers high. The drawer pulls out toward you and the files are accessed easily. This type of file system can also be locked for added security.

Closed File System

According to Health Insurance Portability and Accountability Act (HIPAA) regulations, patient files should not be accessible by other patients or persons in the dental office. To ensure the privacy of patients in this regard, a closed filing system can be used.

STORING FILES

As mentioned earlier, patient records in the dental office must be kept for a period of time, even if they are inactive or closed, as they may be requested for a legal investigation or malpractice suit. Most dental offices store the patient's chart permanently and either use an off-site storage location or have storage facilities in the office.

How a patient's chart is stored depends on the status of the patient. In most dental offices, each patient chart will be considered either active or inactive, both of which are open files, or files that are likely to be needed. **Active patients** are those who attend the dental office for regular care appointments and have been seen in the past 2–4 years, with the timeframe varying between practices. **Inactive patients** are those who have not been into the dental office for 5 or more years, again, with the timeframe varying from practice to practice. Active files are kept in the primary filing system. Inactive files are kept separate from the active files, in an out-of-the-way, yet accessible area, as some patients may return without warning. Inactive patients have not visited the dental office over a long period of time likely because they either have a phobia of the dentist and return infrequently when discomfort occurs or for other reasons such as working out of the state or country. In this situation the patient's file is not closed and therefore may need to be accessed.

However, patients who have left the practice because they have moved or have transferred to another dental office, the dentist has terminated the relationship, or because the patient is deceased, has terminated his or her verbal contract with the dentist. The charts of these patients are considered closed, as they will not likely be needed. Charts that are closed typically must be kept in storage and accessible and not disposed of for 10 years from the date of the patient's last visit. Closed charts can be stored either in a storage area in the dental office or at an off-site storage facility. These charts belong to the dentist, and because the dentist is responsible for them, they must be stored properly.

> **checkPOINT**
>
> 3. What is the difference between an active and inactive patient files?

Files other than patient charts, such as the accounts receivable or accounts payable files, must also be kept for a certain number of years. It is important that you familiarize yourself with the legislation regarding this in your state. The office manager is generally responsible for the maintenance of the financial records of the practice; however, the office administrator must be knowledgeable of their whereabouts in case they need to be accessed. Items in these categories include cancelled checks, receipts for equipment, insurance documents, and tax records. Generally these types of documents are stored in the storage area used for storing paper records, which may be on-site or off-site from the dental office.

TRANSFERRING PATIENT RECORDS

When patients leave the dental office and continue their oral health care with another dentist, it may be necessary to provide their dental history information to their dental office. The patient's chart is the property of the dentist and legally belongs to the dentist, but the information belongs to the patient. If an authorization for information release is on file from the patient or the patient's legal guardian, the information can be released. Never release the original chart or the documents in the original chart. Always make a copy of the information required and supply the copies to the office requesting the information.

Besides a patient's new dental office, other organizations may request copies of dental files, including the following:

- Insurance companies
- Legal representatives
- Other dentists or physicians
- Patients

All requests should be in written form and should include the patient's name, address, date of birth, and social security number. If a caller is requesting the information, after you have received the written request, never release the information over the phone unless the caller has already submitted a written request and you are sure the person you are revealing the information to is the person who requested the information. Usually, a nominal fee is charged for providing this information, as it can be time-consuming to retrieve the chart (especially if it is an inactive patient), photocopy it, and prepare it for mailing.

> **checkPOINT**
>
> 4. How should a patient request his or her dental chart information?

When a patient's chart is being subpoenaed by a court of law, the original documentation must be provided. State legislation regarding this type of situation allows for the temporary release of the documentation from the dental office and provides the protection necessary for the privacy of the information.

If a patient is requesting to make copies of his or her patient chart, the decision about what to provide the patient is up to the dentist. There are state laws that govern this area, particularly when the patient is a minor. Familiarize yourself with pertinent legislation and office policies.

ELECTRONIC FILING

Increasingly, dental offices are relying on the filing of information on computers, either in addition to or in place of standard files. In your role as dental administrator, you likely will be responsible for maintaining such information on a computer. For instance, the dental charts may be computerized. In such cases, the dental software program you are using will provide the necessary organization system for maintaining accurate files. In any case, the following guidelines should assist you in maintaining your computerized records:

1. *Organize files by creating categories:* Creating a file labeled "letters" will be helpful for placing all written communication into for easy access later.
2. *Keep everything in one place:* For instance, in Microsoft Windows, you can place all documents in the "My Documents" folder. Spreadsheets, letters, or PowerPoint presentations should be placed here. This will make it easier to find things and to run backups.
3. *Create folders:* These are like the drawers of a filing cabinet. Use language you will understand to name your folders. Avoid abbreviations; this will create frustration for you when you are looking for a file if you cannot recall the meaning.
4. *Create folders within folders:* Create other folders within these main folders. For instance, a folder called "Invoices" might contain folders called "2004," "2005," and "2006." The goal is to have every file in a folder, rather than having a bunch of files listed.
5. *Be consistent in naming files:* If you are creating invoices for the ABC company and you name it abc_company, be consistent and do not name the next one ABC_Company.
6. *Be specific:* Give files logical, specific names and include dates in file names, if possible. The goal when naming files is to be able to tell what the file is about without having to open it.
7. *File as you go:* The best time to file a document is when you first create it.
8. *Back up your files regularly:* Whether you are copying your files onto another drive or onto tape, it is important to set up and follow a regular back-up regimen.

For computerized dental records, maintaining storage of patient files is performed relatively easily and requires a small amount of office space. Any documents that are originally in hard copy can be scanned and stored electronically. Then, all documents can be grouped together to make one file.

Chapter Summary

The patient chart in the dental office is integral to the continued care of the patient. Proper maintenance and storage of patient charts is an important responsibility of the dental office administrator. Various filing systems are used in the dental office. Familiarity with different systems is necessary to be efficient when filing. Understanding the process, guidelines, and implications of patient record retention and release will assist the office administrator in proper maintenance of patient records. The privacy of the patient must be protected at all times. Furthermore, following the guidelines in place regarding patient record storage and maintenance speaks of quality patient care.

Review Questions

Multiple Choice

1. **Which is not a step to follow to ensure accurate filing?**
   a. Sorting
   b. Recording
   c. Conditioning
   d. Storing
2. **Putting the charts into the order you are going to file them in is referred to as**
   a. sorting.
   b. recording.
   c. conditioning.
   d. storing.
3. **Which of the following names would be filed second using an alphabetical system?**
   a. Jamey Jamerson
   b. Jane Jameson
   c. James Janeson
   d. John Janeson
4. **A geographical filing system means that items are filed by**
   a. location.
   b. spelling.
   c. subject.
   d. oldest.
5. **Inactive patient charts are charts for patients who**
   a. see the dentist infrequently.
   b. have not seen the dentist in over a year.
   c. have not seen the dentist in over 5 years.
   d. have terminated the dentist-patient relationship.
6. **Patient requests for chart copies**
   a. must be in writing.
   b. must include name and date of birth.
   c. cannot be performed verbally.
   d. all of the above.
7. **Advantages to the alphabetical filing system include all of the following except**
   a. easy browsing to find the patient chart.
   b. the alphabet is understood by everyone in the dental office.
   c. cross referencing is not required.
   d. the letter labels on the charts are always color-coded.
8. **An advantage to using the numerical filing system is**
   a. the number labels on the charts are always color-coded.
   b. numerical filing is a popular method to use.
   c. patient identity is easily protected.
   d. cross referencing is not required.
9. **Which of the following patient charts would be considered a closed chart?**
   a. Mr. Jones has not been in the dental office for a checkup in 3 years.
   b. Andy Smith is moving to England for 2 years but will be returning to the dental office.
   c. Debbie Jones has transferred to another dental office for care.
   d. Mrs. Williams has been to see the dentist once in the past 2 years.
10. **When a patient's chart is being subpoenaed by law,**
    a. the original copies must be submitted.
    b. photocopies of the chart must be submitted.
    c. the request must come from the patient.
    d. the chart must be checked for accuracy.

Critical Thinking

1. A patient has called and requested his child's dental chart information. He would like to see the original chart and has asked you to send the whole chart over to his new dentist. What is the process you should follow?
2. Explain which filing system you would prefer to work with in the dental office and discuss the advantages and disadvantages of the system.
3. Discuss the advantages of maintaining an organized filing system on the computer.

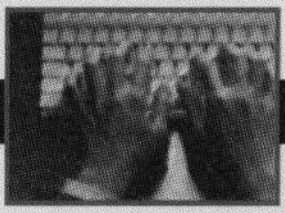

HANDS-ON ACTIVITY

1. Write an office policy regarding the retention and storing of patient charts in the dental office, including the process to follow should a patient request his or her chart information.

2. Make a list of your classmates and place their names in alphabetical order. Next, ask a classmate to assign each name a random six digit number and place them in numerical order.

Web Sites

www.filingsystems.com

Filing systems and accessories available
http://www.ada.org/prof/resources/topics/hipaa/index.asp

HIPAA resource on patient chart filing requirements

chapter THIRTEEN

Inventory

OBJECTIVES

After completing this chapter, you should be able to do the following:

- Spell and define key terms
- Describe the difference between clinical, administrative, and capital supplies
- List the main aspects of supplies that must be considered when ordering
- Explain what an invoice and statement is and the information found on it
- Explain what a backordered item is
- Describe and demonstrate how to use a manual inventory system
- Describe and demonstrate how to use a computerized inventory system

KEY TERMS

- inventory
- clinical supplies
- disposable items
- reusable items
- administrative supplies
- capital supplies
- expiration date
- invoice
- backordered item
- statement
- credit memo
- manual inventory system
- computerized inventory system

OUTLINE

In the dental office, supplies are constantly used in both the clinical and administrative areas and thus must be continually ordered. Supplies vary in their purpose and use, and some items are used once, whereas others are reused. Depending on the size of the dental office, one or two team members may be responsible for keeping track of supplies and replenishing stock. This responsibility may be delegated to one clinical team member for the clinical areas and one administrative team member for the administrative areas. The dental office assistant is responsible for maintaining administrative supplies. Developing and maintaining an inventory system that tracks supplies is important for ensuring that items are not depleted at times when they are required. Thus, this chapter presents the primary types of supplies used in the dental office, considerations to take when ordering such supplies, how to work with suppliers, and developing and managing a manual or computerized inventory system.

SUPPLIES IN THE DENTAL OFFICE

Inventory consists of all the items held available in stock for any area of the dental office, including all clinical and administrative items. There are three main types of supplies found in the dental office: clinical, administrative, and capital.

Clinical Supplies

Clinical supplies are supplies used for clinical procedures in the dental office. Anything that the dentist or hygienist requires for use to carry out treatment is considered a clinical supply. Clinical supplies are used frequently in the dental office. In fact, treatment cannot be carried out without the use of supplies. In the clinical area, two types of supplies are most often used:

- disposable items
- reusable items

Disposable items are those that are used once and then thrown away. Gloves, masks, rubber dams, fluoride trays, and cotton-tipped applicators are just some examples of disposable items in the dental office (Fig. 13-1). Compliance with infection control guidelines is a primary reason why many items used in the clinical area of the dental office must be disposable. Items in the dental office that can be reused to carry out treatment, or **reusable items,** are those that can be sterilized or disinfected (Fig. 13-2). Reusable items include dental instruments such as a mirror, explorer or scaler, curing lights that can be wiped with a disinfectant and a barrier applied for reuse, and most intraoral instruments used by the dental hygienist. Box 13-1 provides some tips on managing inventory.

checkPOINT

1. What are disposable items? What are examples of disposable items?

Administrative Supplies

Administrative supplies are supplies that are used in the administrative area to carry out administrative tasks and duties to facilitate patient care. The dental office administrator is responsible for either ordering the needed administrative supplies himself or herself or reporting the need for such supplies to the employee responsible for ordering inventory. Administrative supplies include everything from pens and paperclips to ink toner and paper for the printer and most items used in the administrative area of the dental office.

Capital Supplies

Besides clinical and administrative supplies, large equipment is also purchased to carry out duties required in the dental office. Supplies found in this category are included in the inventory list but are not replaced on a regular basis like the clinical and administrative supplies. **Capital supplies** in the dental office include items such

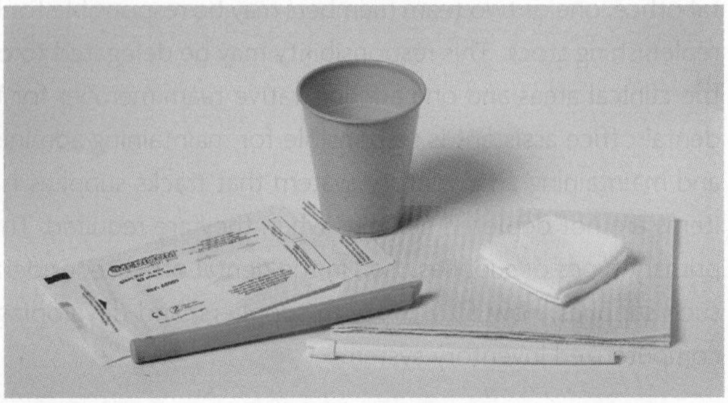

FIGURE 13-1
Disposable items in inventory.

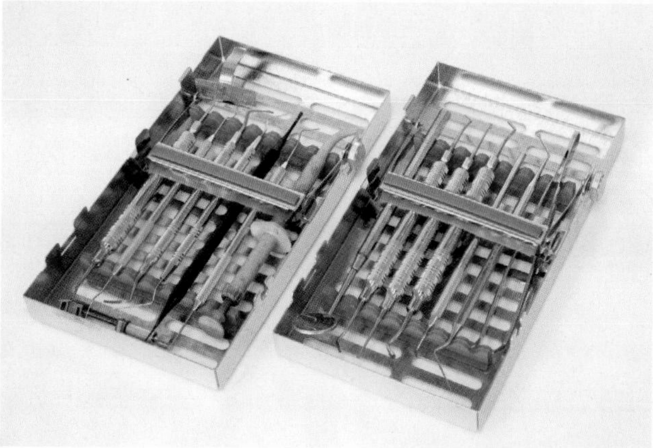

FIGURE 13-2
Reusable items in dental inventory.

as the dental operatory, which includes the dental chair and the stools that the dentist and assistant use. Generally, capital supplies are larger financial purchases, which the dental office makes very infrequently. A significant portion of all capital supplies is purchased when a dental office is set up for the first time. However, there may be an addition to the capital supply list on a yearly basis, as computers are acquired and older equipment is replaced.

checkPOINT

2. What are capital supplies?

ORDERING

The dental office administrator is often responsible for ordering supplies for the dental office in both the administrative and clinical areas. A good rule of thumb to remember is not to wait until the office has run out of a particular item, but to replenish stock as it decreases.

To maintain the supply of stock in the dental office, it is important to determine criteria for reordering supplies. There are many aspects involved that dictate when to order and how much of an item should be ordered. These criteria are as follows:

- expiration of items
- storage space available
- usage of items
- product promotions

BOX 13-1
Inventory Control Guidelines

1. One clinical person and one administrative person should maintain the shared responsibility of inventory supply maintenance.
2. Set aside time on a weekly basis to assess the inventory on hand and determine what supplies need to be ordered.
3. Decide on a minimum amount of supplies that are to be kept on hand before ordering additional supplies to replenish. If supplies have an expiration date, keep a minimum on hand to avoid expiration before using them.
4. Keep a file of promotional fliers that arrive in the office to consult before ordering to ensure optimal pricing for supplies.
5. Encourage staff members to make suggestions regarding new items or supplies for use in the dental office.
6. When placing an order, ask for samples of different or new items for trial in the dental office.

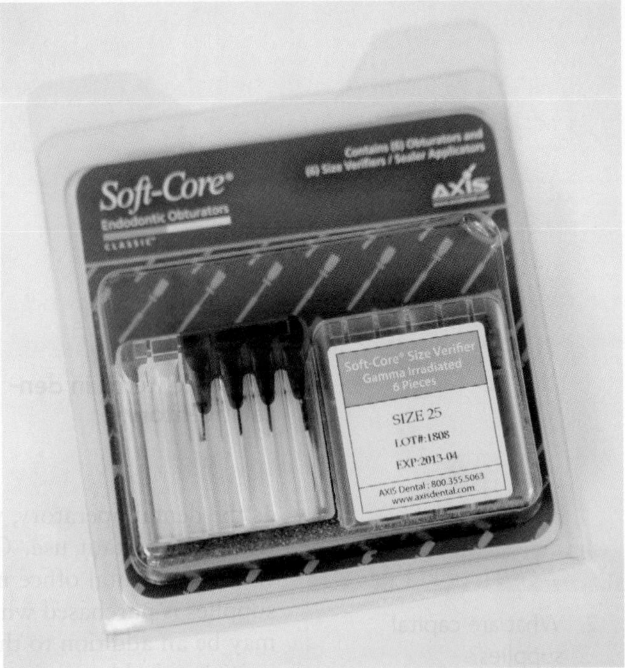

FIGURE 13-3 **Products with expiration dates.**

Expiration Dates

Certain supplies in the dental office are ordered on an "as needed" basis. Usually these items have **expiration dates,** which mean that the item should be used before it becomes ineffective. It is not advisable to purchase a large amount of items that may expire before use. Expired items have to be disposed of, which means that the order was not very cost-effective for the dental office. Examples of products that have expiration dated include dental radiography film, anesthetic cartridges, impression materials, cements, and teeth-whitening material (Fig. 13-3). Keeping items stored in the recommended temperate zone will help maintain the shelf life of the product. For example, if the manufacturer recommends a cool, dry environment, the items should not be placed near a radiator or in an area where heat exposure is high. Such exposure will shorten the usage life of the product, possibly making it ineffective prior to its expiration time.

Storage Space Availability

Most of the supplies ordered in a dental office are stored in cupboards and drawers in the dental operatory. This is because most items must be kept close at hand for use by the dentist and clinical staff. Figure 13-4 is a picture of the typical operatory cupboard and drawer space available. There are not usually large amounts of space dedicated to storing supplies, and, therefore, they must be ordered frequently.

Frequency of Use

The frequency with which certain supplies are used is an indication of how much to order and when to order the item. For example, medical gloves are used daily and frequently. A case of gloves may last about 1 month or less, depending on the number of clinical members and patients in the clinic per day. Gloves do not have an expiration date, but they also require considerable storage space.

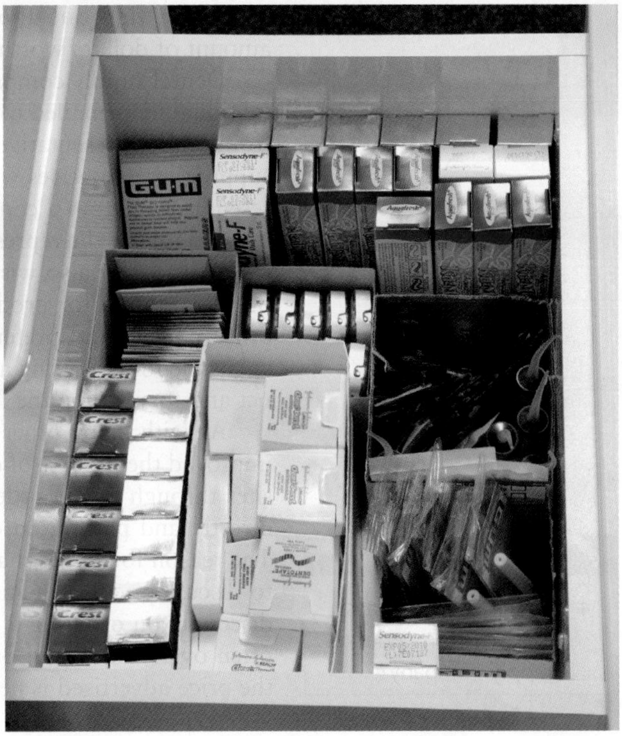

FIGURE 13-4 Dental storage drawers and cupboards.

> **checkPOINT**
>
> 3. What criteria dictate when to order and how much of an item should be ordered?

Product Promotions

Dental supply companies often have items that they offer at a special price, often called monthly promotions. If the item is a frequently used supply and will be used in a timely manner, the promotion is a cost-effective decision for the dental office. If the item is not used often and may expire before its use, the item is not cost-effective.

WORKING WITH SUPPLIERS

Many different dental supply companies are available for purchasing supplies. Some dental offices order a large portion of their dental supplies from one supply company. However, not all dental supply companies carry the same items or every item the dental office needs. So, it may be necessary to purchase supplies from several companies.

The quality of goods is important and should be high on the list of qualifications for selecting a supplier. A good deal on certain items or the least expensive price may mean lower quality. It is never advisable to compromise on the quality of items, because the quality of the dentistry the patient receives is also compromised. If the material offered for sale by the supplier is at a much lower price than what other suppliers offer it for, check that the item is not closer to its expiration date or that the product does not contain similar quality ingredients.

Consider the reputation of the dental supplier as well during the selection process. Ask other dental office administrators what supplier the office does business with and why that company is preferred over the others. Consider calling dental supply companies that are located in the state, or close to the state, the dental office is located. A company that is nearby may not have problems with getting items to your office because of geographical concerns. If the representative from the dental supply company comes into the dental office, ask about discounted savings for bulk purchases. If the dental office will be ordering a certain amount of supplies each year, find out about a price break for ordering a minimum or maximum amount of dollars worth of supplies.

Dental supply companies often keep in contact with dental offices through promotional fliers mailed to the office, telephone calls to check on inventory, and visits from sales representatives from both distributors and manufacturers. Often, dental supply representatives will visit the dental office on a regular basis. If the sales representative is from a company that the office regularly orders from, having a list of items ready for the representative to order is advantageous for both parties. The representative may also wish to speak with the dentist about a new product available or a promotion for products currently used in the office. Depending on the dental office policies and preference of the dentist, the office administrator is usually responsible for collecting any information available regarding the promotion or product and forwarding the information to the dentist.

As with many other areas of dental practice, technological advances have also improved the process of ordering supplies. Most dental supply companies have Web sites through which orders can be placed directly. However, phoning the company directly and placing an order is still the most common method in most practices. The reason for this is that the employee placing the order will have the opportunity to discuss prices of items with the salesperson and request any samples for use or discounts on ordering a certain number of items. A busy order desk employee can often overlook special pricing that is available, and, therefore, requesting items at the price advertised is necessary to ensure a cost-effective inventory supply.

checkPOINT

4. What are three ways to order from a dental supply company?

Invoices

The **invoice** is a legal document given to the customer or client listing goods or services provided, along with prices and terms of sale. The seller must retain a copy as a record of sales. The customer must retain a copy as a record of purchases and expenses. It is a record of the amount of money due or how much has been paid by the customer. The invoice can be sent with the order when it is shipped or mailed separately to the dental office.

The invoice can be divided into three sections: the head, the body, and the bottom. Figure 13-5 is a sample invoice.

Invoice Head

In the first section of the invoice, the following information can be found:

- The name and address of the seller. Often, this is in the form of a letterhead.
- The word "invoice" should be present. This is important to distinguish between an invoice, packing slip, or statement.
- An invoice number. Each invoice from the same supplier should have a different number.
- An invoice date.
- Payment terms and how the invoice can be paid.
- The customer's name and address.
- How the goods were shipped.

Invoice Body

A description of the goods is provided in the middle portion of the invoice. The information regarding the items shipped includes the following:

- The quantity ordered and shipped
- Price per unit or item and total amount for individual items
- The supplier's item number and description of goods shipped
- Items not shipped and backordered
- In the case of services, a brief summary of the work completed and the hourly rate or amount charged for services

DentalBrands For Less!

Invoice

Date	Invoice #
11/28/2007	26058

Bill To	Ship To
Girtel Guy S Dr 204-7125 109 Street NW, Edmonton, AB T6G 1B9 Canada	Girtel Guy S Dr 204-7125 109 Street NW, Edmonton, AB T6G 1B9 Canada
780-435-5300	780-435-5300

B.O. No.	Terms	Due Date	Ship Via	Rep
	Credit Card	11/28/2007	ICS	

Business Hours:
Mon - Fri 9:00AM - 18:00PM
Sat - Sun CLOSED

Qty	Description	Rate	Amount
1	Rely - X Unicem TR (3M-ESPE)	199.95	199.95T
1	Film IP-21 Insight Adult Size #2 (KODAK)	54.95	54.95T
1	Soflex Disc Refill 2381SF (3M-ESPE)	39.95	39.95T
1	Soflex Disc Refill 2381F (3M-ESPE)	39.95	39.95T
1	Soflex Disc Refill 2381M (3M-ESPE)	39.95	39.95T
1	Soflex Disc Refill 2381C (3M-ESPE)	39.95	39.95T
1	Soflex Disc Refill 2382SF (3M-ESPE)	39.95	39.95T
1	Soflex Disc Refill 2382F (3M-ESPE)	39.95	39.95T
1	Soflex Disc Refill 2382M (3M-ESPE)	39.95	39.95T
1	Soflex Disc Refill 2382C (3M-ESPE)	39.95	39.95T
1	Saphora $50 Gift Card	0.00	0.00
	Business Number: 855776209		
		GST	34.47
		Total	Can$608.97

Please make payment available for the mention due date.

To pay this invoice with credit card, Please call 1-888-441-0443.

Prepared By: ____________ Verified By: ____________

DENTAL BRANDS FOR LESS INC.
200 VICEROY ROAD UNIT #6
CONCORD, ON
L4K 3N8

Phone #	Fax #	Toll Free #
905-669-9329	905-669-3728	1-888-441-0443

FIGURE 13-5 Product invoice.

> ✓ checkPOINT
> 5. What does the middle portion of the invoice include?

Invoice Bottom

The lower portion of the invoice includes the following:

- The subtotal amount owing for all items shipped
- Any tax charged and the amount owed after tax
- Forms of payment accepted
- Information regarding return policies and restocking fees

Backorders

Items that are not in stock at the time they are ordered are considered to be ordered but will be shipped at a later date. This type of item is considered a **backordered item** and will be indicated on the invoice. When the backordered item arrives, you should receive a separate invoice for it. Backordered items are not billed to the office until they are shipped. It is the responsibility of the dental office administrator to ensure that the invoice reflects billing for items that are actually received in the office.

Shipping Methods

Manufacturers and dental supply companies use various shipping methods for dental products. Regardless of the method used, the invoice should always reflect how the items were shipped. Dental supply companies often use a courier method to send items, since some items are sensitive to temperature and to the time en route to the office. For example, items that must be kept in a cool environment would be sent by a refrigerated courier truck, or items that have expiration dates would be sent by overnight courier. Usually, items are shipped from the supply company's warehouse as soon as they are ordered and can take anywhere from 1 day to 1 week for arrival at the dental office.

Statements

Typically, a statement will be sent to the dental office on a monthly basis from the dental supply company. Figure 13-6 is a statement. A **statement** is a listing of all the invoices that have been billed to the dental office from that supply company within a 30-day period, as well as any outstanding amounts from earlier periods. It is the responsibility of the dental office administrator to receive the statement and match the invoices to the statement to ensure that the total invoice amounts reflect the statement total. Some office policies reflect a monthly supplier payment period, using the monthly statement as the payment remittance document. This is done to ensure that any items that were returned to the supplier are reflected on the statement in the form of a **credit memo,** which reflects a credit on the account. If the credit is not showing, the supplier must be contacted and the amount deducted from the statement before paying. Payment to suppliers is discussed in Chapter 17.

> *Administrative* TIP
> When returning an item for credit to the dental supply company, always telephone the company and inquire as to its procedure for returning items. The company will inform you of the process to follow in order to ensure credit on the dental office account. If an item has been returned to the dental supply company and the monthly statement does not reflect credit to the account, contact the supply company directly to ensure that a credit is forthcoming.

INVENTORY SYSTEMS

The inventory system in a dental office keeps track of how many items are used in a particular time frame and provides a financial picture for the dentist of where the supply expenses are incurred. Keeping track of supplies and ordering a sufficient amount at the appropriate time are key to maintaining the inventory in a dental

Nobel Biocare Canada Inc.
9133 Leslie Street, Unit 100
Richmond Hill, ON L4B 4N1

SOLD TO
VENDU À

Dr G.S. Girtel
204-7125 109 Street
Edmonton AB T6G 1B9

Customer No. 560808
N° du Client

Statement of account from
Relevé de Compte du
06/30/2008 to/à 07/27/2008

9133 Leslie Street, Unit 100
Richmond Hill, ON L4B 4N1
Telephone/Téléphone (905) 762-3500 1 (800) 263-4017
Fax/Télécopieur (905) 762-1540

PLEASE CHECK THE INVOICE TO BE PAID, SEPARATE THIS SLIP AND INSERT WITH PAYMENT.
VEUILLEZ VÉRIFIER LA FACTURE, DÉTACHER CE BORDEREAU ET L'INSÉRER DANS UNE ENVELOPPE AVEC VOTRE PAIEMENT.

Page 1 / 1

Customer No. 560808
N° du Client

INVOICE NO NUMÉRO DE FACTURE	INVOICE DATE DATE DE LA FACTURE	KEY CODE	AMOUNT MONTANT	PAYMENT	DESCRIPTION	INVOICE NO NUMÉRO DE FACTURE	AMOUNT MONTANT
Clearing procedures from 06/30/2008 to 07/27/2008							
3510368160	06/20/2008	01	98.18			3510368160	98.18
AUTH#033533	07/09/2008	15	98.18-	98.18-		AUTH#033533	98.18-

Open items at 07/27/2008
No open items at key date 07/27/2008.

Balance of account 07/27/2008 Solde du Compte	0.00	Total Total	0.00

	to 0 days	1 to 30 days	31 to 60 days	over 61 days
Net due in				
Overdue since				

Transaction types: 01 = INVOICE 05 = REFUND 06 = BALANCE OWING 11 = CREDIT 15 = PAYMENTS
Types de Transactions: 01 = FACTURE 05 = REMBOURSEMENT 06 = BALANCE DUE 11 = CRÉDIT 15 = PAIEMENTS
After due date penalty interest of 18% may becharged to your account.
Après la date d'échéance, des frais d'intérêt de 18% pourraientêtre chargés à votre compte.

Nobel Biocare Canada Inc. 9133 Leslie Street, Unit 100 Richmond Hill, ON L4B 4N1 Telephone Téléphone (905) 762-3500 1 (800) 263-4017 Fax Télécopieur (905) 762-1540

Brånemark System® PROCERA® Replace

FIGURE 13-6 Statement.

office. For example, ordering dental impression materials should be done prior to the last use of the material. Waiting until the item is completely used leaves the office without the item and will result in frustration because of the lack of availability and inability to provide treatment.

Because of the number and types of supplies used continually in the dental office, it would be futile to try in order to track the actual usage of each item. For example, medical gloves are used on a continual basis throughout the day, when a patient is receiving treatment, during instrument sterilization, and during laboratory and operatory cleaning. Thus, keeping tabs on when and where the gloves are used would not be an efficient use of time. However, the rate of usage of gloves can easily be surmised by keeping track of the number of boxes of gloves in the inventory system. Supplies that are consumed on a daily basis are usually ordered on a regular schedule, such as monthly or bimonthly, or as the supply becomes depleted.

Depending on the type of inventory system used in the office, it still must be maintained by one or two persons. Having too many people involved in the maintenance of the system can lead to errors. Both computerized and manual inventory systems are used in dental offices, the main difference being the format of recording the information into the system used.

Manual Inventory System

A **manual inventory system** involves handwritten entries on a card or page to track supplies and is maintained by one or two people. Each inventory card must include information such as the name of the product, a product or item number, the quantity ordered, the date the item was received, the item price, and the price when ordered in bulk, as well as an indication of the expiration date, if the product is one that expires.

To maintain the inventory in a manual system that makes use of product cards, identifying features that signal the decrease in supply must be put in place. One approach involves using a card file, much like a recipe card file, for keeping cards alphabetically ordered for all supplies in the dental office and placing color-coded tabs on the card of the item that requires replenishing. For example, imagine that a product is getting low and that an order must be placed. The person who is responsible for maintaining the inventory system would place a particular colored tab on the card to signal that ordering is required. When the order has been placed, the tab is changed to a different color to indicate that the item has been ordered. When the order is received, the colored tab is removed and the amount received and the date the order was received are recorded on the inventory card. Items that are on backorder may be given a different color tab on the card. Items that have expiration dates may be written on a different color card to draw attention to the expiration date. For example, if the inventory system uses white-colored cards for each item, products that have an expiration date might have their information recorded on green cards. When all the cards are filed in alphabetical order, there will be green cards interspersed among the white ones, indicating a product that has an expiration date. Paying attention to products with expiration dates is important because once a product expires, it becomes ineffective and therefore unusable in the dental office. Items that expire are ordered more frequently to ensure their use in a timely manner. If a large order of items that expire is not used, it is a financial loss for the dental office since the items will likely be disposed of. To avoid an oversupply of items that have expiration dates, these items should be ordered on an "as needed" basis. That is, smaller quantities of these items should be kept on hand by ordering the items as the supply runs down. This means that these items will be ordered more frequently and in smaller quantities. As the office administrator you may notice that dental supply companies have monthly specials that require a bulk purchase of certain items offered at a lower price. Check to make sure that the item in question is not one that has an expiration date that occurs prior to the time the office may use the item.

Alternate methods of maintaining a manual inventory system might include removing the card of the item that requires reordering from the card system and placing it in a box marked "to be ordered," and, when the order arrives, the card is placed back into the inventory card system. The individuals responsible for the inventory system would be able to communicate with other staff members effectively to inform them that certain items have been reordered by indicating this on the card. That is, it would be written on the item card when an order was placed and the quantity ordered.

Another system may include keeping a master listing of all supplies that are ordered and used in the dental office in a certain period of time, such as on a monthly basis, and updating the list when supplies are reordered. Maintaining the master list by updating it monthly may not be as accurate as the card system since an increase in the use of one type supply for 1 week may not accurately reflect the amounts shown on the master list. For example, if the dentist decided that for the month of June the office would offer a teeth-whitening special, and the master list showed a certain number of whitening kits available at the beginning of the month, if the special was successful and the supply of kits was depleted by the middle of the month, the master list would show an inaccurate amount of whitening kits available.

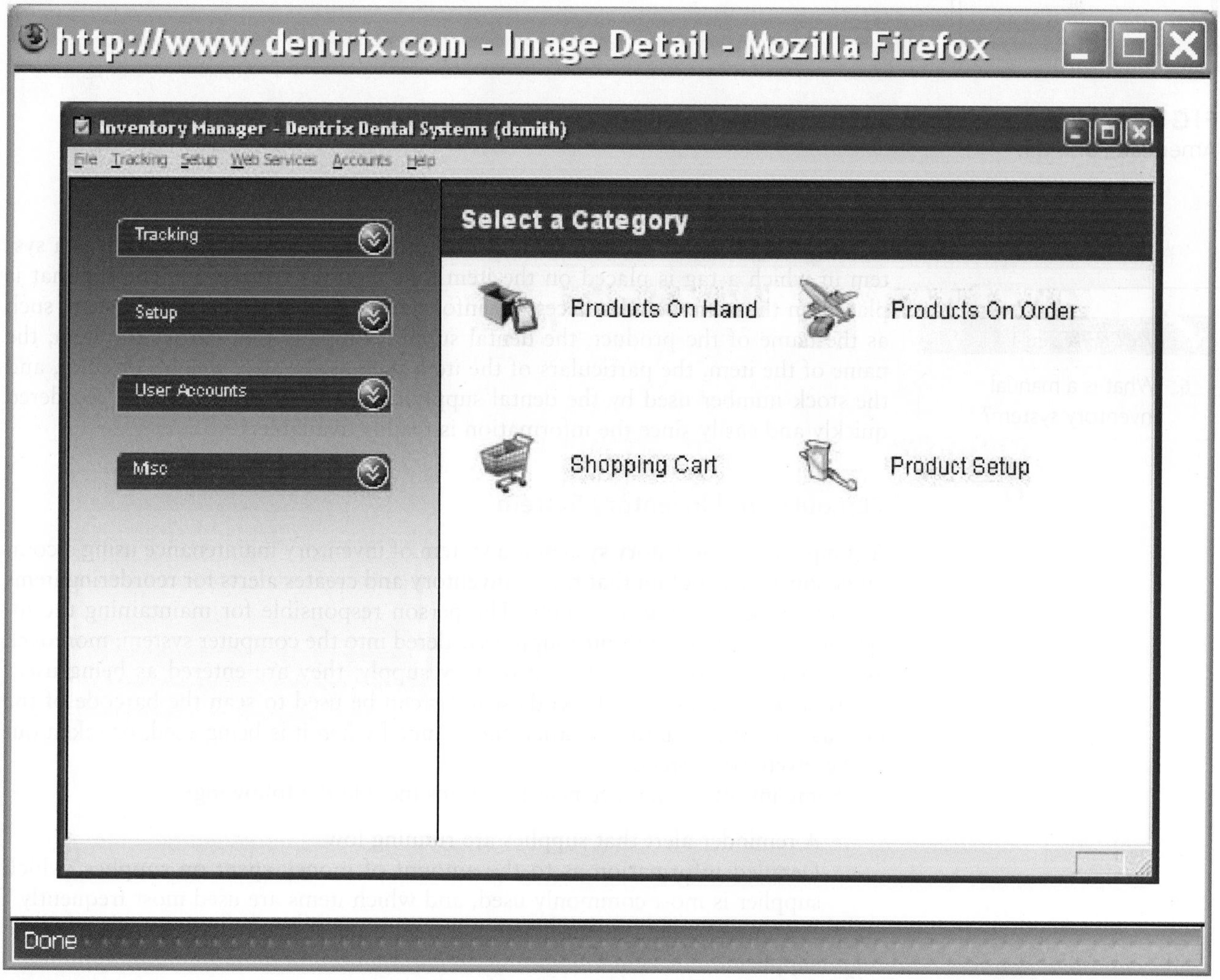

FIGURE 13-7 Inventory management system. DENTRIX image courtesy of Henry Schein Practice Solutions, American Fork, UT.

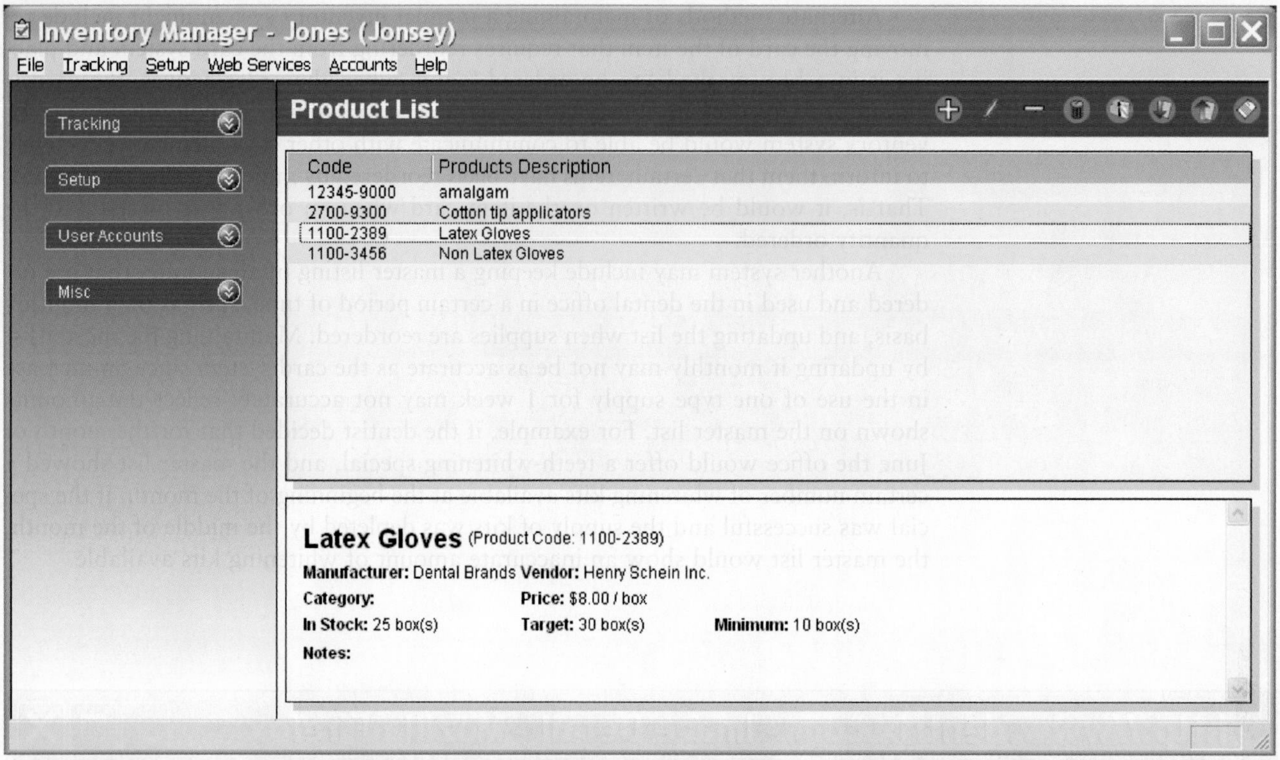

FIGURE 13-8 List of products available. DENTRIX image courtesy of Henry Schein Practice Solutions, American Fork, UT.

checkPOINT

6. What is a manual inventory system?

The "tag system" used in some dental offices for reordering materials is a system in which a tag is placed on the item that requires reordering. The tag that is placed on the item includes necessary information needed to reorder the item, such as the name of the product, the dental supply company that carries the item, the name of the item, the particulars of the item such as the size, weight, or color, and the stock number used by the dental supply company. The item can be reordered quickly and easily since the information is readily available.

Computerized Inventory System

A **computerized inventory system** is a system of inventory maintenance using a computer software program that tracks inventory and creates alerts for reordering items when they become low in supply. The person responsible for maintaining the inventory would manually enter supplies ordered into the computer system; moreover, as the items are removed from inventory supply, they are entered as being used. Alternatively, the use of a barcode scanner can be used to scan the barcode of the item as it is entered into inventory and scanned when it is being used, or taken out of the inventory system.

Some inventory management programs include the following:

- A reminder alert that supplies are running low
- Detailed information as to the amount of money spent on supplies, which supplier is most commonly used, and which items are used most frequently
- Automatic order replenishment when an order is marked as received from the supplier

A computerized inventory management system provides an efficient way to keep track of inventory and provides an accurate picture of the stock on hand and the

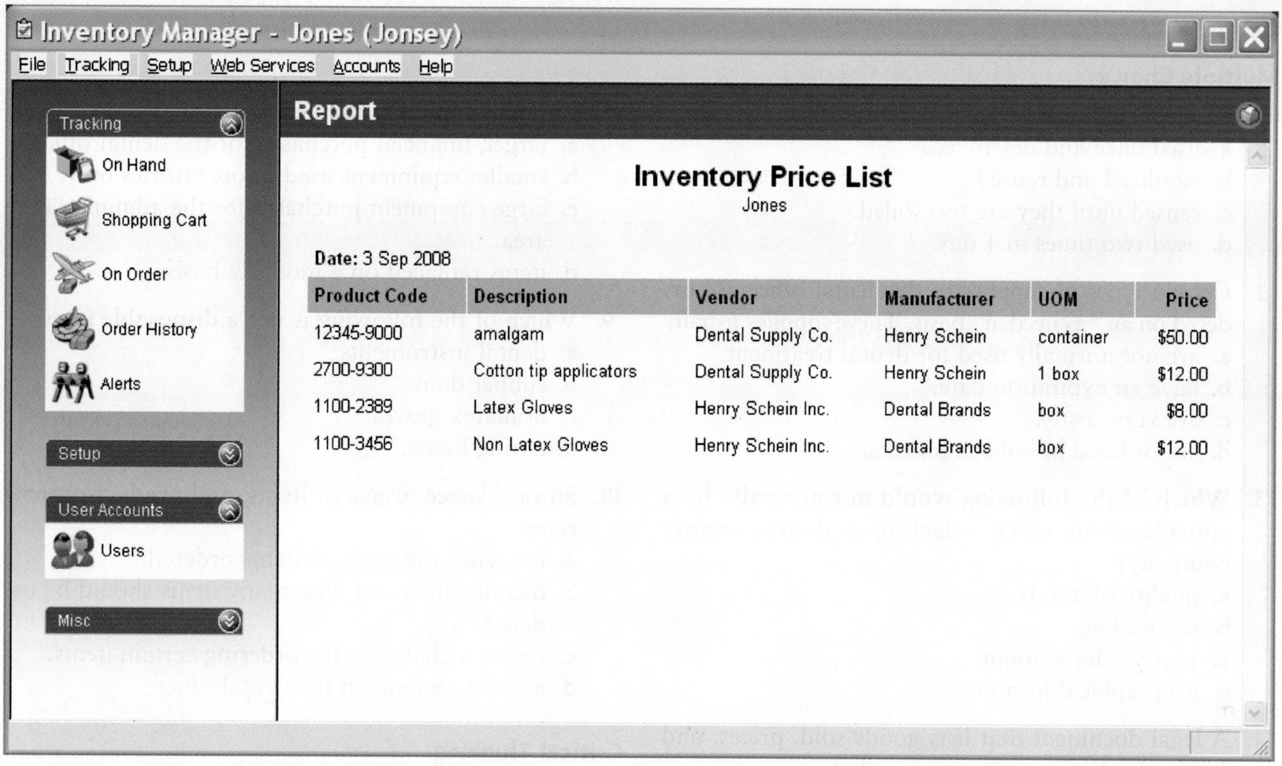

FIGURE 13-9 Inventory reports. DENTRIX image courtesy of Henry Schein Practice Solutions, American Fork, UT.

stock required. In a very busy dental office where a large number of supplies are used on a continual basis, a computerized inventory system is most effective for efficiency and maintenance of inventory.

The inventory management system in DENTRIX (Fig. 13-7) is designed to monitor and track the inventory in the dental office. Each practitioner in the dental practice can access the list of products available (Fig. 13-8). The inventory software enables online Internet ordering of supplies that updates the inventory status of items quickly. The DENTRIX program will automatically make changes to the on-hand items in inventory when certain procedures are billed on completion. The program also allows for inventory reports to quickly and easily be generated and printed (Fig. 13-9).

checkPOINT

7. What is a computerized inventory system?

Chapter Summary

Using both administrative and clinical supplies in the dental office occurs on a continual basis in the dental office. The use of supplies and whether they are classified as reusable or disposable items depend on the purpose of their use. The dental office administrator may be responsible for maintaining the inventory in a dental office. Along with ordering supplies through the dental supply company, the dental office administrator must be competent in reading and understanding the terminology used on an invoice and the monthly statements that arrive in the dental office. Keeping track of inventory in the dental office can be accomplished through the use of either a manual or computerized inventory system.

Review Questions

Multiple Choice

1. **Reusable items are**
   a. used once and destroyed.
   b. sterilized and reused.
   c. reused until they are too soiled.
   d. used two times in 1 day.

2. **Certain types of supplies in the dental office are ordered on an "as needed" basis. These supplies usually**
   a. are not normally used for dental treatment.
   b. have an expiration date.
   c. are very costly.
   d. are ordered in bulk shipments.

3. **Which of the following would not normally be a consideration when selecting a dental supply company?**
   a. quality of goods.
   b. reputation.
   c. yearly sales amount.
   d. geographical location.

4. **A legal document that lists goods sold, prices, and terms of sale to a customer is called**
   a. a waybill.
   b. an inventory list.
   c. an invoice.
   d. invoice head.

5. **Which of the following is true about backordered items?**
   a. They are paid for when ordered.
   b. They are shipped at the time they are ordered.
   c. They are not billed for until they are shipped.
   d. They are more costly compared to other items.

6. **Which is true about manual inventory system?**
   a. It can maintain itself.
   b. It requires one or two persons to maintain.
   c. It is preferred over other systems.
   d. It is difficult to identify when stock is low.

7. **An advantage of a computerized inventory management system is that**
   a. it monitors and tracks inventory in the dental office.
   b. it leaves little room for counting errors.
   c. the program makes inventory changes as procedures are completed.
   d. the program is user friendly.

8. **Capital supplies in the dental office refer to**
   a. larger, financial purchases for the dental office.
   b. smaller equipment used in operatories only.
   c. large equipment purchases for the administrative area.
   d. items replaced on a monthly basis.

9. **Which of the following is not a disposable item?**
   a. dental instruments.
   b. rubber dams.
   c. nonlatex gloves.
   d. curing lights.

10. **Storage space, usage of items, and product promotions**
    a. influence the types of items ordered.
    b. dictate when and how many items should be ordered.
    c. create a challenge for ordering certain items.
    d. are not an issue in the dental office.

Critical Thinking

1. What advantages are available with a computerized inventory system over the manual inventory system?

2. What disadvantages can you anticipate occurring with a manual inventory system? How could those disadvantages be overcome?

3. You have been asked by the dentist to order teeth-whitening kits because the dental supplier is having a sale this month. What considerations will play a part in your order placement?

HANDS-ON ACTIVITY

1. Select five items from the classroom you are in and create an inventory card for each item. Compare your cards with a partner and decide how the inventory cards would be grouped according to different criteria.
2. The office manager has asked for your assistance in developing a policy regarding supply ordering. Write up a policy outling the considerations for ordering clinical items in the dental office.
3. Use the Internet to develop a list of dental supply companies in your area. Select two or three items sold by the companies and compare the costs. Decide which company would be more desireable and explain why.

chapter FOURTEEN

Technology *in the* Dental Office

OBJECTIVES

After completing this chapter, you should be able to do the following:

- Spell and define key terms
- Identify the different types of computers found in the dental office
- List various types of peripherals used with computers
- Describe common administrative applications used in the dental office
- Describe the clinical applications of a computerized practice management program
- Explain how to use the Internet effectively in the dental office
- Discuss the ethical considerations involved in computer use
- Demonstrate the use of proper ergonomics when working at a computer
- Identify other pieces of equipment commonly found in the dental office and demonstrate how to use them

KEY TERMS

- laptop
- tablet PC
- desktop
- central processing unit
- computer system
- peripheral
- monitor
- Internet security system
- cookies
- viruses
- search engine

The role of computers in the workforce today has become central to daily operations. The dental office is no exception. In both administrative and clinical areas of the dental office, the computer plays a central role. For dental office administrators, the computer acts as the daily schedule, accounts receivable and payable center, and the patient financial file. The computer aids the dentists in taking and interpreting radiographs, taking

OUTLINE

intraoral photographs, and providing patient education. As a dental office administrator, you must be confident in using dental practice management software as well as other computer software.

The purpose of this chapter is to develop your skills and knowledge of computers and both administrative and clinical applications in the dental office. Note that the coverage of administrative applications here is merely an overview, with more detailed coverage of individual applications—such as communication, patient record management, recall and recare systems, appointment management, electronic filing, inventory, insurance claims filing, and financial transactions—being integrated throughout the book in the chapters corresponding to these topics. Moreover, this chapter presents Internet basics, ergonomics, and guidelines on performing basic computer tasks. Finally, you will learn about the use of other common equipment in the dental office.

THE COMPUTER

Computers come in many shapes and sizes (Figs. 14-1 and 14-2) to accommodate the many preferences and uses for computers in the dental office. For example, a **laptop** or **Tablet PC** may be preferred by the dentist for use in the operatory, whereas the front desk may be best suited for a **desktop** computer. Regardless of the style of computer, there are certain elements that they all have in common.

Hardware

Computer hardware includes all of the physical core and peripheral components that make up the computer or that may be linked to and used with the computer. These include core components, such as the processor and internal drives, essential peripherals, and optional peripherals.

Core Components: Processor and Internal Drives

Probably the most important part of the computer is the central processing unit (CPU). A **CPU**, housed within the computer's case, is the minute circuitry imprinted on silicon chips that processes computer language data and instructs the operation

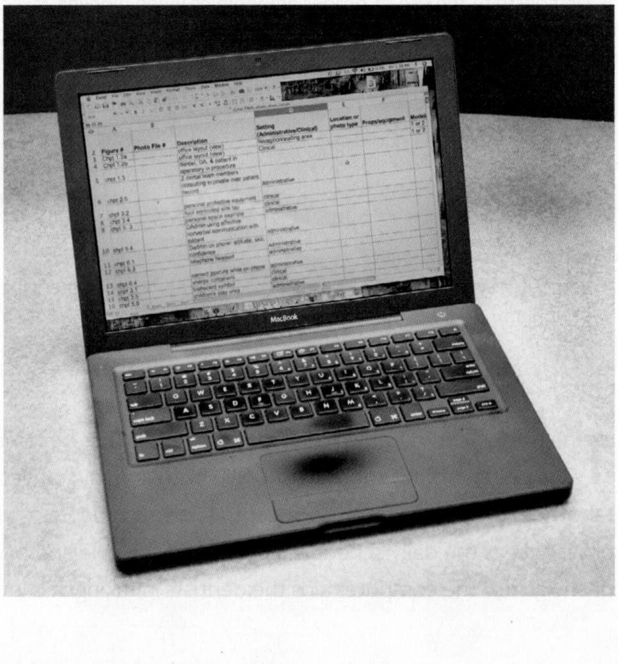

FIGURE 14-1 Laptop computer.

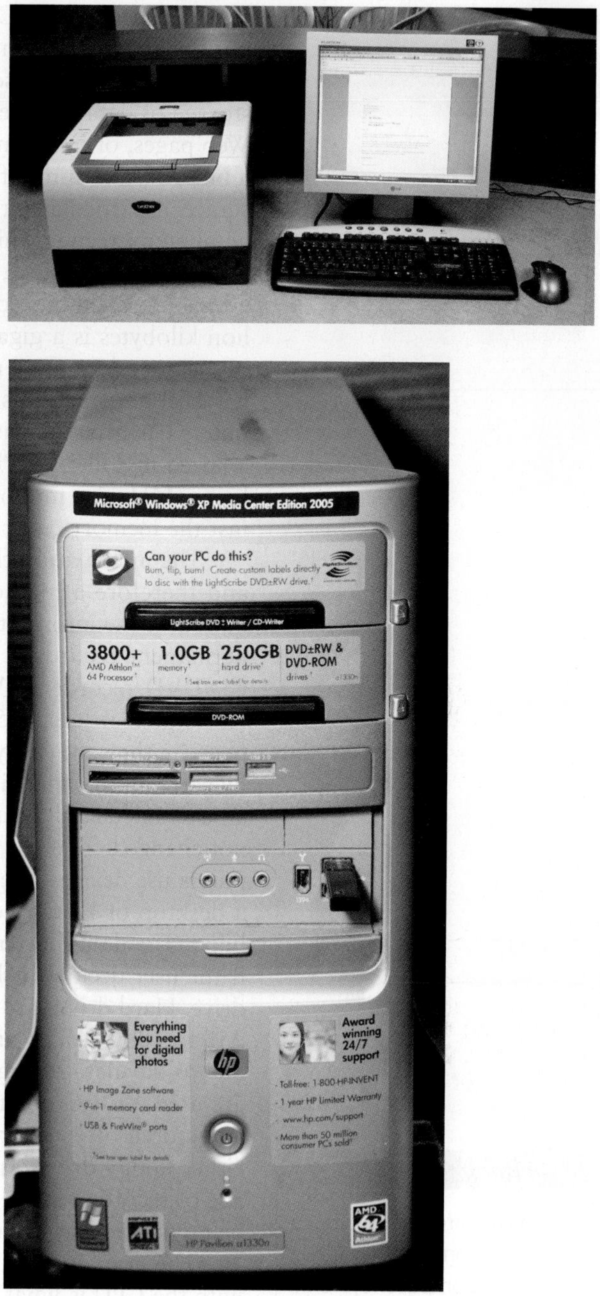

A

B

FIGURE 14-2
Desktop computer.

of the computer. The speed at which these silicon chips can analyze data and run the computer varies. Computer CPUs are rated with a number that refers to their clock speed, or the basic number of commands or "cycles" that they can perform per second (hertz). With modern processors, these speeds are so fast that they must be measured in billions of cycles per second or gigahertz (GHz). Furthermore, a single CPU can have multiple cores or processors within their architecture that all run at gigahertz speed. These CPUs are termed dual core or quad core chips, depending on the number of cores included. The computer can use each one of these cores either together for one program or separately when running more than one program at a time. Effectively this is like having many computers running within one case to help speed up the multitasking that is so necessary when using a computer in today's dental environment.

The speed of the CPU is an important factor governing the speed of a computer, but the amount of memory that is included is equally important in determining the applicability of the usefulness of the machine. Memory is used in a computer for storage of data that needs to be constantly changed, such as pictures on the screen, Web pages, or mathematical calculation results. The smallest memory part is called a bit. You can think of a bit as a light switch. It can be either on or off, so, if for instance, a particular bit in memory is set to on, that may mean one small dot on the computer screen is white, when it is off, that dot may be black. The place that bit is located, or its address, determines what it does. The CPU keeps track of all of these addresses. Eight bits equals one byte, 1024 bytes equals one kilobyte (kB) and a million kilobytes is a gigabyte (GB). Computers can run quite well with one gigabyte of memory, but many modern computers have up to 16 GB of memory. As memory has become much less expensive in recent years, the amount seen in modern computers has been increasing dramatically. Less important than size, memory also has a speed just like a CPU, but it is usually rated much slower and is rated in megahertz (MHz) or millions of instructions per second. This number determines how fast the memory can change what is being held in its addresses.

The information that is contained in the computer's memory is not permanent, and therefore a method to permanently record and recall the information is required. If the information is to be read-only, and not changed, it can be stored as a permanent record on a compact disk (CD) or digital video disk (DVD) using a CD/DVD recorder. DVDs make excellent archival storage media. Most manufacturers give at least a 50-year predicted life for the data on a DVD, they are inexpensive, they are easily stored, and they can carry a lot of data. One DVD can easily carry all the financial and appointment data for 10 years of the daily activities of an average dental office. But data can be written only once to most DVDs and then not changed. To store data permanently, but still have the ability to change it, computers use devices referred to as hard drives. Hard drives can be internal, or within a desktop or laptop computer, or they can be external, which adds to their portability. The data that are typed into a computer first are stored in memory, and then if the user decides to keep the data, it is written to metallic plates within the hard drive. Hard drives are rated on their size. Common sizes for hard drives range from 250 to 1000 MB or one terabyte (TB). Internal hard drives are usually used for the day-to-day data storage operations of the dental office, whereas portable hard drives are used for backup at the end of the day. Monthly backups can be burnt to a DVD and stored off-site for security and fire protection. Some older computers may use either floppy drives or zip drives. These storage devices are good for archival storage of records but tend to be slower and more cumbersome to use, and so they are being phased out quite rapidly.

The combination of the essential peripherals and optional peripherals along with the CPU is what makes up the entire **computer system.**

checkPOINT

1. What are the components that make up a computer system?

Essential Peripherals

A **peripheral** is a type of computer hardware that is added to a computer in order for the intended use of the computer to be fulfilled. Peripheral devices are normally viewed as optional items that are connected to a computer. Peripheral devices are connected to a computer through a port, or bus, such as a Universal Serial Bus (USB) port. Items such as monitors or keyboards are not usually considered peripheral items since they are not truly optional; that is, it is impossible to use the computer without them. They are referred to here as essential peripherals. Box 14-1 lists some guidelines for properly caring for peripherals.

Essential peripherals consist of the following:

- monitor
- keyboard
- mouse

BOX 14-1
Care of Peripherals

Use the following guidelines regarding the care of peripherals in the dental office to maintain their use:

- Place a dust cover over the peripheral at the end of the day or when it is not to be used again for some time. Dust can be damaging to the insides of the peripheral if allowed to accumulate.
- Wipe the peripheral on a weekly basis using an anti-static cloth and solution designed for computers and peripherals. Always spray the cloth with the solution and then wipe; never spray the peripheral directly.
- Never touch a computer monitor with your fingers, especially if the monitor is a liquid crystal display (LCD) monitor. The oils secreted from human skin can be damaging to the screen and may shorten the life of the monitor.
- Keep backup drives or disks stored in a protective case. Maintaining the proper care of these items will prolong their use and ensure that they are effective when needed. Backup drives and external hard drives should be stored in a safe place, where they will not be exposed to harsh temperatures.
- Do not eat or drink around computer peripherals. Food and beverages accidentally spilled on them can cause permanent damage.

MONITOR A **monitor** is the visual display screen used with the computer. The various sizes and shapes available in monitors are designed to address the different needs for monitors. A CRT monitor (cathode-ray tube) is a bulkier style monitor, which uses the same technology as used in most televisions to display the information on the computer screen. An LCD monitor, or liquid crystal display, also known as a flat-panel monitor, is a thin, modern-looking computer monitor that takes up much less space at the computer area. Graphic professionals still use CRT monitors as they are said to have truer colors and less glare and cause less distortion of images. These graphic series monitors can be very expensive, are found only in sizes up to 27 inches, and are not often seen in a dental office. The benefits of size and price have all but caused the replacement of the CRT monitor in most office situations with LCDs. LCD monitors can be found in sizes from 14 inches to more than 60 inches (measured diagonally) although practical sizes range from 20 to 24 inches. They are much less expensive than comparably sized CRT monitors. These monitors create a small "footprint" or amount of spaced used on the desk, and so allow for more room for other items. It should be noted that smaller, older CRT monitors may be found in some dental offices, and when due for replacement, they should be disposed of at the proper facilities, as they contain recyclable materials.

KEYBOARD To enter information into the computer such as patient information, a keyboard is required. There are several different keyboards that may be considered for the dental office. The standard keyboard has a cord that attaches it to the keyboard input on the outside of the computer's case. This keyboard usually has alphabetic and numeric keys, function keys, editing and navigation keys, and a numeric keypad. Manufacturers may also add multimedia keys to control playback of music or movies. The keys on the keyboard may be in straight rows or may be in a more ergonomic, curved pattern that may help some people with problems like repetitive stress injuries. Some keyboards are wireless and do not require a physical connection to the computer. This can be very handy if the keyboard is some distance from the computer case. Washable and sterilizable keyboards should be strongly considered for the dental office where the possibility of cross-contamination of surfaces is possible. These keyboards can be wiped down or cleaned with antibacterial sprays without worry of ruining the mechanical aspects of the keyboard.

Mouse The mouse started to become a standard input device for computers in the 1980s. Early mouse devices had a mechanical mechanism based on a rolling ball that allowed the user to move an arrow or other pointing device on the screen and select and move different items. Very soon after the introduction of the mouse, the mechanical parts, which tended to be prone to failure, were replaced with optical parts that could detect the movement of the mouse over a surface with great accuracy. The optical mouse and its components, either a light-emitting diode or a laser, proved to be much more accurate and much more reliable and required less cleaning than the mechanical mouse and so has largely replaced it. The mouse may be attached to a USB port or a mouse port on the computer case or more conveniently may be wireless. Wireless mice will require battery replacement or battery recharging from time to time. Typically a mouse has a left and right button and a scroll wheel. After moving the pointer, or focus of attention on the screen, by moving the mouse, the new area under the pointer can be selected by pressing the left mouse button. This is termed "point and click." The right mouse button generally is used to perform an action on this area of focus. The scroll wheel quite commonly allows movement through lists or through pages in a rapid fashion by rolling the wheel with the finger. Clicking twice in quick succession on the left mouse button can access different functions. This action, termed "double clicking," usually will select an item and allows the user to perform an action on the selected item. As you can see, the term usually is used quite often here as every program that is used may have different mouse responses and requirements. Programmers have made an attempt at standardization of responses to mouse gestures, but the software manual should be consulted with regard to what mouse actions will provide the proper required response for the user.

checkPOINT

2. What are essential peripherals? List three examples.

Optional Peripherals

Optional peripherals are those that, while not necessary, extend the capabilities of the computer. Peripherals make day-to-day necessary procedures easier to accomplish, such as printing statements for patients, sending dental claims electronically, and obtaining information for patient charts. Optional peripherals include network cards and modems, printers, scanners, speakers, external hard drives and backup devices, and digital cameras.

Network Card and Modem Most dental offices have access to the Internet and the ability to communicate with other computers in the office, which is made possible through the use of a modem. A modem is a device that encodes and decodes the digital signal of a computer to send it as electrical information. Modems are available in various speeds, which means that the faster the speed the modem can provide, the faster the transmission of information. The type of connection to the Internet, which the modem provides, can vary between telephone (dial-up) or a cable system (high-speed Internet). Because some dental programs and dental insurance providers insist on communicating with dental offices by way of older dial-up modems that use regular telephone lines, it is sometimes necessary to have a computer that has this capacity. Newer computers have forsaken this type of modem, and so a telephone modem quite often has to be purchased as an add-on to the system. This modem can be purchased in an external or internal configuration. The external modem will plug into a modem port on the back of the computer, while an internal modem will fit into a card slot inside the computer. A telephone line is then plugged into the modem. Because the speed of dial-up modems is limited to not much more than 56 thousand pieces of data per second, or 56 Kbps, newer broadband modems have taken their place. These newer modems can be as fast as 1 billion bits per second. DSL modems, cable modems, and satellite modems allow the user to send larger files such as radiographs or pictures to other computers in a reasonable amount of time. This is not possible or is at least not practical with dial-up modems. The concept is the same, however, in that the computer must encode and decode data to send it to other computers. Even computers that are networked within the same office must have a network card that operates as a modem to "talk" to other computers. These network cards can be wired to each other with a cable that looks like a thick telephone line (RS232) or they can be wireless. A wireless modem can be attached externally or internally to a computer to provide wireless access for several computers in one office. Wireless cards and access must be configured with security measures to prevent unwanted access to computers or to data on those computers.

Printer The printer is a commonly used peripheral and is used in the dental office for such tasks as printing out patient statements, claim forms and submission results, daily and monthly reports, and daily schedules. The printer is especially important for offices that maintain hard copy files of important documents that are created or received electronically.

The two primary types of printer used in the dental office are the ink-jet and laser printers. The ink jet printer uses liquid ink that is sprayed on the paper in the form of very small dots to form an image. The laser printer uses a powder called toner that is heated on to the paper to form its image.

The ink jet printer is very versatile. It can print very good text documents and can also print photographs that will rival the output of professional photography labs. Printing radiographs or images of teeth is easily accomplished. The pages can be printed fairly quickly, and ink jets print color very well. The initial cost of an inkjet printer tends to be quite low, but the cost of replacement inks can be very expensive and the cost per page of most ink jets is quite high.

Laser printers print excellent text documents, in most cases exceeding the quality of ink jets. In general, laser printers print single and especially multiple pages faster than ink jet printers. Color laser printers are available, but they do not print color or black and white photographs very well. It is not practical to use a laser printer to print patient photographs or radiographs. The cost per page of laser printed output is less than with an ink jet, and toner cartridges tend to last longer than ink cartridges.

The solution for many offices is to have at least one ink jet printer and at least one laser printer. In this way, the laser printer can be used to print day-to-day and important documents at a fast speed. When color or graphic output is required, the ink jet can be used. Printers can be attached to the office network so that they are accessible from any computer on the network. Some printers will even attach to the network wirelessly, so they require no physical connection to the system.

Some practice management programs may require a specific type of printer to be used for printing.

Scanner The scanner is a peripheral device that is used to make digital copies of documents for storage on and output from the computer. Paper forms can be scanned with the scanner, and the resultant scanned document can be sent by e-mail, reprinted as many times as necessary, or stored for future reference. If a document is scanned, a program called an OCR or optical character recognition program can be used to make the document editable in a word processing program. Many scanners can perform the functions of a copier, and this is one of their more common uses. Many ink jet printers have scanners built into them, making the copying process very easy. These so-called "three in one" ink jet printers can also fax documents, making it an easy job to scan a document, save a copy, print a duplicate, and fax it to someone, all with one peripheral.

Speakers Speakers allow a user to interact with a computer by playing audible sounds. At first it may seem like speakers have no practical application in a dental office, but they can be quite useful. Speakers for most computers can be very inexpensive and require very little desk space and so they should not be ruled out as superfluous. For many applications used on the computer, there is an audio cue when the user has made an error, or when a message arrives. This audio cue can be very helpful to the operator. If a computer is used for patient education or entertainment, speakers are a necessity, especially if the educational materials are in the form of a video presentation. Speakers can enhance the usefulness of a computer and make it more pleasant to use.

External Hard Drive and Backup Devices Using a backup device to save computer system information is a necessary procedure in the dental office. Computers are machines, and they can break down, sometimes losing all of their data. The loss of data that can occur will be a very serious problem. It is also important to have a copy of all vital data in case of fire, flood, or theft. It can be easily imagined what will happen if all medical, financial, and appointment data are lost. It will bring most modern dental offices to a standstill. Several types of backup devices are available. An external hard drive is a stand-alone drive that may be easily connected, disconnected, and moved from computer to computer. External drives come with varying storage capacities from a few gigabytes to many terabytes. Larger drives can easily contain all the information that is stored on the hard drive of a computer. Typically, the external hard drive is connected to the computer with either a USB cable or a firewire cable. The most common method is USB as it is found on most computers. Firewire is not as commonly found, although it transfers data more quickly. Patient and financial files kept on the computer are typically saved to a backup hard drive at the end of each day and should be taken home with a staff member.

Other methods of backing up the information include recordable compact disks (CD-ROMs), zip drives, or recordable DVDs. Smaller amounts of data can be stored on flash drives. A USB flash drive is a small device, sometimes called a thumb drive because of its small size. It is plugged directly into a USB port, and the computer recognizes it as a disk drive. They are handy for moving photos or documents from one location to another. They have no moving parts and so are very durable, and the capacity of these drives is getting bigger every year. Some flash drives have capacities over 64 GB. Keeping saved information off-site is necessary, should there be a fire or flood and the information is required for insurance purposes.

Digital and X-Ray Cameras Technologically progressive dental offices may use peripheral equipment such as digital cameras and digital x-ray or intraoral cameras. These peripherals are usually found in the clinical areas. However, a camera used to take patient pictures is usually the responsibility of the dental office administrator. The digital x-ray is used by the dentist and clinical staff to diagnose disease, establish the health of the oral and perioral structures, and provide patient education. They must be available to the office administrator in order that they can be forwarded to insurance companies or a specialist's office. For this reason, the office administrator should be aware of what x-rays are available, and what their limitations are, how to access them, how to e-mail them, and how they are stored and recovered. Likewise, the intraoral camera is used for many of the same purposes, taking pictures of oral and perioral structures for diagnosis and education. Again, the office administrator should be aware of the benefits and limitations of intraoral photographs and how the camera works.

✓ checkPOINT

3. What are optional peripherals? List three examples.

Applications

In addition to understanding the computer hardware used in most dental offices, it is also important that you understand the most common programs or software applications that are used in the dental office. The applications used in the dental office may be divided into two categories: administrative applications and clinical applications.

Administrative Applications

As noted earlier, detailed discussion of the various components of dental practice management software is integrated throughout this book, where appropriate. Provided below is a brief overview of these programs. Also provided is an overview of other, more general administrative applications, such as word processing applications, spreadsheet applications, e-mail, and backup management.

Word Processing Several different word processing programs are available for use in the dental office. Some practice management programs have simple text processing programs integrated into their structure, but for more advanced uses, it is important to be familiar with a more full featured program. To write formal letters to other doctors, lawyers, or patients, it is often necessary to have the features of these products. The manuals that come with these programs should be consulted to provide familiarity with the program.

Spreadsheets Spreadsheets are useful programs for the office administrator to learn to use. Modern spreadsheets allow the user to display and perform calculations on numerical data in several different ways. They can be used to make a list of accounts receivable, petty cash purchases, inventories, or any other purpose where a chart or form is required. The spreadsheet has become a very versatile program as it can also display data graphically in the form of charts and graphs. A smart office administrator will become familiar with spreadsheets, as they are a useful addition to their armamentarium.

E-mail For the modern dental office, it is essential that an e-mail program be adapted and learned by the office administrator. E-mail can be used to communicate with patients, other dentists, and insurance companies. Many patients prefer to get appointment reminders, make appointments, or get notified of the result of predeterminations all by e-mail. It is easy to send digital x-rays to other dentists for referral, and insurance company correspondence is quite often accomplished by e-mail. Composing a good letter and learning how to retrieve and send e-mail have become essential skills. All operating systems on computers today have an e-mail program that comes with the system.

Backup Management The practice management program usually includes in its software a method of keeping an up-to-date copy of the software program and its contents. The backup system can be done through the use of an external hard drive as discussed earlier in the chapter. In some cases, a dental management program will have automatic backup that can be directed to an external drive. In other cases, the backup must be performed manually. Usually this can be set in the program preferences, but it is best to refer to your software manual or software professional for advice on this topic. It is also sometimes possible to back up only certain data components in order to save space. Decisions should also be made as to how many backups are kept. For the most part, the most recent backup is the most important, but keeping a few other copies, but certainly no more than five, may be prudent in case of errors, or data corruption. The backups should be done on a schedule, either automatically by the program itself or manually by the operator. In busy offices, daily backups should be the rule, but weekly backups may be enough for a smaller office. The general rule of thumb is that you should back up frequently enough so that if the data are lost before the next backup, retrieval and reentry will not be a problem

Performing Basic Computer Tasks There are several basic computer tasks that should become second nature to the effective office administrator. It will be assumed that the reader has a basic understanding of turning a computer on and off, using a mouse, opening a program or document, and typing on a keyboard. If this is not the case, then a beginning book on the operating system you are using would be an intelligent purchase. It is important to learn as well how to create a folder, how to create a text document, how to cut and paste between documents, and how files can be deleted or retrieved. These skills should be part of the basic armamentarium. There are, however, some tasks that should be performed on a daily or monthly basis to keep the computer running smoothly and cleanly, and having a neat appearance.

Every day, after the computer is turned on, the following tasks should be performed. If it does not happen automatically, any antivirus programs should have their definitions updated. An e-mail program should be opened to check for incoming e-mails. Any urgent e-mails should be answered and any documents that require typing should be finished. Any seldom used or frivolous icons on the desktop should be removed. At the end of the day, a backup should be performed if one does not occur automatically. There may be other tasks that you like to perform daily, and it may be prudent to keep a written list so that they are not forgotten.

On a monthly basis, the disk drive should be defragmented. This is a process by which the hard drive optimizes itself for the best performance. This process may take as long as a few hours but can be left at the end of the day to happen over night. Unused or unneeded files should be removed, but care should be taken to avoid removing critical files. It may also be necessary to check on a monthly basis for program updates. Many programmers will issue updates to their programs that may contain important improvements to the program. It is a good idea to check for these updates for the programs you use most often by visiting the Web site of the program manufacturer on a monthly basis.

Clinical Applications

The clinical application of the dental software program is designed to assist the dentist, hygienist, and dental assistant in providing the patient with detailed, effective dental health care. The components most commonly used by the clinical staff in a dental software program are charting, digital imaging, and the use of other peripherals.

Charting The main use of the computerized system in the clinical areas is for charting purposes for the dentist and the hygienist. Figure 14-3 is an example of a computerized dental chart for a patient. Each tooth in the dentition of the patient can be clearly seen and any of the surfaces requiring restoration easily viewed. An anatomical view of each tooth is used in order that an accurate charting of the dentition is displayed. Electronic charting varies depending on the software used, but generally, work that is required is indicated in red, work that exists is indicated in blue. Extracted teeth have an X through them, and teeth with root canal therapy have a line in each root. Beyond this, there are specific differences from program to program, and these differences should be learned by consulting the user's manual or learning from other staff members. It is important that an office administrator learn to read a dental chart, as there is little time in the day for the dental assistant or dentist to explain the meaning of each item on the chart. Charts of the patient dentition are important medical records, are private, and will be stored within the patient's file on the computer. These charts can be viewed by any member of the dental team on his or her computer but should be considered a private part of patient records.

Digital Imaging Most digital imaging software that is part of the practice management program is compatible with most or all digital cameras. This is an important aspect to consider before purchasing the software program, since the incompatibility of software digital imaging devices will limit the software or digital devices that can be used. Digital imaging devices used in the dental office consist of digital

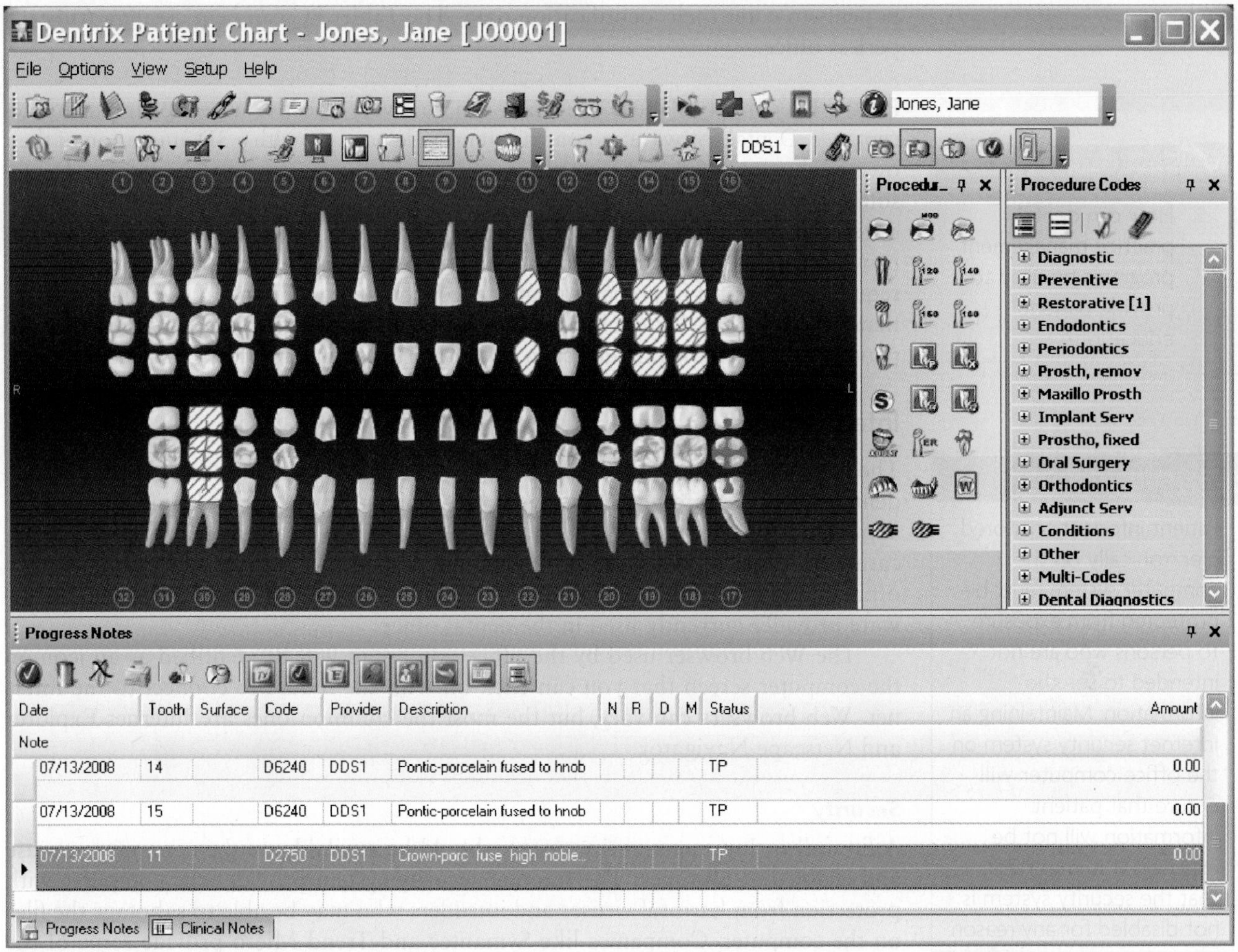

FIGURE 14-3 Tooth charting. DENTRIX image courtesy of Henry Schein Practice Solutions, American Fork, UT.

cameras, digital x-ray sensors, intraoral cameras scanners, and Web cams. A good dental imaging software component of the program will allow the following:

- Link images to the patient's chart and manage them by allowing categorization of images
- Make notes directly on the image as well as adding or subtracting colors to the image for educational purposes
- Use patient images to explain and describe treatment and provide a rendition of the image of what it would look after treatment
- Protect images automatically, which prevents irreversible altering of the image

> **checkPOINT**
>
> 4. What are two features of a digital imaging system that are advantageous to the dentist?

PERIPHERAL INTEGRATION Some dental practice management programs support the integration of peripherals commonly used in dental offices. A popular peripheral used by dentists is the Tablet PC, which is a handheld notebook computer that recognizes handwriting and speech or voice commands and is optimized for wireless network connections. The Tablet PC is particularly useful in the dental office because of its great portability, wireless connection to the network, and ease of use while examining a patient. Using a stylus directly on the screen to enter charting information is a simple, fast, and effective method of getting data into the computer without using paper forms or a keyboard. The surfaces of most tablets can be disinfected, making them ideal for use in the operatory. Some offices use Tablet PCs for patients to enter their identification data. The Tablet PC can help create a truly paperless office.

Patient Education Patient education can be a very effective aspect of treatment acceptance. Dental software programs can provide patients with a 3D animation of their own teeth to explain and have them understand the treatment they require. Dental software programs also include a stock of images and educational shorts on procedures and recommendations for treatment. Educational leaflets, or pamphlets that provide patients with information regarding procedures they may be curious about or require, are helpful in preparing patients for the procedure and answering questions that they may have. Patient images can also be included with treatment plan letters to patients or as a marketing device in encouraging patients to accept treatment.

> **checkPOINT**
>
> 5. How can dental practice management programs be used to provide patient education?

> **legal TIP**
>
> Patient information stored electronically on the computer system must be protected from exposure to persons who are not intended to see the information. Maintaining an Internet security system on the office computer will ensure that patient information will not be exposed. It is important that the security system is not disabled for any reason.

Internet Basics

The Internet, or the World Wide Web, is a household term in today's society. In the dental office, the Internet is used by both administrative staff and clinical staff. The administrative staff may need to access the Internet for various reasons, such as locating addresses of insurance companies and patients, ordering supplies online from office and dental supply companies, and contacting the help desk of the dental software provider currently used in the dental office.

The Web browser used by the office you are in will be identified as an icon on the computer screen that you can click on with the mouse to connect to the Internet. Web browsers can vary, but the most the common ones are Internet Explorer and Netscape Navigator.

Security

A firewall or Internet security system should be available on the computer you use and enabled at all times. The **Internet security system** provides the computer with protection from harmful viruses and intruders who may be able to sabotage the files on the computer. Companies like Symantec and Trend Micro provide some of the more commonly used security systems. AVG and Zone Labs provide very good free programs for security, but they may not be as fully featured as the pay programs. It should be remembered that these programs should have their software and virus definitions updated on a daily basis, in order that they may keep up with the constantly changing world of computer security.

Additional security measures include using sites that are approved by the dental regulating bodies and following Health Insurance Portability and Accountability Act (HIPAA) guidelines on transferring patient information. These sites often have what is called a secure sockets layer. This means that as the information is transferred from the dental office computer, it becomes scrambled so that it is incomprehensible for anyone who intercepts it. When it arrives at the correct site, the information is unscrambled and easily legible.

Keeping the Internet security system on at all times may deny the acceptance of **cookies** on your computer. A cookie is a small file that is placed on the hard drive of your computer by a remote site and that contains information that can identify or control your computer in certain ways. Not accepting cookies may make certain Web pages fail to appear or prevent them from operating correctly.

HIPAA requires that passwords be used to access computerized patient information. From time to time, the passwords should be changed to ensure that information is protected. **Viruses** can be very destructive to a computer system. A virus is a small file that may be transferred to your computer system with the intent to sabotage or annoy. The effects of a virus can be as annoying as shutting your computer down periodically or as destructive as erasing your entire hard drive. Viruses can enter your computer system in different ways, such as when downloading information from the Internet or opening an attachment in an e-mail. A worm is a specific type of virus that enters through an e-mail. Opening e-mail attachments at work should be avoided, particularly if they are sent via personal e-mails! Use the following guidelines when using the Internet at work:

- Do not open e-mails from unknown addresses or suspicious Web site addresses.
- Keep the Internet security system enabled at all times while the computer is on and ensure that the virus protection software is updated as notified.
- When downloading information from the Internet, download only information that pertains to work. Do not download information for personal use.
- Change all passwords on a regular basis.

checkPOINT

6. What is a cookie and how can one be avoided?

Internet Searches

Finding the information you need on the Internet is done through the use of a **search engine.** A search engine allows you to enter a search term and then collects all the sites that match your search terms. Examples of common search engines are Google, Yahoo, and Excite.

Limiting the number of responses you receive on your search is important (Box 14-2). Being specific in the terms that you enter to begin your search is important to avoid wasting time. The Internet can provide hundreds of thousands of Web sites containing information you need if the terms you enter are too general. For example, if you are looking for information on tooth-whitening toothpastes and you enter the search term "toothpaste," you would find innumerable Web sites containing information about toothpaste, from definitions of toothpaste to discussion of ingredients. Entering the terms "whitening toothpaste" will provide a comprehensive list of sources to gather information on whitening toothpastes. When searching for information regarding dental products or procedures, it is a good time saver to begin with searching dental association Web sites for information on the product or topic or going to manufacturer Web sites.

If you are surfing for information that will be used in the dental office for patient information, make sure to print out a copy of the information that will have the name of the Web site on it. Also, make every effort to find information provided by credible Web sites, or Web sites that represent reliable sources of information on the dental industry. Credible Web sites include your local dental association Web site or a well-known dental product supplier, such as Oral-B or Colgate.

checkPOINT

7. How does one gather information quickly and accurately on the Internet?

Computer Ethics

As a dental administrator, you should use the computer professionally as a tool for proficient and efficient work at all times. HIPAA provides comprehensive guidelines for the uses of computers for storing, viewing, and transferring patient information;

BOX 14-2
Tips for Searching on the Internet

1. Select a search engine.
2. Choose one or two words in your query to narrow your search down.
3. If a long list of sites is displayed, refine the search further by entering another key word.
4. If no sites are listed after your initial search, check the spelling of your search terms and try again.
5. Always view more than one site before making a final decision about the information you have found.
6. Download the information or print the information necessary.

adherence to these guidelines ensures the privacy of the patients in the practice. Use the following guidelines in the dental office regarding the use of computers:

- Never leave patient information displayed on the computer when you are not present in the area.
- Always close the screen when you are not in front of the computer.
- Assign separate passwords and log in names for each employee.
- Not all employees should have access to all administrative functions allowed on the computer, such as writing off charges or changing billing or payment information.
- Never use a computer when another employee is logged in under his or her own name on that same computer. Ask the employee to log off or sign off and then use the computer.
- Never access your personal e-mail or download personal information while you are at work.
- Always enter information into the computer with extreme care, making sure that you are entering the information into the correct patient account and using the correct codes. Never stop entering information half way through a transaction.
- Keep the information you read and send by e-mail in the dental office confidential by respecting patient confidentiality and not discussing the information outside of the dental office.

Ergonomics

Because you will be spending a lot of time sitting in front of a computer, it is important that you practice proper body positioning and proper typing style and that a rest period is obtained at regular intervals.

While sitting in front of the computer, you should adjust your chair so that your back is straight, and your neck and back muscles are relaxed. Arm supports should be adjusted so that your arms form no less than a 90 degree angle at the elbow. If the back of your chair is adjustable, it should be adjusted to create gentle support for your pelvis and neck. Feet should be flat on the floor, and the height of the chair should be adjusted so that your thighs are approximately level with the floor.

While typing, your elbows should be above the level of the keyboard. This will prevent fatigue and numbing of arms that can occur from prolonged posturing of your arms at an angle to the work surface. You should sit close to the desk in order that your elbows can be close to your body. Wrists should not rest on the table or keyboard when typing, as this will cause stress on your wrists. Use your whole arm to support your hands and fingers.

Make sure, during the day that you take time away from your desk, and take time away from the computer. While entering data or typing for a long period of time, make sure you look away from the screen every so often and let your eyes focus on a more distant object. During breaks or lunch periods, make sure you get up from your desk and walk around. Gently stretch and rotate your neck if you have been sitting in the same position for a long time.

If you start to exhibit any symptoms of back pain, neck pain, or repetitive stress injury, check your posture and your rest periods, and make sure you are doing the right thing. It may be prudent to request an ergonomically correct chair for your workstation if you cannot work with the chair you have now.

OTHER OFFICE EQUIPMENT

Many offices that you may work in may have several other office machines that you will have to gain familiarity with in order that you can efficiently use them when the need arises. The manuals for these machines should be made available and should

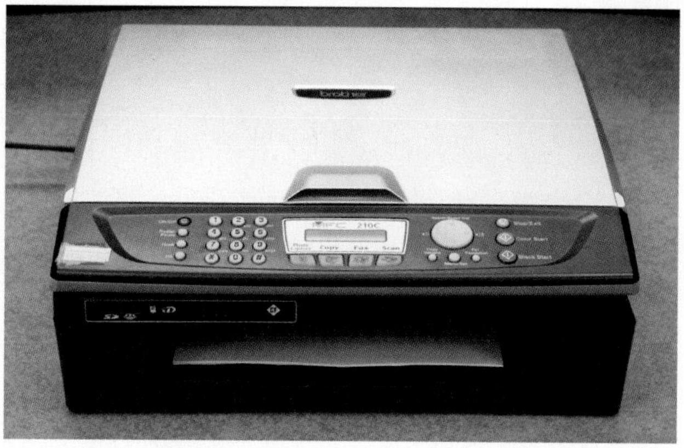

FIGURE 14-4 Fax machine.

be consulted to gain expertise with each type of equipment. If the manuals are not available, most companies have online manuals in the form of pdf documents that can be downloaded and printed.

Fax Machine

Although many computers can provide the services of a fax machine, the ease of sending a paper document over telephone lines that a fax machine provides cannot be denied (Fig. 14-4). When sending a fax, always take care that fax numbers are entered carefully. Sending medical or dental records to the wrong phone number can have embarrassing or serious consequences. A cover letter should always be included before each fax in order that the receiver of the fax knows its source, the length of the fax in pages, who else received the fax, the phone number of the sender, and the date that the fax was sent.

Copier

It is quite often easier to use a dedicated copier rather than a scanner or a fax machine when making a large number of copies of a document, although in recent years, office supply stores and copying companies provide very cost efficient copying services for larger numbers of copies. For single copies, most fax machines or computers with scanners can copy documents quickly and easily.

Postage Machine

A postage machine is a very convenient method for providing postage for the large quantities of mail that goes out of a dental office. A postage machine prints a metered amount of postage directly on an envelope after postage is purchased for the machine over the phone line or Internet. Generally they are very easy to operate, and the manufacturers are normally more than happy to provide online or phone support for their use.

Shredder

A shredder is an important part of keeping patient records private (Fig. 14-5). Quite often, confidential information will appear on items that need to be recycled or thrown away. A heavy-duty shredder is of paramount importance in protecting the confidentiality of these records by rendering them unreadable. Remember, even phone notes that you have taken while conferring with a patient should be shredded. The shredded material can be recycled when necessary.

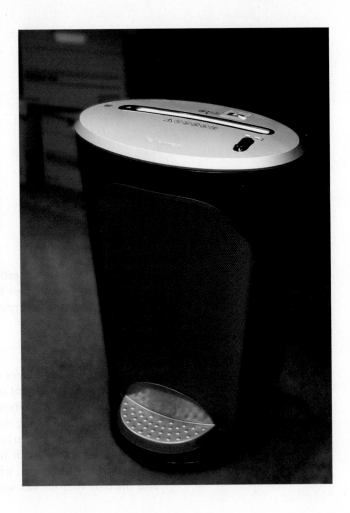

FIGURE 14-5
Shredder.

Calculators

A printing calculator is a useful part of the office equipment on the front desk. Quick additions on patient estimates, verification of deposits, or quick confirmation of order totals can be done without resorting to paper and pencil.

Point of Sale Terminals

Many dental offices have adopted terminals that allow the patient to easily and quickly use credit cards or debit cards to make payments on their accounts. These machines are quite specific to the financial institution that supplies them, and so the instruction manuals should be consulted for their use. Training courses and advice are usually provided free of charge from the company that supplies the terminals. Great care should be taken to provide accuracy when using the terminals, and privacy should be available while patients are entering private codes or pin numbers into the terminals.

Chapter Summary

There are many different types of computers used in the dental office. Desktop computers are more commonly used in the administrative areas, whereas laptops and Tablet PCs may be found in the clinical areas. Although the type and use of a computer may vary, the core components and peripherals needed for the computer are common among them. Peripherals include essential items such as monitors, keyboards, and mice and optional items such as network cards and modems, printers, scanners, speakers, external hard drives and backup devices, and digital x-ray and camera equipment.

The use of a computerized practice management program, along with other common administrative programs, will assist in the maintenance of patient flow in the dental office. Becoming proficient in both the clinical and administrative components of the computer program will assist the dental office administrator in ensuring complete and accurate patient records and maintenance of patient dental care. Competency using computers and confidence with computer programs is essential.

Moreover, dental office administrators should be familiar with using the Internet effectively, understand the ethical considerations of computer use in an employment setting as well as the HIPAA applications regarding computerized patient records, and practice proper ergonomics. Finally, dental administrators should be familiar with the use of other common office equipment, such as copiers and fax machines.

Review Questions

Multiple Choice

1. **A spreadsheet is primarily used to**
   a. arrange text in a format suitable for printing and to create letters.
   b. format numbers in a layout suitable for calculations and analysis.
   c. create presentations to show to the patients for their education.

2. **A USB flash drive**
   a. can hold any kind of data and plugs in to a port called a USB port.
   b. can hold digital images only and plugs in to a port called a firewire port
   c. can hold only numerical or text data and plugs in to a port called a flash port.

3. **Which of the following is true about computer modems?**
   a. An external modem is always slower in speed than an internal modem.
   b. A modem always requires an attachment to a phone line.
   c. A computer must have a modem to get e-mail from the Internet.

4. **A good dental imaging software component of the program will allow the clinician to**
   a. link images to the patients' chart and manage them by allowing categorization of images.
   b. allow for notes to be made directly on the image.
   c. use patient images to explain and describe treatment.
   d. all of the above.

5. **The Internet security system provides the computer with**
   a. cookies that appear when you want.
   b. a history of Web sites visited in the past.
   c. protection from harmful viruses and intruders.
   d. none of the above.

6. **Which of the following is not a guideline for proper computer use?**
   a. Assign separate passwords.
   b. Never use the computer when another employee is logged in.
   c. Always treat all patient information entered into the computer with extreme care.
   d. Using screen savers is at the discretion of the dentist.

7. **Which of the following is considered a clinical application of dental software**
   a. word processing
   b. spreadsheets
   c. charting
   d. internet searches

8. **Administrative applications in dental software include all but which one of the following**
   a. back up management
   b. digital imaging
   c. email
   d. spreadsheet applications

9. **The Tablet PC in the dental office is an example of**
   a. computer peripheral
   b. patient education
   c. administrative application
   d. back up management

10. **Ergonomics in the dental office refers to**
    a. proper hand and back positioning
    b. correct posture
    c. proper posture while typing
    d. all of the above

Critical Thinking

1. Is there a difference between the handling of a digital x-ray and a physical x-ray as far as patient privacy is concerned. What special considerations might have to be thought of with regard to the privacy of digital x-rays?

2. If a fax has been sent to a specialist's office, what should be done with the original cover sheet that was sent with it? Is it important to keep it or to shred it?

3. If an e-mail is sent to a patient, should a hard copy always be printed out for the patient chart? Compare and contrast how the answer may be different in offices with different philosophies on the use of paper.

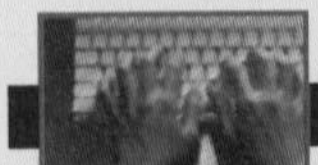

Hands-On Activity

1. Locate the Web site of the state dental association in your area. Navigate throughout the Web site as if you were a patient wanting to locate a dentist close to your home.

2. Search for three different Web sites for dental offices in your state. What components of the Web sites do you find useful? What components would you like to change?

part FOUR

Financial *Management*

chapter FIFTEEN

Dental *Insurance*

OBJECTIVES

After completing this chapter, you should be able to do the following:

- Spell and define key terms
- Explain the purpose and design of dental insurance
- Describe various group plans and individual plans
- Describe Medicare and Medicaid and identify who may be covered by these programs
- Discuss dental indemnity insurance
- Explain the components of dental preferred provider organizations and dental health maintenance organizations
- Describe what is involved in filing insurance claims
- Explain the procedures involved in submitting claims electronically and manually
- Discuss the procedure codes used in the dental fee guides

KEY TERMS

- dental insurance
- preventive dental care
- group
- subscriber
- employee
- group member
- dependent
- carrier
- provider
- provider identification
- insured
- self-funded
- eligibility
- benefit booklet
- dental indemnity insurance
- deductible
- coinsurance
- usual, customary, and reasonable fee
- fixed fee
- managed care
- dental health maintenance organization
- network
- capitation
- dental preferred provider organizations
- direct reimbursement plans
- individual practice associations
- assignment of benefits
- coordination of benefits
- primary insurance
- secondary insurance
- birthday rule
- electronic data interchange
- predetermination of benefits
- explanation of benefits

OUTLINE

Dental insurance provides coverage for individuals that provides assistance with paying and protection from the cost of dental treatment. In the United States, dental insurance and health insurance usually are bundled together in the benefit package provided by one's employer. Additionally, individual dental insurance plans are available for purchase through insuring agencies.

Most people in the United States have healthcare insurance. Healthcare or medical care insurance is designed to cover the costs involved with diagnosing and treating medical illnesses. For most, medical insurance is provided as a benefit and partially funded by an individual's employer, with the employee contributing to the funding. In the United States today, certain large insurance companies, such as Blue Cross and Blue Shield, offer health insurance plans in every state. However, many Americans are covered by entirely self-funded insurance plans or are covered by tax-funded plans, such as Medicare and Medicaid, or are uninsured. According to the most recent statistics provided by the National Coalition of Health Care, in the year 2005 there are currently almost 47 million Americans without health insurance.

Dental insurance operates somewhat differently from health insurance. Dental insurance is primarily designed to provide coverage for the costs involved with **preventive dental care,** which includes regular routine care, such as examinations, radiographs, and dental cleanings. Most dental insurance plans provide coverage for both preventive and major treatments, with patients required to assume a larger portion of the costs for major procedures, such as crown and bridge placement, than for preventive procedures.

As a dental office administrator, a large portion of your time will involve discussing dental insurance coverage with patients and colleagues and filing insurance claims, which require an in-depth understanding of dental insurance and the differences between plans. An understanding of the terminology associated with dental insurance coverage is also necessary for you to competently explain coverage to patients and provide information to patients that concerns their dental coverage. Thus, this chapter presents information on types of dental insurance plans available and guidelines on how to file insurance claims.

checkPOINT

1. What types of dental care do dental insurance plans typically cover?

CANADIAN PRACTICE: PUBLICLY FUNDED HEALTHCARE

The health insurance program in Canada is also referred to as a Medicare system of health insurance where all provinces and territories represent an interlocking set of healthcare plans. Through this system all Canadian residents have access to hospital or physician services that are prepaid through healthcare premiums paid to the provincial government. The provinces and territories in Canada each manage their own healthcare plan but not without the involvement of the Federal Government, which administers national principles, financing, and delivery on the basis of the guidelines of the Canada Health Act. In Canada, dental insurance is a benefit that is usually provided through employer benefit plans; although health insurance is a publicly funded benefit, supplementary healthcare is required to cover other healthcare services.

Moreover, just as in the United States, individual dental insurance plans are available for purchase through insuring agencies.

Most people in Canada have healthcare insurance. Medical insurance in Canada provides both hospital and physician services for patients and does not require payments from deductibles or copayments for insured services.

THE FUNDING OF DENTAL CARE: WHO PAYS?

Dental care may be funded in several different ways. In the dental office, you will come across patients who have dental insurance through employer-, organization-, or association-sponsored group plans or individual dental plans. Other patients will have coverage through such government-sponsored programs as Medicare and Medicaid. Some patients will not have any insurance and thus will be responsible for paying all of their dental care expenses. Each of these types of coverage is discussed below.

Group Dental Plans

Patients who take part in a group dental plan have dental benefits that are sponsored by their employer, the union they are members of, or an association they belong to. The **group** is the employer or organization that provides the dental plan. The person who has coverage in his or her name under the group dental plan is considered the **subscriber, group member,** or **employee.** The patient with dental coverage can also be a **dependent** of the subscriber or employee. A dependent is normally a family member of the subscriber, such as a spouse or child. The insurance company that carries the dental plan is referred to as the **carrier.** The carrier is responsible for paying the dental claims and collecting the premiums. The dental claim, which is created when a patient receives treatment, is usually sent directly to the insurance company from the **provider.** The provider is the dentist who provides treatment. Each dentist is identified to the insurance company by a **provider identification** number, which is included on the dental claim form.

Dental insurance plans provided through an employer or other organization can be either **insured** or **self-funded.** Insured benefit plans are ones in which the employer or other organization pays a portion of the monthly premiums to an insurance company on behalf of the employee or group member. The insurance company then processes the dental claims and pays the dental provider. Box 15-1 lists the roles of the various participants in this process. A dental benefit plan that is self-funded is a plan in which the employer collects premiums and, instead of providing the insurance company with the funds, invests the funds; all dental claims are then processed and paid by the employer. The employer pays the claim to the dental office on employees' behalf. Self-funding group benefit plans have been increasing in popularity.

It is important to remember that group dental plans vary greatly in the type of treatment coverage provided and the amount of treatment cost covered. This means that patients will be eligible for different services. Knowing patients' **eligibility** for the treatment required will be necessary before beginning treatment. Eligibility refers to the fact that some services will be covered by the insurance plan and others may not, depending on certain criteria set out within the plan. For example, a dental benefit plan must stipulate that a certain number of hours worked must be completed before eligibility for benefits occurs. Each dental plan outlines eligibility

BOX 15-1
Dental Insurance Roles

Employee/Subscriber/Group Member (Patient): pays premiums (usually deducted from paycheck)

Employer (Group Administrator): collects premiums from employee (pays to carrier)

Carrier (Insurance Company): collects premiums from group administrator; pays dental claims

Provider (Dental Office): receives payment from insurance company

checkPOINT

2. What does eligibility mean?

requirements that the patient must meet to have certain treatments covered. Some patients may provide you with a **benefit booklet,** which they receive when they become plan members. Often, the terminology used in the benefit booklet regarding dental benefit eligibility may not be familiar to patients, and the office administrator will be asked to decipher the information. All dependents of the employee are bound by the same terms of eligibility requirements as the employees or subscribers of the dental benefit plan. Children of the plan member often have benefits that they are eligible for but the plan member is not, just by virtue of their age and the restrictions outlined in the plan. For example, some dental plans outline an age limitation on coverage for services such as fluoride treatment. That is, if the patient is over a specific age as set out in the dental plan, fluoride treatment is not a covered benefit. Orthodontic services are also a benefit that may be provided under the plan for children and not necessarily for the plan member. Children who are full-time postsecondary students up to a certain age may also be eligible for certain benefits under the employee's dental plan.

You may be required to confirm a patient's dental coverage if you are not in a dental office that uses electronic submission of dental claims. In this case, you must telephone the insurance company and inquire as to the breakdown of coverage for the patient. Maintaining a list of up-to-date phone numbers of insurance companies will be beneficial for efficiently carrying out the task of confirming a patient's eligibility. The name of the insurance company, and often the telephone number, can be found on the dental benefit card or form the patient presents. Figure 15-1 provides an example of a dental claim form.

Administrative **TIP**

When a patient informs you that he or she has dental insurance, it will be necessary for you to collect the patient's dental plan identification numbers to have on file for claims processing. Patients may bring written information with them to the appointment regarding their dental coverage that can assist the patients in making decisions regarding the financial aspects of their dental treatment. Electronic claims processing is also useful for predetermining patients' financial responsibility for treatment. For example, if a patient has a dental plan that provides coverage for teeth cleanings once every 12 months, yet the patient would like his or her teeth cleaned once every 6 months, you can explain that the insurance plan he or she currently has will provide coverage once per year for teeth cleanings. Making patients aware of their financial responsibility prior to treatment commencement will avoid misunderstandings.

Individual Dental Plans

An individual dental plan is a plan that is purchased by an individual directly from an insurance company. The individual pays the premiums to the insurance company directly, and the insurance company accepts claims and pays the provider directly. Individual dental insurance coverage plans are not necessarily better or worse than group dental coverage plans. As more individuals become engaged in self-employment, individual dental insurance plans are more prevalent. There are various individual dental insurance plans available that are designed to suit the specific needs of the person subscribing to the plan.

In some cases, individuals who already have some dental coverage through their employers will choose to purchase an individual dental plan to supplement their employer-sponsored plan. This is because dental insurance plans provided through employers may change as employee contracts are updated and negotiated, and may not be adequate for the patient. Thus, an employer-sponsored dental insurance plan and an individual dental insurance plan can be held by one patient.

Medicare and Medicaid

The U.S. Social Security Act outlines provisions afforded to citizens of the United States who qualify for assistance under guidelines set out by the State. Medicare and Medicaid are two areas under the Social Security Act that provide coverage to citizens for dental care. **Medicaid** is a joint funded program between the State and the Federal government that provides additional coverage for health and dental services for low-income families. The specifications of a patient's eligibility for Medicaid are

TO: Great West Life

Canadian Dental Association

Canadian Life and Health Insurance Association Inc.

STANDARD DENTAL CLAIM FORM

PART 1 DENTIST	UNIQUE NO. 590255300	SPEC. 0	PATIENT OFFICE ACCT NO. 1560

I HEREBY ASSIGN MY BENEFITS PAYABLE FROM THIS CLAIM TO THE NAMED DENTIST AND AUTHORIZE PAYMENT TO HIM/HER.

X

SIGNATURE OF SUBSCRIBER

PATIENT
Dawna Hawkeswood
11022 - 64 Avenue
Edmonton, AB
T6H 1T5
Claim # 14780

DENTIST
Dr. Guy Girtel
#204, 7125-109 Street
Edmonton, AB
T6G 1B9
PHONE NO.7804355300

FOR DENTIST USE ONLY - FOR ADDITIONAL INFORMATION, DIAGNOSIS, PROCEDURES OR SPECIAL CONSIDERATIONS.

*** Please Pay Dentist ***

DUPLICATE FORM []

I UNDERSTAND THAT THE FEES LISTED IN THIS CLAIM MAY NOT BE COVERED BY OR MAY EXCEED MY PLAN BENEFITS. I UNDERSTAND THAT I AM FINANCIALLY RESPONSIBLE TO MY DENTIST FOR THE ENTIRE TREATMENT. I ACKNOWLEDGE THAT THE TOTAL FEE OF **$156.26** IS ACCURATE AND HAS BEEN CHARGED TO ME FOR SERVICES RENDERED. I AUTHORIZE RELEASE OF THE INFORMATION CONTAINED IN THIS CLAIM FORM TO MY INSURING COMPANY / PLAN ADMINISTRATOR. I ALSO AUTHORIZE THE COMMUNICATION OF INFORMATION RELATED TO THE COVERAGE OF SERVICES DESCRIBED IN THIS FORM TO THE NAMED DENTIST.

X

SIGNATURE OF PATIENT (PARENT/GUARDIAN)

OFFICE VERIFICATION

DATE OF SERVICE DAY	MO.	YR.	PRO-CEDURE CODE	INTL. TOOTH CODE	TOOTH SURFACES	DENTIST'S FEE	LABORATORY CHARGE	TOTAL CHARGES
8	8	2008	23322	46	MO	156.26		156.26

FOR CARRIER USE

ALLOWED AMOUNT	INC	%	PATIENT'S SHARE

CHEQUE NO. | DATE

DEDUCTIBLE | PATIENT PAYS | PLAN PAYS

CLAIM NO.

THIS IS AN ACCURATE STATEMENT OF SERVICES PERFORMED AND THE TOTAL FEE DUE AND PAYABLE, E & OE.

TOTAL FEE SUBMITTED $156.26

INSTRUCTIONS FOR CLAIM SUBMISSION

BEING A STANDARD FORM, THIS FORM CANNOT INCLUDE SPECIFIC INSTRUCTIONS ON WHERE IT SHOULD BE SENT, DEPENDING ON WHO IS THE CARRIER FOR YOUR PLAN. YOU CAN OBTAIN DETAILS FROM EITHER YOUR PLAN BOOKLET, YOUR CERTIFICATE OR FROM YOUR EMPLOYER.
IF YOUR PLAN REQUIRES SUBMISSION DIRECTLY TO THE CARRIER, PLEASE SEND THIS FORM WITH ONLY PARTS 1, 2 AND 3 COMPLETED TO THE CARRIER'S APPROPRIATE CLAIMS OFFICE.
*IF YOUR PLAN REQUIRES SUBMISSION TO YOUR EMPLOYER, PLEASE DIRECT THIS FORM TO YOUR PERSONNEL OFFICE/PLAN ADMINISTRATOR WHO WILL COMPLETE PART 4 AND FORWARD THE FORM TO THE CARRIER.

PART 2 - EMPLOYEE/PLAN MEMBER/SUBSCRIBER

1. GROUP POLICY/PLAN NO. 55400 DIVISION/SECTION NO. ______
2. YOUR NAME (PLEASE PRINT) Hawkeswood, Stuart J.

EMPLOYER Merit Contractors
YOUR CERT. NO. OR S.I.N. OR I.D. NO. 900003146 For Dep. # 01

NAME OF INSURING AGENCY OR PLAN Great West Life
YOUR DATE OF BIRTH 06/06/1963 DAY MONTH YEAR

PART 3 - PATIENT INFORMATION

1. PATIENT: RELATIONSHIP TO EMPLOYEE/ PLAN MEMBER/SUBSCRIBER Spouse
   DATE OF BIRTH 08/08/1962 IF CHILD INDICATE: [ ] STUDENT [ ] HANDICAPPED
   IF STUDENT, INDICATE SCHOOL ______
   PATIENT I.D. NO. ______
2. ARE ANY DENTAL BENEFITS OR SERVICES PROVIDED UNDER ANY OTHER GROUP INSURANCE OR DENTAL PLAN, W.C.B. OR GOV'T PLAN? [X] NO [ ] YES
   POLICY NO. ______ SPOUSE DATE OF BIRTH ______
   NAME OF OTHER INSURING AGENCY OR PLAN ______
3. IS ANY TREATMENT REQUIRED AS THE RESULT OF AN ACCIDENT? [X] NO [ ] YES
   IF YES, GIVE DATE AND DETAILS SEPARATELY.
4. IF DENTURE, CROWN OR BRIDGE, IS THIS INITIAL PLACEMENT? [ ] NO [ ] YES
   GIVE DATE OR PRIOR PLACEMENT AND REASON FOR REPLACEMENT.
5. IS ANY TREATMENT REQUIRED FOR ORTHODONTIC PURPOSE? [X] NO [ ] YES
6. I AUTHORIZE THE RELEASE OF ANY INFORMATION OR RECORDS REQUESTED IN RESPECT OF THIS CLAIM TO THE INSURER / PLAN ADMINISTRATOR AND CERTIFY THAT THE INFORMATION GIVEN IS TRUE, CORRECT, AND COMPLETE TO THE BEST OF MY KNOWLEDGE.

DATE 25/02/2009 DAY MONTH YEAR

X

SIGNATURE OF EMPLOYEE/PLAN MEMBER/SUBSCRIBER

PART 4 - POLICY HOLDER/EMPLOYER (FOR COMPLETION ONLY IF APPLICABLE. SEE ABOVE*)

	DAY	MONTH	YEAR
1. DATE COVERAGE COMMENCED			
2. DATE DEPENDENT COVERED			
3. DATE TERMINATED			

4. CONTRACT HOLDER

DATE		
DAY	MONTH	YEAR

AUTHORIZED SIGNATURE

(POSITION OR TITLE)

COPYRIGHT 09/03 ALL INFORMATION RECORDED ON THIS FORM IS CONFIDENTIAL Page 1

FIGURE 15-1 Dental claim form.

determined by the state in which the coverage occurs. For this reason, being familiar with guidelines for coverage in the state you are in will be helpful in your dealings with patients who qualify for such assistance. Under the terms set out within the Medicaid program, the dental office must accept the payment provided by the program as full payment of services, which means that collecting any unpaid amounts from the patient is not permitted. Also, obtaining preauthorization from the Medicaid program office is required before starting any treatment. Finally, patients who qualify for Medicaid may have insurance coverage through their employers. In this situation, the employer-provided coverage is the primary coverage and Medicaid is the secondary coverage. Medicaid is somewhat different from Medicare in that **Medicare** is a program that focuses on the provision of additional health and dental coverage for senior citizens, which generally includes citizens 65 years and older.

Uninsured Patients

Not all patients who frequent the dental office have dental insurance. Depending on the financial policies in place in the dental office, patients without dental insurance are responsible for the full amount owing for their dental treatment at the time of their appointment. The acceptance of dental insurance as partial or full payment for service is at the discretion of the dental office. Offices that do not accept dental insurance as a form of payment utilize a fee-for-service approach to collecting fees for treatment. The main advantage to using a fee-for-service approach is that the accounts receivable balance remains at a minimum. One of the disadvantages of using this method centers around the need for a third party credit company to be available to patients. To assist patients in accepting services, a third-party company that specializes in extending credit to patients is made available for the patient through the dental office. The patient applies for credit to the company, and the dental office is provided with payment in full. The contract is between the patient and the third party creditor. This is advantageous to the dental office in that the accounts receivable balance is minimized. A disadvantage to the dental office with this method is that the dental office must provide the patient with information on the third party company and facilitate a relationship between the company and patient until all information has been provided.

As a dental administrator, you will encounter many patients who wish to accept treatment but must deal with roadblocks such as finances and time. The following are some general tips to keep in mind when assisting patients who do not have dental insurance:

- Always be prepared to discuss payment plans with patients prior to treatment acceptance. The office you work in may have policies and procedures in place regarding payment plans and tools available for you to develop a payment plan for patients. Payment plans allow patients to accept, follow through, and complete treatment using a plan that works well for both the office and the patient.
- Always provide a prioritized breakdown of the treatment. A prioritized breakdown outlines the more urgent issues to be addressed first; this allows the patient to see what needs are more urgent and assists in decision making when it comes to treatment selection. In other words, although cost may be an issue, outlining which treatment is necessary at what stage focuses on the benefits of treatment.
- Never assume that the patient will be concerned solely with the cost of the treatment. Providing the patient with an explanation of the benefits of accepting a specific treatment and how it contributes to cost-savings in the future will facilitate decision making. For example, providing the patient with an explanation regarding the importance of having a teeth cleaning before beginning treatment for prosthetic placement would be a responsibility of the dental administrator.

TYPES OF INSURANCE PLANS

The type of coverage provided in any one insurance plan can differ. For example, a patient who has dental benefit coverage from her employer may not have the same dental coverage as that of another employee from the same company. Since the coverage held by each patient can vary widely in the type of coverage, each patient must be treated as an individual. Figure 15-2 provides an example of the type and frequency of coverage that may be available to a patient who has made the choice to purchase individual dental insurance. Not all patients will be fully familiar with their level of coverage. They may present you with information about their plan, or you may need to contact the insurance company. Your understanding of insurance plans and service frequencies is essential for effective communication with patients. The information provided in Box 15-2 will assist you when contacting an insurance company to obtain information for patients regarding their insurance coverage.

Dental insurance plans may be divided into two main types: indemnity and managed care. These are discussed below.

Fee-for-Service (Dental Indemnity Insurance)

Dental indemnity insurance is a fee-for-service insurance plan. What this means is that the patient pays the dental provider for the treatment rendered and then submits a dental claim directly to the insurance company for reimbursement. The patient may not be reimbursed for the full amount paid to the provider. The insurance contract between the insured and the insurance company outlines the criteria of the amount or percentage the insured can expect to receive for specific treatment. If the

Dental

- Dental coverage is for fillings, cleanings, scalings, examinations, polishing and certain extractions
- Recall visits every 6 months

	Percentage Paid	To a maximum of (per anniversary year)
Year 1		
On your first $1,200 of eligible services	60%	$720
Total benefits payable for the first anniversary year		$720
Year 2 and beyond		
On your first $500 of eligible services	90%	$450
On your next $700 of eligible services	60%	$420
Total benefits payable for your second and subsequent anniversary years		$870

The following six dental services have a combined maximum of $1,250 per 3 year period. For oral surgery, periodontics and endodontics (root canal), benefits are available beginning Year 2; for orthodontics, crowns, bridges and dentures, no benefit is available until Year 3. The payment percentage increase from the effective date of the contract is as follows:

	Anniversary Year 1	Anniversary Year 2	Anniversary Year 3 & beyond
Oral Surgery	0%	60%	80%
Periodontics	0%	60%	80%
Endodontics (Root Canal)	0%	60%	80%
Orthodontics	0%	0%	60%
Crowns, Bridges	0%	0%	60%
Dentures	0%	0%	60%

Coverages are designed to coincide with your current provincial Dental Association Fee Guide for General Practitioners. The Flexcare DentalPlus coverage will be adjusted to match any increases in the fee guide.

FIGURE 15-2 Individual dental insurance plan.

BOX 15-2
Information Required When Contacting an Insurance Company

When calling an insurance company, have this information in front of you (this can be found in the patient's chart):

- Name of subscriber and patient (if different)
- Patient's date of birth
- Policy number
- Division number
- Certificate number
- Date of service

Also, be sure to get answers to the following questions:

- What is the annual maximum allowed for the patient? Is there a separate annual maximum for basic and major services?
- Is the anniversary date of the policy on a calendar year?
- What is the frequency and amount of the deductible?
- What dental fee guide does the plan base reimbursements on?
- How many units of scaling and polishing are covered per year?
- What percentage of coverage is allowed for the following:
  - Diagnostic services
  - Preventive services
  - Restorative services
  - Endodontic services

fee charged by the dental office is greater than the amount that the insurance company will reimburse, the difference is the responsibility of the patient. In return for receiving the monthly premiums paid by the plan member, the insurer reimburses (indemnifies) the plan member if covered procedures are incurred. It is common for the plan member to pay a **deductible,** which is a set dollar amount that the plan member must pay on a set basis. For example, the patient may pay a $50 deductible once per year, which is deducted from the reimbursable amount to the patient. The patient may also pay a **coinsurance** amount. The coinsurance amount is a percentage of the expenses that the patient is financially responsible for. For example, the insurer may reimburse the provider for 80% of the fee charged, and the patient is responsible for the 20% of the fee that is not reimbursed. After the deductible and the coinsurance amounts are satisfied, the patient receives reimbursement for the remaining expenses.

*check*POINT

3. What does fee-for-service mean?

Typically, fee-for-service insurance plans reimburse the plan member and calculate benefits by using one of three methods:

- usual, customary, and reasonable fees
- schedule of benefits
- fixed fee

Usual, Customary, and Reasonable Fee

Usual, customary, and reasonable (UCR) fee method of reimbursement involves the insurance company reimbursing the patient either the dental provider's fee or the UCR fee, whichever fee is less. The insurance company devises the UCR fee by determining, first of all, the **usual fee** charged by the dental provider for the service. The insurance company obtains the information regarding the fees that have been filed by the dental office and charged to other patients. **Customary fees** are those fees that are charged for the same service by similar dental providers in the same geographic area. A **reasonable fee** is one that is greater than what is usually charged by the dental provider because of exceptional circumstances but is considered to be reasonable by the insurance company if it is justified by the dental provider. For example, if a root canal therapy procedure was much more difficult or time consuming, the dentist might charge a higher fee to cover costs of extra material used and exceptional time spent.

This type of insurance plan is one most commonly dealt with in the dental office, since it allows for plan members to select the dentist of their choice. That is, the plan does not outline which dentist the subscriber must attend. Challenges that arise from this type of plan most often occur between the dental office and the patient. The fee-for-service plan reimburses the patient on the basis of the fees used in the plan agreement. The fees often used in the plan agreement are less than the amount charged by the dental provider. The patients are then responsible for the difference between what they are charged and what they are reimbursed for. This type of plan can lead patients to feel that their dentist is charging too much, when in reality, there are no two dental offices that charge the same fees. Fees charged are based on what the dental office deems as appropriate on the basis of overhead costs, the experience of the dentist, and the type of treatment rendered. The fees reimbursed by insurance companies also vary greatly between insurance companies.

Schedule of Benefits and Fixed Fee

Dental insurance plans that use a schedule of benefits or table of allowances use a defined list of benefits that are reimbursed for a specified amount. The fees charged by the dental provider are usually different from the amount the insurance company reimburses. **Fixed fee** schedule plans are plans that use a set dollar amount that they will reimburse the dental provider for specific fees. Plans that use this type of reimbursement method are usually social assistance dental plans (Medicare and Medicaid). The dental provider must accept payment in full for treatment rendered for patients using these dental plans, based on state or federal governmental regulation.

> **checkPOINT**
>
> 4. What is a schedule of benefits?

Managed Care Plans

The rising cost of health and dental care has required employers to offer **managed care** programs, which are designed to provide access to health and dental treatment by offering a lower cost alternative to traditional health and dental insurance plans. Under managed care insurance plans, the type of dental treatment and the frequency it can be received is limited. Dental health maintenance organizations (DHMOs), dental preferred provider organizations, direct reimbursement plans, and individual practice associations are all examples of managed care programs.

Dental Health Maintenance Organizations

More common in the United States, a health maintenance organization (HMO) acts as both insurer and provider of health services. Instead of reimbursing a patient for payment of health services at the insurance plan's reimbursement rate, the provider of the health service is paid an amount regardless of the treatment rendered. In a managed care system, unlike in traditional insurance systems, the contract is between the insurer and the provider and the patient is much more limited in the choice of doctor. The contract outlines what amount of money will be paid for treatment.

DHMO insurance plans are very similar to traditional medical HMO insurance plans. **DHMO** are organizations of dental providers who provide dental treatment to members of the dental plan. The dental providers have contracted to provide services to the plan members. Under this contract, the dental providers are paid a set amount of money per patient, regardless of the treatment provided or the fees the provider charges. With this type of dental coverage, the choice of dental providers is limited for the covered member to the dentists who are under contract to the DHMO. Patients who have insurance coverage through DMHOs are encouraged to use the **network** of providers, including dentists and dental specialists, under contract to the DHMO. Patients who chose to see a provider outside of the network are financially responsible for the fees that are incurred with that provider. DHMOs do not pay the dental providers a fee for each service provided. The providers are paid on the basis of the number of members enrolled in the dental health plan. When a patient's insurance plan pays providers on a per capita basis, this is referred to as **capitation**. This means that the dentist receives a fixed rate payment per member regardless of the treatment provided.

It is your responsibility to be familiar with the DHMO and the other dental providers in the network that the patient is a member of. You can find this information on the patient's identification card and by calling the phone number that is on it to contact customer service.

Dental Preferred Provider Organizations

Dental preferred provider organizations are similar to the medical PPO insurance model. A medical PPO is a health benefit program that has a contract with a third party, such as an insurance carrier or self-insured employer with a purpose of providing members with services at prenegotiated reduced rates through contracted providers. The PPO contracts with dental providers to provide dental services to their plan members at a reduced fee rate. A dental office may become a member of the PPO network to maintain patients in the practice who are members of the PPO or as a method of attracting new patients. Patients who are members of the PPO are charged the reduced fee as per the PPO contract. Patients who are not members of the PPO are charged the dental provider's regular fee.

The main difference between PPO dental insurance and HMO dental insurance is that PPOs allow patients more freedom in selecting their dental provider. The premiums that the plan member pays are usually lower if they choose a dental provider from the PPO's network; however, patients can choose to see a provider outside of the network and still be reimbursed, although the reimbursement rate will not be as high.

Direct Reimbursement Plans

A **direct reimbursement plan** provides reimbursement to the plan member from the employer of the self-funded plan. Patients who have coverage through a self-funded plan are free to choose the dental provider of their choice. The plan member pays the dental provider directly for the fees that are charged, and the employer reimburses the employee a percentage of the fees paid, based on the plan specifications. There is no insurance company involved in a direct reimbursement plan.

Individual Practice Associations

Dentists and dental associations may form a collective organization to take part in contracts of providing dental treatment to specific plan member populations, which are referred to **individual practice associations**. These dental providers practice out of their own offices yet provide treatment to specific plan members on a per capita basis, as well as providing care to patients who are not enrolled in any specific dental insurance plan on a fee-for-service basis.

FILING INSURANCE CLAIMS

If you are employed in a dental office that accepts dental insurance as a form of payment, you will deal predominantly with dental insurance companies for payment of dental treatment, whether the claim is filed electronically or mailed to the insurance company. Dental offices that deal directly with the patient's insurance company to obtain payment for treatment rendered are said to accept **assignment of benefits.** This means that the patient is assigning his or her insurance benefits to the dental office in payment of the treatment received. The patient usually pays for the portion of treatment that is not paid for by the insurance carrier at the time of the appointment. Electronic submission of dental claims allows the dental office a quick

checkPOINT

5. Why is it necessary to obtain correct insurance information from the patient?

response from the insurance company regarding its coverage of the treatment and the patient's share. This allows the dental administrator to collect the patient's portion immediately.

Some dental offices do not accept assignment of benefits and collect the full amount owed for treatment at the time of the appointment. The dental office administrator can still submit a claim either electronically or manually on the patient's behalf, and the insurer will reimburse the patient directly.

Obtaining the correct insurance information from patients is necessary to ensure that claims are filed accurately and payment is received in a timely manner. To ensure accuracy of claims submission, request that the patient provide you with his or her dental insurance identification card; you can then record the information in the patient file or take a copy of the card to be kept in the patient's chart. Each visit, ask the patient whether there have been any changes to the dental insurance coverage you have on file. Patients may change jobs, may not come in to the dental office for quite some time, and then forget to inform you of any changes. It is the responsibility of the dental office administrator to maintain up-to-date information regarding insurance coverage of the patient. Claims that are rejected by the insurance carrier will delay payment to the provider or patient. Table 15-1 outlines various reasons for claim rejection by an insurance carrier and the actions you can take to rectify them.

legal TIP

Insurance companies must also adhere to guidelines regarding the privacy of client information. The patient must provide verbal or written permission to the insurance company in order for the insurance company to discuss the patient's insurance coverage and treatment information with the dental office representative. Speak with the patient to ensure that this permission has been given before contacting the insurance company; otherwise, no information will be obtained for the patient.

Coordination of Benefits

Some patients may have more than one dental insurance plan that they are eligible to receive benefits from. For example, a patient may have coverage as a subscriber under the dental plan provided through his employer and may also have coverage as a dependent under his spouse's dental insurance plan. Having two insurance plans means that **coordination of benefits** will apply to this patient. The plan to which the patient is the subscriber is considered the **primary insurance** plan. This is the insurance plan that will pay for a portion of the services first. The spouse's plan, to which the patient is a dependent, is known as the **secondary insurance** plan and will then consider payment for the remaining amount. Coordinating the benefits from both insurance carriers is the responsibility of the dental office administrator, particularly if the dental provider accepts assignment of benefits.

When a patient has both primary and secondary insurance coverage available to her, and she has children who are also eligible for these benefits, when a claim is submitted for the child, the **birthday rule** must be followed. The birthday rule refers

TABLE 15-1 Claim Rejection Reasons and Corrections

Reason	Correction
The patient's coverage is no longer valid.	Confirm the information with the patient, and contact the insurance company while the patient is in the office to correct the errors.
A procedure code used is not recognized.	Check whether the code being submitted is up-to-date and accurately reflects the procedure.
Procedure codes are not an eligible benefit under the plan.	Bill the patient for the charges for these procedures.
Bad data are detected (data are incomplete).	Correct data errors and resubmit the claim.

Administrative TIP

If a patient does not have her dental insurance card with her but has written down some identification information that she is quite sure is accurate, depending on the office policies in place in the office, you can call the insurance company to confirm that the identification numbers you have received are accurate. Attempting to submit a claim that does not have accurate information on it will result in a rejection notice. Confirming patient information with the insurance company while the patient is present in the dental office is helpful, particularly if the insurance company representative requires verbal authorization from the patient to provide information to the dental office.

checkPOINT

6. Who does the birthday rule apply to?

only to dependents (children) of the parents who both have dental insurance: the insurance plan of the parent whose birthday occurs first in a calendar year is the primary plan. For example, Mrs. Smith has a birth date of March 13; Mr. Smith's birth date is November 2. Since the month of March occurs first in the calendar year, the primary plan would be Mrs. Smith's. Note that the age of the parent is not the consideration, but when the birthday occurs in the calendar year.

Each patient for whom the dental office submits a dental claim must be the only patient on the claim form. You cannot put more than one patient on one claim form. For example, if a family of 3 comes into the dental office and each person receives treatment, each person in the family must have a dental claim form completed, regardless of age. Figure 15-1 provides a sample of how a completed dental claim form would appear prior to submission to the insurance company for payment.

Electronic Claims Submission

Most dental offices submit dental claims electronically to insurance companies. There are still some cases in which dental claims must be mailed to the insurance company. A dental office that has a computerized dental practice management program and a modem can submit claims electronically. Submitting claims electronically to the insurance company reduces the amount of time it takes to receive payment for dental claims. Computer program updates occur on a regular basis to ensure compatibility between the practice management program and the insurance company's submission software.

Electronic data interchange is the electronic interchange of business information using a standardized format. In other words, electronic data interchange is a process that allows the dental office to send information (dental claims) to the insurance carrier through electronic means rather than mailing the claim. It is similar to an e-mail program or a text messaging system. Since the electronic program is sensitive to the accuracy of information on the claim form, all fields must be completed and accurate. Some practice management programs will not allow submission of a claim that is incomplete. Some insurance companies that receive claims electronically and reject them because of inaccuracy will accept the claim only if it is mailed in after the correction is made. Claims that have information such as radiographs or photographs attached, or predeterminations, must be submitted manually through the mail or courier and cannot be submitted electronically.

Predeterminations

When a patient with dental insurance requires major dental services and the patient would like to have his or her insurance benefits cover the cost, it is often required by the insurance company for the dental provider to submit a **predetermination of benefits.** This means that the dental administrator will put together an itemized estimation of cost for dental treatment that a patient requires. A predetermination of benefits is not a request for authorization to begin treatment. The dental provider, together with the patient, has determined the best course of treatment for the patient. The patient has dental insurance that may cover some or all of the cost of the treatment and, according to the regulations of the dental insurance the patient has, a predetermination of benefits must be submitted before starting the treatment.

Estimate for Dental Treatment

Date: January 4, 2006
Patient's Name: Jane Smith
Address: 1234 Oak Street Edmonton, KY 90012-9876
Telephone: (H) 555-1234 (W) 555 — 4321

Treatment	Time	Fee
Porcelain Bridge Tooth #13-15	2 appts	**$1100**
Laboratory Fee		**$600**
		$
		$
		$
TOTAL FEE		**$1700**

This is an approximation of costs only. Circumstances can arise which may increase or decrease the cost of treatment either before or during the treatment process. This estimation is valid for 30 days from the date it was created.

FIGURE 15-3 **Estimate for dental treatment.**

Most dental plans require a predetermination of benefits to be submitted for any treatment costing more than $500.00 or any major restorative dental work such as crowns, bridges, or implants. The dental administrator itemizes the treatment required along with the cost for treatment and attaches radiographs or photographs and submits the information to the insurance company. The insurance company employs staff members who have practical experience in the dental industry, such as dentists, dental hygienists, and dental assistants, who are familiar with scenarios for treatment and the exceptional circumstances that sometimes surround them. These dental professionals consider the criteria of the individual's dental insurance, such as the percentage of coverage and the frequency allowed for the type of treatment considered. Once a decision is made, the response will be sent to the dental provider and the patient.

Patients who do not have dental insurance coverage for treatment that they require are often provided with a treatment cost estimate before beginning treatment. A treatment estimate provides patients with a breakdown of the cost involved and the number of appointments required for the treatment to be completed. A treatment estimate given to patients before booking their appointments will eliminate misunderstandings about cost and the financial responsibility of the patients. Figure 15-3 is a sample treatment estimate.

legal TIP

According to the regulations under HIPAA, submitting claims electronically to the insurance carrier requires consent from the patient. Asking the patient to provide consent for this process involves informing the patient that his or her personal information will be sent electronically to the insurance company on his or her behalf and only for the purposes of submitting dental claims for treatment that has been completed. Obtaining written consent from patients for electronic submission is recommended.

Explanation of Benefits

Once the claim has been received by the insurance company or claim administrator and paid, an **explanation of benefits (EOB)** is sent to the dental provider along with the payment. Normally, a copy of the EOB is also sent to the patient. Figure 15-4 provides an example of an EOB. The EOB provides information regarding how much is being paid on the claim, who is receiving the payment, as well as any deductible or copayment information. The responsibility of the dental office administrator is to ensure that the payment received from the insurance company matches the claim that was submitted. In other words, the EOB must accurately reflect payment for the correct patient on the correct date of service.

ALBERTA BLUE CROSS®

TM The Blue Cross symbol and name are registered marks of the Canadian Association of Blue Cross Plans, an association of independent Blue Cross plans. Licensed to ABC Benefits Corporation for use in operating the Alberta Blue Cross Plan.

ABC 10196 (R05/2002)

EXPLANATION OF DENTAL BENEFITS

Statement ID 6561710	Document Source EDI		Paid To DR. GUY GIRTEL	Date October 21, 2003	Cheque 4798831
Subscriber Group 20389	Section FCC	ID 4135043-22	Subscriber Name Geraldine T Irlbacher-Girtel	Provider ID 590255300	Provider Name Dr. Guy Girtel
Reference 200328895638		Patient ID 4135043	Patient Name Geraldine Irlbacher-Girtel	Patient Birthdate 1970/01/19	Paid Amount $283.45

Service Date	Submitted Procedure	Allowed Procedure	Tooth Code	Tooth Surface	Submitted Amount Prof	Submitted Amount Lab	Allowed Amount Prof	Allowed Amount Lab	Ineligible Amount	Plan's Portion Prof	Plan's Portion Lab	Other Insurer	Paid Amount	Messages	
2003/10/15	01202	01202			46.49	0.00	41.06	0.00	5.43	90%		0.00	36.96	1659	841
2003/10/15	11114	11114			185.98	0.00	164.00	0.00	21.98	90%		0.00	147.60	1659	841
2003/10/15	02142	02142			30.93	0.00	27.32	0.00	3.61	90%		0.00	24.59	1659	841
2003/10/15	11101	11101			44.18	0.00	39.00	0.00	5.18	90%		0.00	35.10	1659	841
2003/10/15	12101	12101			22.08	0.00	0.00	0.00	22.08			0.00	0.00	841	236
2003/10/15	41301	41301			49.75	0.00	43.55	0.00	6.20	90%		0.00	39.20	1659	841

236 This claim is only eligible if the patient was not older than 20 years of age and a dependent of the cardholder at the time of service. Our records indicate the patient's age was 33 on the date of service.
841 The balance of this claim has been forwarded to your Spending Account for consideration.
1659 The eligible amount for the professional fee is based on the fee schedule in effect for this plan.

RECEIVED Oct 23/03

PLEASE SEE THE REVERSE SIDE FOR ADDITIONAL INFORMATION. INQUIRIES SHOULD BE MADE WITHIN 30 DAYS. PAGE 1

FIGURE 15-4 Explanation of benefits.

BOX 15-3 Dental Fee Code Categories

Diagnostic: D0100-D0999
Preventive: D1000-D1999
Restorative: D2000-D2999
Endodontics: D3000-D3999
Periodontics: D4000-D4999
Prosthodontics, Removable: D5000-D5899
Maxillofacial Prosthetics: D5900-D5999
Implant Services: D6000-D6199
Prosthodontics, Fixed: D6200-D6999
Oral Surgery: D7000-D7999
Orthodontics: D8000-D8999
Adjunctive General Services: D9000-D9999

PROCEDURE CODES

Accurate recording and reporting of dental treatment is ensured by a set of codes that provide a consistent format for all dental providers to use when billing insurance companies for dental treatment provided. The American Dental Association provides its dentist members with the *Code on Dental Procedures and Nomenclature* (the Code). The Code is reviewed and revised on a regular basis to reflect the changes that occur regularly in the dental industry.

It is the responsibility of the dental office administrator to become familiar with the fee codes to be used. The procedure codes used for dental treatment are divided into categories. Each category makes use of a specific set of numbers. Box 15-3 outlines the code categories used in the United States.

Each category of codes refers to a specific area of services provided by the dental provider. For example, a porcelain crown is a restorative procedure, and the specific code for this can be found in the Restorative category. The first digit of the procedure code refers to the category that the procedure falls under. The digits that follow refer to the subclass that the procedure falls under.

Each dental office has a copy of the Code currently in use, which provides a detailed listing of all procedure codes. The codes used and fee amounts charged in each dental office vary between states, and even among dental offices in the same city. The guide provided by American Dental Association is designed to provide a guide for dentists and not a set fee amount for services.

CANADIAN PRACTICE: DENTAL FEE GUIDE

In Canada, each provincial regulatory body provides its members with a *Dental Fee Guide* (the fee guide). The fee guide provided is designed to give dentists a guide by which to set their individual practice fees and is not intended to act as a fixed schedule of fees. Although the price of a procedure may vary between dental offices, the code used for a specific procedure will be the same. Below are the code categories used in Canada:

00000–09999: Diagnostic
10000–19999: Preventive
20000–29999: Restorative
30000–39999: Endodontics
40000–49999: Periodontics
50000–59999: Prosthodontics, Removable
60000–69999: Prosthodontics, Fixed
70000–79999: Oral & Maxillofacial Surgery
80000–89999: Orthodontics
90000–99999: Adjunctive General Services

Chapter Summary

Most dental patients you will encounter will have some type of dental insurance coverage. There are many different types of group, individual, fee-for-service, and managed care plans available. Being familiar with each type of plan and having the knowledge that there are various plans available will prepare you for dealing effectively with different guidelines within each plan. Filing accurate claims within the time limits specified by the patient's plan is necessary and will be easily achieved if you become familiar with the dental plan for each patient, as well as the procedure codes provided in the *Code on Dental Procedures and Nomenclature*.

Review Questions

Multiple Choice

1. **Dental insurance is designed to**
   a. cover some of the costs of dental treatment.
   b. provide coverage for some of the costs of only preventive dental care.
   c. pay for most of crown and bridge work.
   d. none of the above.

2. **The dollar amount that the plan member must pay at the start of every calendar year of the plan is referred to as**
   a. a coverage penalty.
   b. a deductible.
   c. treatment fee.
   d. coverage credit.

3. **Dental offices that deal directly with insurance companies to obtain payment for a patient's treatment**
   a. are fee-for-service.
   b. accept assignment of benefits.
   c. are indemnity coverage offices.
   d. provide discounted rates.

4. **An itemized estimate of costs for treatment submitted to an insurance company is a(n)**
   a. coverage request.
   b. estimate for payment.
   c. predetermination of benefits.
   d. explanation of benefits.

5. **The category of codes that refers to orthodontic work is**
   a. D8000-D8999.
   b. D9000-D9999.
   c. D4000-D4999.
   d. D2000-D2999.

6. **Dental indemnity insurance is**
   a. delegated under state law.
   b. a fee-for-service insurance plan.
   c. an insurance plan provided by the federal government.
   d. an insurance contract between the patient and the dentist.

7. **All dependents of the employer under the insurance plan**
   a. are bound by the terms and eligibility requirements of the plan.
   b. have a separate agreement with the coverage provider.
   c. must provide proof of age on an annual basis.
   d. always have age restrictions imposed on them.

8. **Which of the following statements is false?**
   a. The insurance company will provide the dental office with the necessary coverage information.
   b. It is the responsibility of the dental administrator to obtain accurate coverage information from the patient.
   c. The patient must provide coverage numbers for himself or herself and any dependents who are patients of the dental office.
   d. Confirming eligibility of benefits can be done electronically.

9. **The birthday rule refers to**
   a. the birthdays of dependent children of plan holders.
   b. the insurance plan of the parent whose birthday occurs first in a calendar year.
   c. the day the plan holder became eligible for coverage.
   d. whether or not the plan holder is eligible for coverage on his or her birthday.

10. **A treatment estimate provides**
    a. a breakdown of only the most urgent treatment.
    b. the cost and time involved in dental treatment for the patient.
    c. only a cost estimate to assist the patient in making a decision.
    d. the best method of making the patient aware of treatment cost.

Critical Thinking

1. Mr. and Mrs. Jones both had their teeth cleaned in the practice today. They both have dental insurance coverage through their employers. Mr. Jones is 3 months younger than Mrs. Jones, with his birthday being in April. Whose insurance company will each patient's claim be submitted to first, and second? If Mr. and Mrs. Jones had their son James, who is 13 years old, in the practice for a teeth cleaning also, which insurance company would you submit James' claim to first and then second?

2. A new patient has come into the dental office for a teeth-cleaning appointment. The patient informs you that he has coverage through his employer plan and through Medicaid. Explain how you are going to determine this patient's eligibility for coverage under the two plans? Which plan will you submit to first?

3. If you were to explain to a new colleague how to distinguish among dental fee category codes, how would you do this?

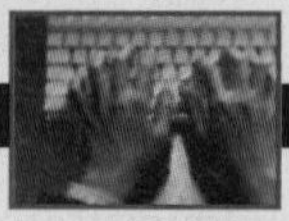

HANDS-ON ACTIVITY

1. List three insurance companies that provide individual plans for patients in your state or province. Use the Internet to perform your search.
2. Use the fee guide in the practice management program to look up the following procedures: Porcelain Crown on tooth 11, 2 units of root planing, Root Canal Therapy on tooth 36. Select three other procedures and ask your classmate to find the codes in the fee guide.
3. Using one of the procedures you practiced finding in question 2, complete an insurance claim form for a patient and attempt to submit the claim form.

Web Sites

Blue Cross Blue Shield
www.bluecares.com

Blue Cross Canada
www.bluecross.ca

American Dental Association
www.ada.org

Canadian Dental Association
www.cda-adc.ca

Government of Canada—Canadian Health Care System
http://www.hc-sc.gc.ca/hcs-sss/medi-assur/index-eng.php

National Coalition of Health Care
http://www.nchc.org/facts/coverage_fact_sheet_2007.pdf

U.S. Social Security Laws
http://www.ssa.gov/OP_Home/ssact/title19/1900.htm

chapter SIXTEEN

Accounts *Receivable*

OBJECTIVES

After completing this chapter, you should be able to do the following:

- Spell and define key terms
- Describe bookkeeping as it pertains to the dental office
- Explain basic concepts of bookkeeping, such as double- and single-entry systems, charges, payments, account adjustments, and fiscal year
- Identify and describe key components of a computer bookkeeping system and demonstrate how to use them
- Describe various components of the one-write system of accounting and demonstrate how to use them
- Explain what is involved with management of accounts receivable
- Describe what is involved in extending credit to patients
- Explain the procedure involved in making a collection phone call
- Discuss the most common methods used for collecting monies owed to the dental office

KEY TERMS

- bookkeeping
- accounts receivable
- accounts payable
- one-write accounting system
- journal sheet
- day sheet
- proof of posting
- ledger card
- credit balance
- discount
- credit adjustment
- debit adjustment
- fiscal year
- overhead
- creditworthiness
- aged accounts receivable listing

OUTLINE

The dental office is a business that must maintain accurate and up-to-date financial records. The financial records of a dental practice are needed to determine the financial health of the business. Moreover, many business decisions are made on the basis of the dollar amount of expenses in certain areas, the amount of accounts receivable, how inventory and cash flow affect the financial picture, and the overall revenue generated by the practice.

To present an organized picture of the business, maintaining organized records is necessary. Maintaining the financial records of the dental practice is usually a shared responsibility between the dental administrator, office manager, dentist, and an accountant. The role each of these individuals plays in the financial record maintenance of the practice varies. The dental office administrator is usually responsible for collecting payment from patients at the time of their appointment and collecting monies owed to the dental office that are outstanding. The office manager is responsible for assisting in the collection of monies and ensuring that suppliers are paid in a timely fashion. The dentist receives reports of the financial status of the practice on a regular basis from the office manager. The dentist also employs an accountant, who receives all the financial information of the practice on a monthly or yearly basis.

In larger dental practices, there may be more than one person involved in the financial record maintenance, or bookkeeping, of the dental practice. In a smaller dental office, the office administrator is the person who maintains the **accounts receivable,** or patient financial records, which is money owed to the practice, and the financial records of the practice, which is money owed by the dental office, or **accounts payable.**

To provide you with the skills you need to effectively manage the accounts receivable in a dental office, this chapter covers some basic bookkeeping concepts, both computer and manual accounting systems, extending credit to patients, and policies and procedures for collecting payment from patients.

BOOKKEEPING BASICS

Bookkeeping is the recording of all financial transactions undertaken by the dental office. The daily financial transactions that occur in a dental office include patient charges and payments and payments to suppliers. Below are some basic bookkeeping concepts to help you better manage the accounts receivable of a dental office.

Double- and Single-Entry Systems

Different bookkeeping systems are used in maintaining accurate records for the dental office. The system most commonly used in bookkeeping is the double-entry bookkeeping system. The accountant employed by the dental office will use this method to develop financial statements of the practice. The double-entry method of accounting refers to a method of tracking what account money is taken from and where the money is applied to. In other words, there are always at least two accounts used to track funds. For example, if a phone bill has to be paid for the dental office, the bank account, or cash account, will show funds being taken from it and the phone bill, or utilities account, will show the same amount of money being transferred into it. The double-entry method of accounting always shows what specific account the money is from and where it is applied.

The dental office administrator will use the single-entry method of accounting for the recording of daily financial transactions in the dental office. This means that transactions are entered as either a positive or negative amount in the accounts receivable or account payable records. The single entry method of accounting is simple and easy to use. One main account, the business account, is referred to and each entry shows money going either in or out of the main business account. Similar to using the checkbook register of a checking account, each time a deposit is made, it is recorded as money going into the account. Each time

checkPOINT

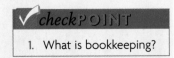

1. What is bookkeeping?

what IF ?

What if a patient asked you to bill the insurance company for her treatment on a date other than the day the treatment was received?

Misrepresenting any part of the treatment or services received is not ethical practice on the part of the dental office administrator. All treatment received is dated for the date on which it was rendered and as such it must be billed for the date on which it incurred. Explain to the patient that you do not have the authority to change any of the information regarding his or her treatment and this includes the date on which it was received.

a check is written, it is shown as money being taken from the account. One entry is written for each transaction.

Charges

A charge is the cost that a patient must pay in exchange for dental care. The charge for the treatment is based on the dental fee guide prices used in the dental office. Each dental office is responsible for developing and maintaining the amounts charged for treatment provided. The fee guide provided by the dental association is a *guide* to be followed by the dental office in setting the fee. Based on the policies outlined in the dental office you work in, there may be circumstances in which discounts may be applied to the fee, which will change the amount of the charge. Regardless, the amount of the charge must be reflected accurately and on the day when they occurred. In managing accounts receivable, charges incurred for treatment must be recorded for the day that the treatment was actually performed. In other words, backdating a charge or waiting for a future date to charge for services is not acceptable practice.

Payments

Patient accounts can be paid in different ways using different forms of payment. Each time a payment is received from a patient or on behalf of a patient account, the payment must be recorded. Patient accounts can be paid by insurance checks mailed directly to the dental office from the insurance company or by patients via cash, credit card, debit card, personal check, or money order. The form of payment should be noted where appropriate, depending on the type of bookkeeping system used (see the section "Bookkeeping Systems" below).

On occasion, a patient's account may be overpaid, or a payment may be made in advance of treatment. This results in a **credit balance** on the patient's account. The office policy regarding credit balances must be consulted. If the insurance company overpays the patient account, the amount must be sent back to the insurance company. If the patient has overpaid his account, it may be necessary to contact him and give him the option of applying the credit to future treatment or receiving a refund of the amount. The office policy will dictate how credit balances are dealt with. Most office policies stipulate a minimum amount that can be refunded to a patient; for example, if the credit balance is less than $50.00, the credit will remain on the patient's account, whereas if the amount is more than $50.00, the amount will be refunded.

Account Adjustments

An adjustment to an account occurs when a **discount** is given to a patient or an account is written off as a result of being uncollectible. A discount may be given to patients for various reasons such as family discounts or seniors' discounts. A dentist may be participating with a particular insurance group in which members in that group receive services at a discounted rate. In any situation in which the patient receives services at a rate lower than the amount normally charged for the service, the amount the patient is not being charged for must be written in the adjustment column. When posting an adjustment in which a reduction in the patient's account balance results, the difference between what the office normally charges for the procedure and what actually gets paid is the amount that is placed in the adjustment column. An adjustment that is made to reduce the patient's balance is called a **credit adjustment.**

Other types of adjustments occur in the dental office, which add to the balance that the patient is responsible for. Adjustments such as this are termed **debit adjustments.** Situations that result in debit adjustments to a patient's account include a check that is returned for nonsufficient funds (NSF) from a patient's bank, an account that has been placed with a collection agency for collection, and refunding a credit balance to a patient. The difference between a debit adjustment and a credit adjustment is that with a debit adjustment, you are adding an amount to the patient's account. For example, a patient has paid $50.00 on her account by personal check and you record the payment and provide a receipt showing that the new balance is now $0.00. One week later, the check is returned to the dental office marked NSF. The $50.00 payment must be undone from the patient's account because it is now in deficit again. You cannot recharge the patient for the services that the check was originally paid for. You must enter the amount of the NSF check in the adjustment column in brackets and provide the description of the adjustment in the description column; in this case, the description will be NSF check. The amount in the adjustment column must be in brackets. In the computer system, the amount will be shown in brackets or in a different color, such as red.

checkPOINT

2. What is a credit adjustment?

Fiscal Year and Month-End Procedures

The accounting of a dental office can be done on a **fiscal year** basis or a calendar year basis. A fiscal year is a 12-month period of time that is set up by the practice's accountant to serve as the timeframe for the yearly accounting of the practice. Usually, the financial records of the month-end procedures are submitted to the accountant to have a year-end financial picture created. A more in-depth view of the components that affect the financial picture of the dental practice will be discussed in Chapters 17 and 18.

At the end of each month, specific tasks must be completed to keep the records of the business accurate; these may be the responsibility of the dental administrator. The following are the most common tasks performed when completing the month-end process.

checkPOINT

3. What are month-end procedures and what are three examples?

- Process statements for outstanding accounts
- Reconcile bank accounts
- Manage accounts receivable by contacting outstanding accounts or send to collection

BOOKKEEPING SYSTEMS

Most dental offices now use computers for tracking of daily financial transactions, although some still use a manual system of bookkeeping. Although a manual system may work fine for smaller offices, larger, busier dental offices will likely have difficulty maintaining it and would be better served by a computer system. Both of these types of systems are described below.

Computer Bookkeeping Systems

Because of the great efficiency they offer in managing business financial systems, dental practice management programs, which often include an accounts receivable component, are the most widely used method of bookkeeping in dental offices today.

Computer bookkeeping software should include elements necessary to maintain an accurate accounts receivable. For example, an accounts receivable ledger must be produced at least monthly, or when needed. The accounts receivable ledger is a listing of patient names, or account identifiers, and the amount of money each patient owes to the practice. The listing should also provide details pertaining to the specific charge, such as the date and type of treatment. The software used should allow the

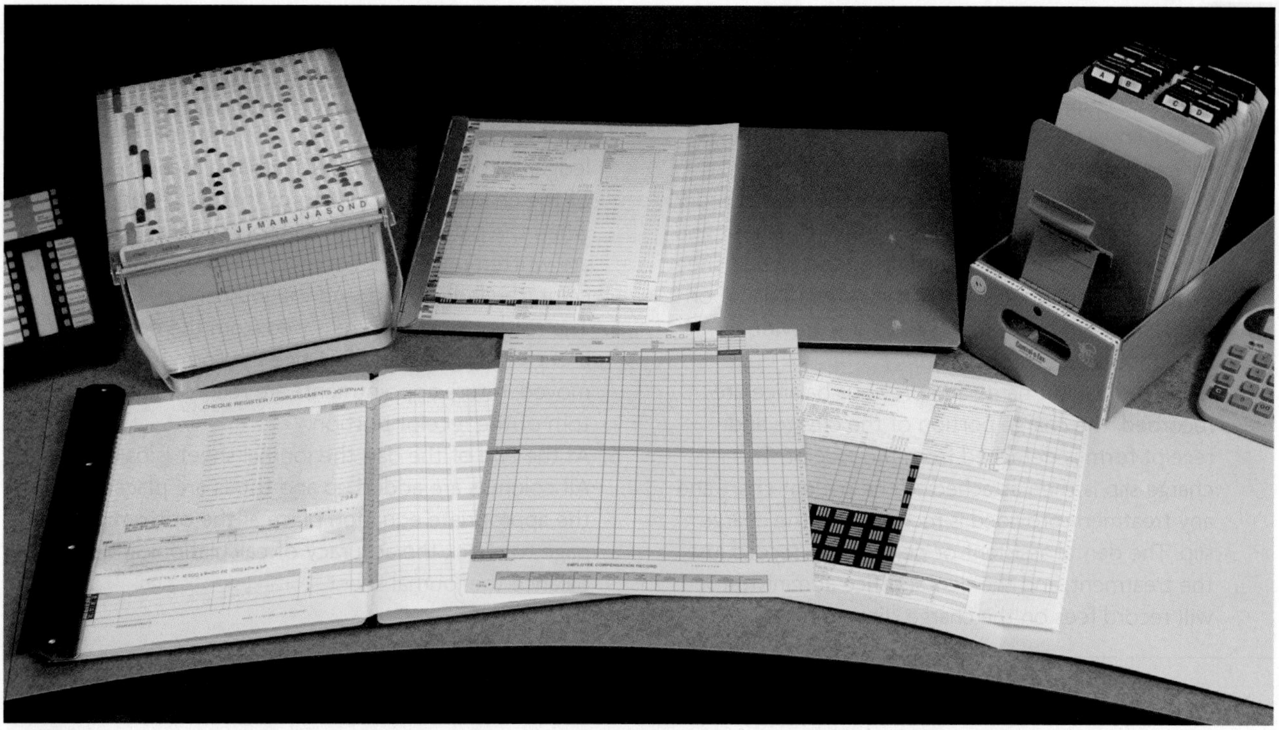

FIGURE 16-1 Peg-board and forms.

ledger to be updated at any time. That is, invoices or charges can be added or payments applied to patient accounts, and these transactions are reflected in the individual and overall balance on the ledger. An accounts receivable software program should also allow you to print off account statements for customers that reflect current and past-due balances.

Manual Bookkeeping: One-Write System

The **one-write accounting system,** or pegboard system, is a manual system of account management that uses a pegboard and carbon forms, on which transactions are recorded. It is termed a "one-write" system because the use of carbon forms enables the recorder to write the information only once and yet have it be recorded on four forms. Figure 16-1 shows the peg-board and the forms that are used in the transaction process. The peg-board is used to keep all forms aligned in order to obtain accurate recording.

Different accounts receivable transactions occur in the dental office throughout the day and must be recorded. Using the one-write system of accounting for each transaction that occurs ensures that the transaction is recorded on the appropriate record. Each time a patient comes into the dental office for treatment and makes a payment or requires an account adjustment to be made, all information can be recorded using the one-write system of accounting. Using the one-write system of accounting can be easily divided into six steps on the basis of the various forms used to record transactions. Procedure 16-1 outlines the steps to take in operating the one-write system. Procedures 16-2 through 16-4 outline how to post a charge, a payment, and an adjustment to a patient account using the one-write system.

There are four forms that are used in the one-write system of accounting: the day sheet or journal sheet, the ledger card, the charge slip, and the receipt form.

PROCEDURE 16-1 *Operating the One-Write System of Accounting*

1. Place the daily journal, or day sheet, on the peg-board. Enter the day's date and record the balance forward from the previous day's transactions.
2. Place the receipt and charge slips in numerical order over top of the day sheet. Place the first receipt and charge slip on the first blank line of the journal sheet. When a patient arrives, enter the patient's name on the charge slip portion as well as any previous account balance information.
3. Once the patient name and previous balance are recorded, the charge portion of the charge and receipt form is detached from the receipt. The charge slip is then attached to the patient chart and any treatment provided is recorded on the charge slip. The dental assistant or dentist may record just the treatment, and the dental office administrator will record fees on the charge slip.
4. When treatment is completed, the charge slip is returned to the dental office administrator. The ledger card is placed underneath the receipt portion of the charge and receipt form that was filled out when the patient arrived. All charges and payments are written once and recorded in three places: the receipt, the ledger card, and the journal sheet.
5. The receipt portion is removed from the peg-board and given to the patient. Once the form has been removed, future appointments are recorded at the bottom of the receipt portion.
6. At the end of the day, the journal sheet is balanced. All columns are added up and totals are placed in the appropriate equation place at the bottom of the page to check the accuracy of calculations and balance the journal sheet.

PROCEDURE 16-2 *How to Post a Charge to a Patient Account?*

1. Once the patient has returned the charge form to you from the clinical area and the information includes the treatment received for the appointment, check for the accuracy of patient name and address against the patient ledger card. The information you are recording on the ledger card and journal sheet must be correct to avoid errors.
2. Place the ledger card under the receipt portion for the patient and record the appropriate charges under the charge column on the ledger card. When using abbreviations under the description column of the receipt and ledger card, be sure to provide an explanation of the procedure for the patient. A photocopy of the ledger card should provide the explanation of the abbreviation at the bottom portion of the card.
3. File the ledger card in the appropriate ledger filing tray. If the ledger card shows a balance owed, it may be filed in a place separate from the other cards. Ledger cards are always filed in alphabetical order.

PROCEDURE 16-3 *How to Post a Payment to a Patient Account?*

1. Place the ledger card pertaining to the patient on the journal page. If the patient is making a payment for services rendered on the charge slip for that day, place the receipt and charge slip over the ledger card.
2. Once the journal card and receipt are in place, write the patient name in the patient name column, the amount being paid in the payment column, and a description of the payment in the appropriate area. Make sure that the posting date is written in the date column of the day sheet. The posting date should be the same as the date the payment was received.
3. Ensure that the description of the payment is accurate and shown correctly. If abbreviations are used, provide an explanation of the abbreviation somewhere on the receipt.
4. Subtract the payment amount from the previous balance amount on the ledger card. The new balance should be shown on the receipt, the patient ledger card, and the journal sheet. If the payment is the only transaction, subtract the payment from the balance. If there are charges for services that day, add the charges to the previous balance and then subtract the payment.

PROCEDURE 16-4 *How to Post an Adjustment?*

1. Using the peg-board and the patient's ledger card, line up the ledger card with the empty line on the day sheet. Record the name of the patient, the previous account balance, and the date of the posting. For credit adjustments, record both the payment received and the adjustment on the same day and on the same line. A debit adjustment may require a new line.
2. Record the amount to be adjusted, either added or subtracted from the patient account, and enter an accurate description of the adjustment.
3. Subtract or add the amount from the patient account and record the new balance of the patient account in the appropriate column.

Journal Sheet

At the beginning of each day, a **journal sheet** or **day sheet** is placed first on the peg-board. The pegs should be on the left-hand side of the board, and the peg notches on the day sheet are placed on the pages to hold it securely in place. The journal sheet is a record of charges and receipts that have occurred throughout the day. There is a great amount of information that is recorded on the journal sheet, which is identified by the column headings at the top of the sheet: charge, payment, balance, previous balance, description, and adjustment. The journal sheet also has a deposit slip, which is detachable from the sheet and used to deposit the day's payments.

The current date is written on the top, and the totals from the previous day are brought forward, that is, written in the first space at the top of each column. The bottom of the journal page provides an area for proof of posting, accounts receivable control, and the daily cash summary. The total of each column is assigned a letter. For example, the total of all charges added up is named column A, the total of all payments is column B, and so on. **Proof of posting** is the balance of transactions at the end of the day. It is common for more than one journal page to be used in the dental practice on 1 day. A series of receipt and charge slips is placed over the top of the journal page.

At the end of each business day, one of the last things the dental office administrator will have to do before leaving for the day is to ensure that all charges, payments, and adjustments that were made throughout the day are accurate and accounted for. A series of equations that involves the totals of the columns ensures a balanced journal sheet. Each column is added up and the balance entered into the equation at the bottom of the page. For example, the proof of posting section uses the following equation: Column D total (previous balance total) "plus" Column A total (total charges) "subtract" Column C (total payments) should equal Column C total (balance column total). The total in the balance column should equal the number arrived at in this equation. If the numbers are different, the journal sheet does not balance. Use the tips provided in Box 16-1 when balancing the journal sheet at the end of the day.

In the event of an overpayment, the amount of the credit is shown on the ledger card and journal sheet as an amount in brackets. For example, if a payment results in a credit balance of $14.00, the balance would appear as [14.00] on the ledger card and journal sheet. The brackets used indicate that the amount is negative, which means that the patient has a credit.

The journal sheet is an important financial document that must be accurate. The journal sheet provides information regarding accounts receivable on a daily basis. As the charges and payments change with each transaction, the accounts receivable total changes also. On a very busy day, it can be easy to make errors on

checkPOINT

4. Where is the form of payment recorded using a manual bookkeeping system?
5. What information does the journal sheet provide regarding accounts receivable?

BOX 16-1
Tips for Balancing a Journal Sheet

- Add the columns one more time to ensure that an addition error is not at fault.
- Review each transaction one at a time, to ensure that numbers have not been transposed or placed in the wrong column.
- Leave the balance sheet for a few moments and do another task and then return and try it again.
- Ask a colleague to review the balance sheet for errors.

the journal sheet. Periodically balancing the day sheet throughout the day can help you avoid having to track down errors at the end of the day when the journal sheet will not balance. The completed journal sheets must be given to the office manager or dentist for review on a daily basis and stored with financial documents for safekeeping.

Charge and Receipt Slip

The charge slip is a small portion of the receipt and charge form, which has preprinted information sections for items such as patient name, account balance, list of treatment received at the appointment, and future appointment times. The format of charge slips can vary, and some are a triplicate form, which means that there are two carbon copies and the original of the form, once they are completed. If the charge slip is in triplicate form, one copy stays in the patient's chart, one copy is given to the patient for insurance billing purposes, and the third copy is also given to the patient as a receipt for their records. Charge and receipt forms are used in conjunction with the patient ledger card. When a patient receives treatment, the charge for the treatment is recorded on the charge form and on the patient ledger card.

> ***check*POINT**
> 6. What information is found on the charge and receipt form?

Ledger Card

The **ledger card** is the written record of financial transactions for each patient. The information found on a ledger card includes the name and address of the person responsible for the account, the patient name, and dental insurance information, if applicable. The top portion of the ledger card provides the patient information, whereas the bottom portion is the record of all transactions on the patient account. The ledger card can be photocopied and used as a statement of account for patients. Providing a photocopy of the ledger card to patients provides them with an up-to-date and accurate record of the information the dental office has regarding their account.

In a manual bookkeeping system, the ledger card is the primary financial record regarding the patient's account. To maintain the accounts receivable, the ledger cards are kept separate from the patient's charts. A ledger tray is used to file the ledger cards in alphabetical order. When a patient calls regarding an amount owed on his or her account, the ledger card can be found quickly and easily, as it is filed alphabetically. Some dental offices will keep ledger cards with outstanding balances in a separate ledger tray. This is so that the cards can be easily photocopied and statements mailed or patients telephoned until the accounts are paid. The system used in the dental office depends on the preferences of the person responsible for collecting payments from patients. However, it is important to keep all of the ledger cards in one area if it is not possible to keep them together in one file tray.

> ***check*POINT**
> 7. What purpose does a ledger card serve?

EXTENDING CREDIT AND COLLECTING PAYMENT

Monies owed to the practice must be collected in a timely fashion. It is the responsibility of the dental office administrator to ensure that balances outstanding on patient accounts are collected. Depending on the office policy, collection of money may be done at the time of the appointment or payment plans may be extended to patients who require them, as well as contacting insurance companies for payment for a patient. It is a task that is necessary on a daily basis, because without it the dental office will not be able to meet the needs of staff and patients. These topics, as well as special instructions on collecting overdue payments, are covered below.

Collecting Payment

The fee schedule used in the office is set by the dentist in conjunction with other members of the dental team. When the fees are set, the dentist must consider the cost of running the dental practice. In other words, if the dentist sets fees too low, the expenses incurred in running the dental practice may not be met. To maintain a sound financial business, components such as rent, utilities, payroll, and insurance must be covered, and this is done through the collection of fees. As discussed earlier in Chapter 15, dental fees charged by the dentist can change as a result of an agreement with an insurance company. In this situation, the dentist must ensure that providing services at a discounted rate will still enable coverage of the **overhead** or expenses in running the business.

Being responsible for maintaining accounts receivable in the dental office is one of the most important tasks for the dental office administrator. Periodically assessing the collection methods used by the practice may be necessary to determine optimal collection. To maintain healthy accounts receivable, guidelines regarding the credit and collection aspects in the dental practice, as outlined in the office policies, must be followed.

Regardless of the policies set by the practice, the very first rule of doing business in the dental office is to discuss the fees in advance of treatment, which is the responsibility of the dental administrator. Patients must be made aware of their financial responsibility for the treatment that they are about to receive. Sending a predetermination to the insurance company will assist in the explanation of the patient's portion of services; however, the patient is ultimately responsible for the account. Never schedule an appointment for a patient who is not aware of his financial responsibility for treatment, and never assume that he is aware of the amount he will have to pay, unless you have discussed this in advance.

To facilitate and initiate a conversation regarding the financial aspects of treatment, the following points can be used:

- Provide all patients with a brochure or printout of the financial policies of the dental office
- Post the financial policies of the dental office in a visible area, where patients will see them
- Collect patient portions at the time of the appointment for all services
- Provide the patient with options regarding payment plans for treatment
- Inform the patient that you will submit a predetermination of benefits to the insurance company before scheduling treatment to determine the financial responsibility of the patient

Collecting fees in advance, or collecting the patient portion for services at the time of the appointment, can be done through the use of a computerized dental practice management program. When dental claims are submitted electronically to the insurance company, a response can be received within minutes and the amount owed by the patient can be calculated and collected at the time of the appointment.

A manual financial system, on the other hand, can create a lot of outstanding patient accounts unless the full amount of services is collected at each appointment.

How the patient chooses to pay for services will depend on the options available at the dental office. Credit cards, debit cards, cash, personal checks, and money orders are payment options that are common in many different businesses. A patient with dental insurance will also have the additional option of having the insurance company submit the payment directly to the dental office. Developing solid collection practices will benefit the dental office administrator and the practice. From time to time, a patient's insurance information may change. As a general rule, each time the patient returns to the dental office, an update of address, employment, and insurance information must be checked. Often, patients may neglect to inform the dental office of changes to their insurance because they themselves have not been asked of any changes. Never assume that patients have not had any changes to their insurance. Keeping patient information current is the responsibility of the office administrator.

checkPOINT

8. What is the most important aspect of maintaining accounts receivable and collecting fees from patients?

Extending options to patients regarding the method of payment accepted can be costly to the dental practice. For example, credit card companies often charge the business a percentage of the amount the patient pays to the dental office when paying by credit card. However, this is a small cost to the dental office for collecting monies owed compared with the cost of possibly not collecting any money at all!

Extending Credit

There will be patients in the dental practice who are not able to pay for their treatment in one payment and will request the option to make payments. The office policy will be the reference in situations such as this. Extending credit to patients is a decision that should not be made lightly. Installment plans should never be determined by the patient, but by the office administrator or office manager. Extending credit to a patient always involves a cost to the dental office. The office administrator must spend time sending statements or making phone calls to the patient, and supplies are needed to maintain the account and contact the patient.

Extending credit to a patient should involve an approval process that should apply to all patients in this situation. The office policy may require that a credit history check be done prior to approval, or there may be a third-party organization that specializes in financing patient treatment. When credit is extended to a patient, a written agreement that is signed and dated by the patient should be used that outlines the following:

- Treatment involved
- Number of appointments required
- Method of payment
- Number of payments due on specific dates

Figure 16-2 is a sample payment plan. A dental office may have payment plan forms that are preprinted and can be easily accessed and completed by the office administrator when required. Alternatively, payment plan forms can be generated on the computer through the use of a practice management program. Interest charges may also be automatically generated on a patient's account on the outstanding balance at the end of each month. This must also be communicated to the patient at the time of the payment plan discussion.

Determining the **creditworthiness** of a patient, the ability of a patient to pay her accounts on time as agreed, can be done by credit history checks or on the basis of past payment performance of the patient. Some dental offices may have policies regarding payment plans that will require a credit check for patients who are new to the practice or who have never had a payment plan in the past. Alternatively, patients who have proven to be consistent with their payments in the past may be extended credit at the dentist's or office manager's discretion. As a dental office

Payment Plan/Financial Arrangement

Date: __January 4, 2006.__

Patient's Name: Jane Smith

Address: 12432 Oak Street Edmonton, AB T6G 1B9

Telephone: (H) (780) 435-5555 (W): (780 998-5555)

Financial Arrangement

Treatment	Time	Fee
PFM Crown – Tooth # 36	2 appointments	**$ 850.00**
PFM Crown – Tooth #46	2 appointments	**$ 850.00**
		$
TOTAL FEE		**$ 1700.00**

Payment Method: ☐ **Interac** ☐ **Cheque** ☒ **VISA** ☐ **MasterCard** ☐ **Amex**

Credit Card# 1234 5678 9000 1234 **Expiry date:** 04/2011

Name of Cardholder Jane Smith

I elect to make a deposit of $ _500.00_ at my first appointment and to pay the balance in monthly installments of $__600.00__ over a period of __two__ months.

Jane Smith *January 4, 2006.*

Patient's Signature Date

FIGURE 16-2 Payment plan form.

administrator, unless you are given the responsibility and authority to extend credit to patients, you should never extend a payment plan to a patient outside of the office policy guidelines. Box 16-2 provides questions that the dental office administrator should be able to answer regarding credit extension in the dental office. If the office policy is in the process of being developed, these questions can assist in developing the financial policies.

Collecting Overdue Payments

In cases in which accounts are unpaid by patients or insurance payments have not been received within a certain time period, usually within a 30-day period, the dental office administrator is responsible for contacting the account holder, using the methods prescribed by the office. Following up with patients who have overdue accounts can be a time-consuming process and requires a quiet, private environment.

BOX 16-2
Questions to Consider When Developing Financial Policies in the Dental Office

- What portion of the services is the patient responsible for at the time of the appointment?
- What forms of payment are accepted by the office?
- Does the office provide payment plans?
- What is the maximum number of months for a payment plan?
- How will the payment plan be documented?
- Who will be responsible for ensuring that the payment plan is adhered to?
- What fees will the patient be responsible for if the payment plan is not followed?
- How will the creditworthiness of the patient be determined?
- Will there be interest charges on the account the patient will be responsible for?

The information discussed over the telephone with patients and insurance companies is confidential and must not be done in presence of other patients. Moreover, telephoning patients and requesting their account be paid is a task that must be handled tactfully and professionally. The dental office policy manual should outline the policies and procedures involved in account collection.

The amount of money owed to a dental practice at any given time by patients and insurance companies can vary depending on the number of patients seen in a month. To determine which accounts are current and which accounts are overdue, a report must be generated on a monthly basis that itemizes all patient accounts according to the amount of time the account has carried a balance. The age of an account is determined by the amount of time the account has been unpaid since the date it was billed. An **aged accounts receivable listing** provides this information. The information found on an aged accounts receivable listing includes the patient name, balance owed, and number of days the account has been unpaid. An account that is current, that is, billed within the past 30 days, will list the account balance in the column that is headed "current." An account that has been unpaid for more than 30 days will be listed under the 30 days column. An account that has been unpaid for 60 days will be listed under the 60 days column, and an account that has been unpaid for 90 days or more will be listed under the 90 days column. As a general rule, accounts that are current and 30 days past due should comprise 75% of the total accounts receivable balance. Accounts that are 60–90 days past due should comprise no more than 20% of the accounts receivable balance, and no more than 5% of the total accounts receivable should be made up from accounts that are 90 days past due or greater. The accounts receivable aging report is a report of the practice's ability to collect the amounts owed by patients.

Accounts that are more than 90 days past due are likely going to be uncollectible accounts; that is, these accounts may be sent to an outside collection agency for collection or written-off. Some accounts may get to this point and will likely be handled by the office manager for collection. Reasons an account may become 90 days past due or greater include the following:

- The patient has moved and neglected to inform the office.
- The patient was unhappy with the service or treatment and has left the practice.
- The patient may have received the insurance payment and has not forwarded it to the office.
- The payment plan was not followed through on.

None of the aforementioned reasons excuses a patient from keeping financial obligations to the dental practice, but they are real reasons as to why the patient account may become outstanding. Be proactive in your collection procedures to maintain the

BOX 16-3
Tips for Maintaining Accounts Receivable

- Discuss fees in advance of treatment with patients.
- Relate the office policy regarding payment plans, payment options, and insurance payment information to all patients.
- Document all fees quoted to patients in their chart.
- Have a signed agreement with patients who elect to use payment plans.
- Telephone all accounts that are past due instead of sending written notice.

accounts receivable. Box 16-3 provides tips for maintaining the accounts receivable in the dental office.

Collection Policies and Procedures

Collecting payments from patients with outstanding account balances can at times be a difficult task to accomplish. There are three ways of collecting outstanding payments from patients:

- Mailing a statement
- Telephoning
- In person at the appointment

Mailing a Statement

Sending an overdue notice or statement to a patient can be done on a monthly basis or whenever the statement is generated from the computer. A message can be selected to print on the statement that informs the patient of the overdue status of the account and how long the account has been outstanding. Some offices provide information regarding forms of payment accepted and the amount of time the patient has to make payment. Other methods include the use of brightly colored stickers that express the outstanding nature of the account. Instead of statements with messages, a form letter may be used by the office that provides a written notice to the patient that his or her account is past due and provides specific information to the patient about the account. If you must develop a collection letter for use in the dental office, keep in mind the following points to include in the letter:

- Explain the reason the patient is receiving the letter, that is, the amount owed, the length of time it has been owing, and the office policies regarding outstanding accounts
- Include the specific charges incurred on the account. This can be done by including an account statement that itemizes all charges on the account
- Include any payments made on the account
- Provide the patient with a deadline of when the office must be contacted or when the account must be paid
- Provide information to the patient regarding the consequences of not adhering to payment deadlines
- Make sure that contact name and phone number information for the office is provided in the letter

Telephone Call

Generally, the most effective method of collecting an account is by telephoning the patient. All patients should receive the courtesy of a statement mailed to them. If the written letter or statement does not solicit payment, a phone call should be made to

PROCEDURE 16-5 *Making a Collection Phone Call*

1. Select a quiet and private area where the telephone call can be made without distraction or interruption. You will need at least 1 hour of time to make phone calls to as many patients as possible in one sitting.
2. Have the following items in front of you: the patients' chart, the accounts receivable listing, and a copy of the patients' statement of account and any financial arrangements agreed to regarding the account.
3. Check to make sure that the patient has not outlined a preference for when and where they would like to be contacted. If so, you must adhere to that request. Select a time and day when the person is most likely to be available to speak to you; this may be evening times or morning hours.
4. Inform the patient who you are, where you are calling from, and why you are calling. Be specific when you speak to the patient and ask for payment: ask "When can we expect payment?" Try to get a specific date. Offer to take a credit card number over the phone to clear the account at that moment.
5. Document your conversation with the patient in the chart and make a note to follow up in the future if necessary.
6. Follow up with the patient by telephoning again if the account has not been paid by the date promised or within 30 days.

legal TIP

When making a collection telephone call to a patient, you may have to leave a message with a family member or on voice mail. In this case, it is important that the information you leave does not mention details related to the patient's account or other personal information. You may leave only your name and phone number and from where you are calling. Leaving personal information for the patient on an answering machine or with another person may place you in a position of violating a patient's right to privacy.

the patient. In any case, if the account is at the 60 past due column, a phone call should be made. Procedure 16-5 outlines the steps to take in making a collection phone call to a patient. The Fair Debt Collection Practices Act in the United States ensures that abusive debt collection practices are not used in the collection of consumer debts. This act allows consumers to dispute a debt or gain information regarding the debt in order to ensure that it is accurate. The guidelines provided under the act ensures that violations by collectors will be met with penalties.

In Person at the Appointment

If a patient is in the dental office, this is the best opportunity to inform her of her account balance and inquire as to when payment can be made. The best way to handle this situation is to give the patient a copy of her statement and ask, "How would you like to pay your account today?" If the person is unable to pay and requests a payment plan, use the payment plan form used in the office. Encourage the patient to make a partial payment on the account if possible. Let the patient know you will make a note on her file regarding the date and form of payment she will be using. Documenting the information while the patient is at the front desk will reinforce to the patient that you are taking her promise to pay seriously and will follow through. Entering the information into the computerized patient chart or manual chart will alert any staff member to the financial situation of the patient's chart.

Collection agencies are used by dental offices when there is difficulty in collecting a debt. That is, a large amount of time and resources have been used in attempting to collect the debt. The size of the collection agency used will depend on the preference of the person selecting the company. Some collection agencies are used specifically by dental offices because of the experience and knowledge the company has regarding the collection of debts based on healthcare treatment. The advantage to using a collection agency is also reflected in the resources that the company has available, such as the phone systems used and the access to the resources needed to locate a person who is evading debt. The collection agency is able to devote a greater amount of time and resources to collecting the debt than the dental office administrator has time for.

Chapter Summary

Maintaining the financial records of the dental practice can be done with a computerized or manual bookkeeping system. Although most dental offices today use a computerized system for maintaining practice finances, the manual system is still in use in some offices. Understanding the manual bookkeeping system allows the dental office administrator to understand more fully the effect of the daily financial transactions on the overall financial picture of the practice. Maintaining accurate financial records depends on the office administrator making sound decisions regarding extending credit to patients who require a payment plan to pay their account, as well as tact and professionalism in collecting monies owed to the practice. Ensuring that accounts are kept up-to-date and managed effectively by the office administrator will ensure a healthy financial picture for the dental office.

Review Questions

Multiple Choice

1. **An adjustment to an account is given**
   a. when a patient asks for it.
   b. when a discount is given.
   c. after the patient leaves the practice.
   d. when a credit balance is used.

2. **Monies owed to the practice are termed**
   a. accounts payable.
   b. accounts receivable.
   c. credit and collectables.
   d. overhead.

3. **A fiscal year-end is a term that refers to**
   a. the month of December only.
   b. the accounting year of the business.
   c. the financial report of the business.
   d. the regular calendar year of January to December.

4. **Account adjustments that add to the balance of a patient's account are**
   a. credit adjustments.
   b. credit balances.
   c. debit adjustments.
   d. debit balances.

5. **It is the responsibility of the dental office administrator to**
   a. ensure that accounts are up-to-date.
   b. manage the accounts receivable.
   c. inform patients of their financial responsibilities to the office.
   d. all of the above.

6. **Which of the following is an example of a debit adjustment?**
   a. A patient makes a cash payment on his or her account and the balance is now $0.00.
   b. A check is returned as NSF from the patient's bank and must be charged to his or her account.
   c. A patient comes in for treatment and it is charged to his or her account.
   d. An account has a credit balance.

7. **The guidelines for ensuring that abusive debt collection practices are not used are set out through**
   a. the Best Debt Collection Act.
   b. the Fair Debt Collection Practices Act.
   c. the American Dental Association.
   d. the Dental Assistants Association.

8. **Which of the following would not be included in the month-end process?**
   a. Process statements for outstanding accounts
   b. Print off daily schedule statistics
   c. Reconcile bank accounts
   d. Manage accounts receivable by contacting outstanding accounts or send to collection

9. **When making a collection telephone call, you should**
   a. leave the details of the call on voice mail.
   b. provide information to family members at their request.
   c. never leave details with a person who is not the patient.
   d. offer to call back without giving any message to be passed on.

10. **Which of the following forms of collecting payment should you be most familiar with?**
    a. telephoning the patient
    b. in office payment collection
    c. letter writing for outstanding balance
    d. all of the above

Critical Thinking

1. How do you find the error in a journal sheet that does not balance?
2. What components of the one-write bookkeeping system are similar to what might be found in a computerized system? What advantages are there to learning the manual system first?
3. How will you address a request from a patient who has an outstanding balance on his account and would like to pay the next time he is in the office?

Web Site

Federal Trade Commission
http://www.ftc.gov/bcp/edu/pubs/consumer/credit/cre18.shtm

chapter SEVENTEEN

Accounts *Payable*

OUTLINE

OBJECTIVES

After completing this chapter, you should be able to do the following:

- Spell and define key terms
- Describe categories of office expenses
- Identify and explain overhead expenses
- Discuss the importance of controlling expenses in the dental office and describe ways to control them
- Describe how to maintain a file of paid invoices
- Explain various forms of payment used in the dental office
- Name the parts of a check
- Describe the difference between the one-write system and a computer system for issuing checks
- Name and describe different types of checks
- Discuss how to maintain petty cash

KEY TERMS

- overhead expenses
- accounts payable
- budget
- stale-dated check
- postdated check
- payee
- order check
- counter check
- traveler's check
- money order
- postal money order
- bank draft
- cashier's check
- certified check
- teller's check
- petty cash

In order for the dental office to run efficiently, all expenses related to running the business must be paid promptly and managed efficiently. These expenses include rent or mortgage, power, water, and clinical and office equipment and supplies. All of these costs fall under the term **overhead expenses.** Overhead expenses are the usual and ongoing expenses involved in running a business. All of the costs that are paid out to various

checkPOINT

1. What are accounts payable and overhead expenses?

suppliers and venders fall under the category of **accounts payable.** In this chapter, we will look at overhead expenses in the dental office and how to manage them, how to pay invoices, forms of payment, writing checks, manual and computer accounts payable systems, and managing petty cash.

TYPES OF OFFICE EXPENSES

There are generally two types of costs in the dental office:

- capital costs
- overhead or operating costs

Capital costs refer to costs associated with large and expensive equipment purchases. For example, a dental operatory, which is very expensive, would be considered a capital cost. Generally, an expense that requires a large outlay of money, more than $1000, is considered a capital cost. Overhead or operating costs are the everyday expenses associated with doing business, such as payroll, administrative and clinical supplies, and utilities.

This section focuses on overhead expenses, defining what they are, how to control them, and how to pay them.

Overhead

As noted above, overhead expenses generally occur on a continual basis and are for services that are essential to the operation of the business. The following items are commonly considered overhead expenses:

- *Administrative supplies*: stationary supplies (pens, paper, ink) etc.
- *Clinical supplies*: any item used in the clinical areas of the dental office
- *Dues*: monies paid to professional associations by the dentist to maintain operation of the business
- *Legal fees*: fees paid to legal professionals such as lawyers in return for providing services such as consultations and filing of corporation documents
- *Medications*: pain relievers, antibiotics, and oxygen or nitrous oxide
- *Payroll*: the gross amount paid to all employees (we will discuss this in detail in Chapter 19)
- *Rent/mortgage*: the rent paid to a landlord for use of office space or mortgage owed to a bank for purchase of property
- *Taxes*: property and business taxes as well as payroll withholding taxes
- *Travel*: expenses incurred as a result of travel for continuing education purposes or the use of vehicles for errands such as banking and supply pickup
- *Utilities*: the costs incurred through telephone, power, water, gas, and electricity

checkPOINT

2. What is the difference between overhead expenses and other expenses?

Controlling Expenses

To maintain the business and a healthy financial picture, the expenses should be controlled. One tool for controlling expenses and pinpointing areas where overspending may be occurring is a budget. A **budget** is an estimation of the expenses for the business for a certain time period. Budgets are developed by reviewing the past year's income and expense results and projecting new figures for the upcoming year based on these figures and on changes in expected expenses for the upcoming year.

Controlling expenses may be the sole responsibility of the office manager, but in a smaller practice the dental office administrator may be responsible for maintaining this also. Box 17-1 provides tips on controlling business expenses.

BOX 17-1
Controlling Business Expenses

- Pay suppliers using a check or credit card. This allows for an itemized list on the credit card or bank statement at the end of the month to compare to invoices paid.
- Assign one person to order and pay for supplies. Too many people with authority to pay suppliers could result in overordering and overpayment.
- Pay suppliers at the same time each month or bimonthly. Keeping track of what was paid and when can be easily maintained when it is done at a set time each month.
- Keep all invoices that need to be paid in a separate file from the main vendor file. Once the invoice or statement is paid, place it in the main vendor file.

Paying Invoices

Expenses related to supplies that are ordered for the dental office are typically billed to the dental office as invoices, which may come with the order or be sent separately. As the dental administrator, it will likely be your responsibility to pay invoices. Although practices vary among offices, most invoices are paid when the monthly statement arrives, as opposed to when the order arrives.

Once the statement arrives, you can match the invoices to it for payment. Keep a separate file for all invoices that must paid. Once the invoice is paid, place it in the vendor file. For example, if Dental Supply Company, Ltd. sent three separate orders this month, you would place the invoice for each of those shipments in a file marked "accounts payable" or "to be paid." At the end of the month when the statement is received, you would match up and attach the three invoices to it and pay the statement balance. You would then mark the statement and the attached invoices "paid" and place them in the vendor file for Dental Supply Company, Ltd. There are different ways a supplier can be paid, depending on the forms of payment accepted by the supplier and the preference of payment by the dentist.

Forms of Payment

Using a credit card or debit card and paying by checks are both generally accepted forms of payment for dental vendors or suppliers. Paying with a credit or debit card can be done quickly and easily over the telephone, or the credit or debit card number can be kept on file by the vendor and the account balance can be paid in full every month, and a receipt sent to the dental office. A credit or debit card is also useful for vendors who will not ship supplies without prepayment of the goods. Using a check for payment is also necessary when vendors do not accept credit cards. The dentist is always involved in and aware of the accounts payable process, as usually he or she has signing authority on the checks and it is the dentist's credit card that is used for making payments. Oftentimes, the vendor will include the option of making a payment online. For example, by going to the Web site of the vendor, you can easily access account information by entering both the log-in and password for the dental office. Once the account is accessed, the credit card information can be entered, a payment can be made, and the account balance can be updated immediately. Usually, the office manager or administrator is responsible for making these payments as they have access to the account information for both payment and ordering. The convenience of paying online allows for the payment to be made on time and at a point in the day when it is convenient for the office administrator to make the payment. A receipt for payment can be printed immediately. It is necessary to obtain a receipt for the payment made in order for it to be matched to the credit card bill for payment.

checkPOINT

3. When is it useful to use a credit card for paying invoices?

CHECK WRITING

Issuing checks to vendors for payment of services or supplies is normally done by one person in the dental office to avoid errors. The person who manages the accounts payable usually writes the check, and the individual with signing authority on the account signs it. As a general rule, if you are responsible for issuing the check for payment, you must provide the person who is signing the check with the pertinent invoice or statement.

Let's now consider the parts of the check and the different types of checks available.

Parts of a Check

Checks generally contain the following elements:

- name, address, and phone number of the account holder
- check number
- account number
- date of issue
- payee
- amount of currency in numbers and written
- signature of the account holder
- bank name and address
- memo

checkPOINT

4. What are a postdated check and a stale-dated check?

what IF?

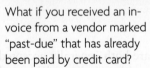

What if you received an invoice from a vendor marked "past-due" that has already been paid by credit card?

Double check the credit card statement to make sure that the payment has been processed. If it has, call the vendor and inform him or her that you have the credit card statement showing that the payment has been processed. You may have to copy the statement and provide the vendor with a copy. If this is the case, make sure that all other information regarding other vendors is not legible and information such as the credit limit and balance owed are not legible.

The name, address, and phone number of the account holder must be displayed on the top left-hand corner of the check or in the center of the top portion of the check. A check that does not have an address or phone number on it should not be accepted. Every check will have a check number; this is for the benefit of keeping track of checks that have been written and a way of checking to see whether any checks are missing. The routing number, unique to each bank, and account number can be found along the bottom of the check as a series of numbers, along with the check number.

The date the check is written should appear in the upper right-hand side of the check in the space provided for the date. A check is generally valid for 6 months after the date of issue, after which time it is considered a **stale-dated check.** A check that is written for a future date is considered a **postdated check.**

The name of the person to whom the check is written, referred to as the **payee,** must be clearly written on the space provided after "pay to the order to." The amount the check is written for must be written in both numbers and words, and both of these numbers must match. The signature of the account holder must appear, legibly, on the signature line on the bottom right-hand side of the check. A signature that does not match the one on file at the bank will lead to the check being returned for signature. The bank name and address should appear on the check on the left-hand side of the check just below the written amount of the check. The last part of the check, found on the lower left-hand side, is a space marked "memo," in which the check issuer may include account information or a brief description of the purchase. Ensuring that the check you are writing (or receiving) is correct is important for accurate bookkeeping. Box 17-2 provides information on what to look for when issuing a check.

Checks used for business purposes are usually attached to a check stub and kept in a binder-style checkbook to keep them all together. The check stub remains in the checkbook after the check is detached and the information on the check stub includes the payee, the amount paid, and the date the check was written.

BOX 17-2
Check the Check

Checks should always be reviewed before being mailed in for payment, or accepted as payment, to ensure that they will not be rejected by the bank. Make sure that:

- The check is not postdated (dated ahead of today's date).
- The check is not stale-dated (dated more than 6 months ago).
- The check is signed.
- The payee is correct.
- The amount in words and the amount in numbers agree.
- Any alterations are initialed by the account holder.

Types of Checks

There are many different types of checks that you will come across during your task as a dental office administrator. Being familiar with all of them will assist you in being effective with both making and accepting payments in the dental office.

An **order check,** the most common form of check, is payable only to the named payee, as it usually contains the language "Pay to the order of." A **counter check** is a bank check given to customers who have run out of checks or whose checks are not yet available. It is often left blank and is used for purposes of withdrawal.

A **traveler's check** is a type of check that is purchased by the payer from a bank or other financial institution, that is available in fixed denominations, and that is generally treated as cash. Traveler's checks are safer to carry than cash, as they require the issuer to sign twice—once when the checks are first purchased and again at the time they are used to make a purchase—which makes them more secure if stolen. Moreover, traveler's checks can usually be replaced if lost or stolen, so they are often used by people on vacation instead of cash.

legal TIP

Checks that are issued for a date in the future, such as postdated checks, are not considered legal tender by the bank. Accepting postdated checks is a courtesy the dental office provides, and not a right of the patient.

A check sold by a post office for payment by a third party for a customer is referred to as a **money order** or **postal money order.** Money orders can also be purchased from any bank for a higher fee than what the post office may charge. A check issued by a bank on its own account for a customer for payment to a third party is called a **bank draft** or **cashier's check** or **certified check.** A bank draft or cashier's check is usually recommended for large monetary amounts. A check issued by a bank but drawn on an account with another bank is a **teller's check.**

Credit cards and debit cards have begun to replace the checks as a form of payment due to ease of use, and an increase of businesses preferring payment methods of this kind instead of personal checks.

PETTY CASH

In the dental office, purchases must be made from time to time that are infrequent and of a small dollar amount. A petty cash account is kept for these purposes. **Petty cash** is an amount of cash kept on hand in the office to pay for small purchases. The office you work in will have specific items that are paid for using the petty cash account. These items may be as follows:

- courier costs
- stationary items
- coffee-room supplies
- taxi fare for patients

These are just examples of what petty cash can be used for. The use of the petty cash is at the discretion of the dentist. If there is a frequently occurring charge that petty cash is used for, it may be more cost-effective to purchase the item in bulk through the accounts receivable process. There is always a set amount of money in a petty cash fund. Each time money is disbursed from petty cash, there must be a petty cash voucher completed that corresponds to the amount of cash disbursed. The voucher represents money spent and has a store receipt attached to it as proof that the reimbursement was legitimate. The amount of money in the petty cash added to the amount of all vouchers should equal the total amount originally placed in the petty cash fund. For example, if the petty cash fund is $50.00, and there is $20.00 in cash in the fund, there should be $30.00 of vouchers in the fund. In some situations, funds are required to purchase an item, which means that the cash is taken out of petty cash before a receipt being produced. In this situation there will be a system in place. This could mean that the name of the person receiving the cash would be written in to the petty cash journal along with the amount received, and when the receipt and change were returned, those would be entered on to the journal to show where the funds were spent.

The following information is typically included on a petty cash voucher:

- voucher number: vouchers are consecutively numbered
- date of the reimbursement
- a description of what was purchased
- the amount paid
- tax amount included in the purchase cost: find this on the receipt
- signature of the person incurring the expense and being reimbursed
- the signature of the person responsible for maintaining petty cash

Usually, one person in the office is designated as the person who maintains petty cash. This person is responsible for making sure that purchases reimbursed with petty cash are legitimate and that all vouchers have a store receipt attached to them. Usually, the petty cash fund is kept under lock and key in a secure place.

The petty cash fund is maintained regularly through the exchange of receipts and vouchers for cash. It is also replenished on a monthly basis; that is, the vouchers and receipts are taken out, and their amounts are recorded on the petty cash disbursements journal or book. Then, a check is written by the dental office for the amount of receipts, and cash is put back into the petty cash fund. To accurately maintain the petty cash fund, the following steps should be taken:

1. Complete a petty cash voucher for reimbursement of expenditure by doing the following:
   - Check the accuracy and authenticity of the receipt received. Is the receipt dated and does it specify what was purchased?
   - Prepare a petty cash voucher and attach the receipt to the voucher.
   - Pay the money owed to the staff member and have him or her sign for it.
   - Place the voucher and receipt into the petty cash tin.
2. Record the transaction in the petty cash book or journal
   - Record entries in chronological order.
   - Details should be the same as those on the voucher.
   - Record the total amount of the voucher in the total column.
   - Tax paid amount is recorded in the tax column.
   - All columns must be totaled and the totals recorded on the last line of the page.
3. Replenish the petty cash fund by cashing the check written for the replenishment.

checkPOINT

5. Why is a petty cash voucher necessary?

ACCOUNTS PAYABLE SYSTEMS

Accounts payable can be managed and checks can be issued using either a computer system or a manual system. These are discussed below.

Computer System

Most dental practice management programs will include an accounts payable component, which may or may not include a check-writing component. In using such a program, when you indicate that you are paying a bill, the computer will prompt you to write a check for the payment or pay by credit card. If you wish to pay by check, you select the prompt for check. The check appears on the computer screen, looking much like a manual check. Once the check is printed, the computer automatically records that the invoice was paid and the date it was paid and records the transaction into the appropriate expense category. If the bill is a regular occurrence, the computer can recall the most recent information for you to verify before allowing it to be printed. Some software programs may even remind you to pay certain vendors at certain periods of time.

Besides programs specific to dental practice management, many general check-writing programs are available. Software programs that facilitate check writing on the computer can be purchased separately or come as a component of the accounting software system used in the dental office.

An advantage of using a computer accounts payable and check-writing programs is that having all of the financial information in one software program will allow for the compilation of financial reports with ease. Another major advantage is the accuracy of the mathematical computations and completeness of the checks that computer programs allow. Having all of the financial information in one place facilitates the completeness of financial records in the dental office.

One disadvantage is that the computer system of check writing can be much more time-consuming than the manual system as a result of operator error and the need for correction. The additional disadvantage of the inconvenience created when the computer system becomes unavailable as a result of technical malfunctions can also lead to delays in the processing of information. During these technical malfunctions or when the computer "crashes," the office administrator may have to refer to a manual method of maintaining the records. Hard copies of documentation can be kept in the dental office, or an electronic backup of all information on the computer system can be accessed from the backup system used in the dental office.

✓ checkPOINT

6. What is an advantage of using a computerized system for accounts payable record keeping?

Pegboard System

The one-write or pegboard system used for accounts payable is part of the same system of accounting as that described for accounts receivable in Chapter 16. A check register sheet is used on the board, along with a ledger card for the employee or vendor for whom the check is being written, as well as a check with a strip of carbon on it so that the information can be written once and recorded in three places. The check register used with the pegboard system contains columns that pertain to different categories. The categories refer to the various headings used by the office for expenses. For example, the column headings may be as follows: rent, telephone, heat, dental supply company 1, employee A, employee B, and so on. When the register is complete for the month, all entries are totaled. The totals are carried forward to the new register for the next month.

Bank deposits that occur throughout the month are also recorded on the check register, and the check register provides an accurate balance of the bank account until the bank statement arrives and can be reconciled. Figure 16-1, in the previous chapter, includes a one-write check register system. The components of the pegboard system used for accounting procedures such as accounts receivable, accounts payable, and payroll are discussed in detail in Chapter 16. You can also refer to the procedure boxes in Chapter 16 for details on how to use the components of the pegboard system.

Chapter Summary

Expenses in the dental office must be paid promptly and managed effectively to run a dental office efficiently. Payment of invoices should be given special attention and controlled by one person in the dental office to control ordering and expenses. Payments can be made using credit cards, debit cards, or checks in most dental offices. Understanding the many parts of a check and the purpose that each part plays will ensure an efficient accounts payable recording system. There are many different types of checks that are used and accepted, such as money orders, counter checks, certified checks, and traveler's checks. The dental office administrator should be able to recognize any of these. Both computer accounts payable systems and the one-write system for issuing checks are used in dental offices. A familiarity with these systems will assist in maintaining accounts payable and petty cash.

Review Questions

Multiple Choice

1. **Which one of the following would not be considered a legitimate office expense?**
   a. clinical supplies
   b. office supplies
   c. personal lunch
   d. travel expense
2. **Overhead expenses are**
   a. unusual costs involved in running a business.
   b. usual costs involved in running a business.
   c. expenses incurred by employees only.
   d. bank charges and payments to vendors only.
3. **A stale-dated check is**
   a. written for a future date for payment.
   b. not a legal form of payment at any time.
   c. 6 months older than the date on the check.
   d. none of the above define the term stated.
4. **Which of the following is one advantage to paying vendor bills online using a credit card?**
   a. The payment to the credit card company does not have to be made until a later date.
   b. The payment applied to the vendor account updates the balance immediately.
   c. The payment can be changed if an error is made.
   d. The vendor can be made aware of the account payment sooner.
5. **Petty cash**
   a. is the amount of cash held by the dentist for personal use.
   b. is the amount of cash kept on hand for small business-related purchases.
   c. should be maintained by two or more people.
   d. is not a valid account in the dental office.
6. **The most common form of check is**
   a. traveler's check.
   b. blank check.
   c. order check.
   d. certified check.
7. **A traveler's check may be safer to carry than cash because**
   a. loss of a traveler's check is not as devastating as losing cash.
   b. a traveler's check requires a signature to use it.
   c. travelers' checks are not as widely accepted as cash.
   d. most people do not carry traveler's checks.
8. **Petty cash can be used to purchase which of the following?**
   a. gas for the dentist's car
   b. lunch for the staff meeting
   c. dental masks
   d. brochures for patient education
9. **Which of the following would be considered an advantage to using the pegboard system of accounting?**
   a. The computer may "crash" causing a delay in information processing.
   b. Information can be written once and recorded in three places.
   c. Operator error can create errors and delays.
   d. Software programs facilitate check writing on the computer.
10. **Which of the following is not a recommended tip for controlling business expenses in the dental office?**
    a. Pay suppliers at the same time each month or bimonthly.
    b. Keep track of what was paid and when should be done at a set time each month.
    c. Allow vendors to automatically charge the credit card.
    d. Keep all invoices that need to be paid in a separate file.

Critical Thinking

1. The dentist has asked you to take on the responsibility of managing accounts payable and petty cash. You must set up accounts for all expense categories. Using a register form, develop the accounts payable and expense categories.
2. An employee has asked you to give her $20 from petty cash in order that she may purchase stationary supplies for the office. What procedure do you follow and how do you follow up to ensure that procedure is adhered to?
3. A supplier calls you and informs you that an invoice has not been paid. All invoices are paid by check on the 15th of each month. What information do you need to check to see whether payment has been sent?

Web Sites

Internal Revenue Service
www.irs.org

Receiver General for Canada (Revenue Canada)
www.cra-arc.gc.ca

chapter EIGHTEEN

Banking

OBJECTIVES

After completing this chapter, you should be able to do the following:

- Spell and define key terms
- Describe the many types of bank accounts used by dental offices
- Identify and explain the bank fees incurred by dental offices
- Demonstrate the procedure for doing a bank deposit
- Reconcile a bank statement
- Identify common methods of electronic banking and describe how the dental administrator can use them to more efficiently manage the dental office's bank account or accounts

KEY TERMS

- business bank account
- checking account
- savings account
- banking fees
- monthly fees
- transaction fee
- overdraft protection
- endorsed
- bank statement
- electronic banking
- online banking
- ATM

OUTLINE

There are many financial transactions that occur regularly in the dental office and in order for the dental office to run efficiently the financial obligations must be met in a timely manner. The dental office administrator must ensure that the financial obligations of the dental practice can be met and must use the resources available to him or her to facilitate this. This means that being aware of the various forms of electronic banking for making deposits to the account and methods for paying bills is necessary for the dental administrator. This chapter discusses the necessity for a business bank account in the dental office and the role that the dental office administrator plays in the maintenance of the account, which includes tasks such as the management of bank deposits and the reconciliation of the bank account statements. Various forms of electronic banking available to the dental office administrator and how they are incorporated into the dental office are also discussed.

BUSINESS BANK ACCOUNT

The **business bank account** is a bank account used for financial transactions of the business, such as deposits received and checks written for accounts payable and payroll. There is normally one person in the dental office, typically the dental office administrator or office manager, who is responsible for ensuring that the bank account is managed accurately on a regular basis.

The bank account used by the dental office will most likely be in place when you begin your employment as a dental office administrator. However, if you are involved in selecting it, the following components should be considered:

- Fees charged by the bank
- Interest paid on balances in the account
- Nonsufficient funds fee
- Overdraft protection

The dentist may have an established relationship with a particular bank and, therefore, with a banking representative who is the designated contact person at the bank. When a concern arises regarding the bank account, the banking representative can be contacted directly for explanation. The dental office administrator or office manager is responsible for making such inquiries. Being aware of the components of the bank account, such as those listed earlier, will assist in understanding some of the costs involved with banking.

Types of Accounts

There are many different types of business banking accounts available for the dental office. The dental office is not limited to using one bank account. There may be more than one account for various reasons. The most common bank accounts used are discussed here.

A **checking account** is a bank account on which checks are written based on the amount of money held in the account. Deposits are made in to the account, and checks are written for payment of bills and payroll. The checking account is the main bank account used in the dental office because it allows for tracking the payments and deposits made on a daily basis.

A **savings account** may also be used by the dental office. The savings account allows money to earn interest at a higher rate than what may be offered with the checking account. The dentist may choose to set aside money for future capital expenses or transfer money not being used to a savings account. The advantage provided by the savings account is that it provides an interest-bearing account and allows for easy access to that money when it is needed. The disadvantage of most savings accounts is that checks cannot be written directly from the accounts. Some banks offer bank accounts that provide both the ease of check writing and an interest-bearing advantage for balances held in the account.

checkPOINT

1. What advantages and disadvantages are there in having a savings account for the dental office?

Bank Fees

Regardless of the type of account used in the dental office, there are usually fees associated with the account. **Banking fees** are dollar amounts charged to the business by the bank for providing banking services. Banks may charge fees for services, which range from a flat-fee, or one-time charge, to fees per transaction. Both of these are discussed next.

Monthly Fee

A **monthly fee** is an amount charged to the business on a monthly basis. The monthly fee can include a certain number of transactions in the account within the month, or it can be based on maintaining a minimum dollar amount in the account.

Administrative TIP

If it is your responsibility to ensure that there are no discrepancies in the bank accounts each month, open the bank statements the same day they arrive in the mail. Perform a quick check of all checks that have been processed, looking for changes to amounts, as well as a review of the bank fees that have been charged. Sometimes new bank fees may occur as a result of changes to the account or because of an unusual transaction. Catching discrepancies early and contacting the bank immediately will rectify small errors before they become big ones.

Some accounts specify that maintaining a minimum balance in the account will allow for the monthly fee to be waived. The monthly fees charged by banks may vary and should be considered carefully when looking to open a bank account.

Transaction Fee

Some banks charge the business a **transaction fee** for each transaction in the business account. For example, each time a check is processed or a deposit is made to the account, the business could be charged 10 cents, with the cumulative total appearing in the monthly statement. For dental offices that conduct numerous transactions each month, such fees can become considerable. When selecting the type of checking account to use in the dental office, it is wise to consider the type of checking accounts available. If the office you are in completes a large number of deposits every month, you should consider a checking account that charges a flat monthly fee for unlimited deposits, for example. As the productivity of the practice changes, it is wise to consider the availability of checking accounts and the charges for services and the impact that the charges have on the overall account balance.

Overdraft Protection

Overdraft protection can be provided by the bank for the business account to allow for checks written on the account to be covered in the event that there are not enough funds in the account to cover them. The dollar amount, or overdraft limit, is established by the bank and is seen as a form of credit given by the bank. This service entails fees, such as a flat fee or an interest amount charged on the amount used.

Nonsufficient Funds Fee

On occasion, a personal check submitted by a patient for payment may be returned from the patient's bank due to nonsufficient funds. The dental office's bank may in turn charge the dental office account for processing the patient's returned check. To compensate for this expense, many dental offices charge patients a nonsufficient funds fee in the event that a check is returned. Management of the dental practice account balance is important to ensure that the practice portrays a healthy financial picture. Just as you would keep track of and manage your own household expenses by ensuring that you do not overspend so that you are not in an overdraft position, the same must be done with the dental practice. Large expenses in the dental office should be planned for, that is, productivity must be maintained to ensure cash flow and then large expenses made after months of planning. If the finances in the dental office are not managed properly and expenses and cash flow are not balances, the dental office could get into a position where checks that are written are not honored by the bank. Ensuring this does not happen is part of the responsibilities of the dental office administrator.

*check*POINT

2. What is overdraft protection?

BANK DEPOSITS

One of the duties of the dental office administrator is making regular bank deposits. Preferences regarding deposits, such as frequency of deposits (i.e., daily vs. weekly) and type of forms used, vary from office to office, so you should become familiar

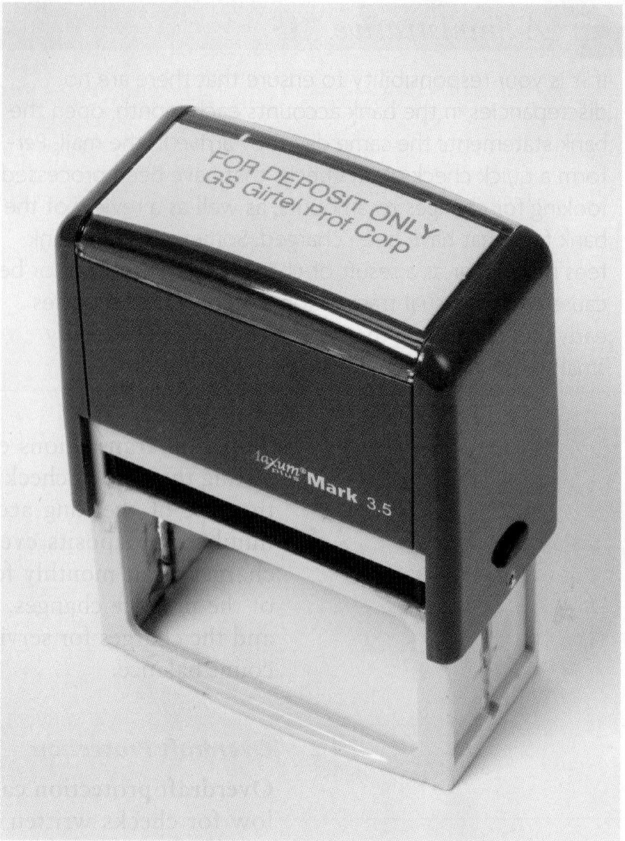

FIGURE 18-1
Deposit stamp for endorsement.

with standard procedure at the office you work in. Covered below, however, are some basic guidelines on preparing checks for deposit and making deposits.

Preparing Checks for Deposit

Checks are received by the dental office from patients, in payment of their account, and from insurance companies, on behalf of patients. Once the checks are entered into the ledger or patient account, they must be **endorsed,** or signed on the back. The checks must then be stamped on the back with a "deposit only" stamp, so that they cannot be used for any other purpose; once stamped, they can only be deposited into the dental office account. This is an important first step to remember, because leaving checks sitting out on the front desk or in any other area of the office without being stamped for deposit could leave them vulnerable to theft. The endorsement stamp (Fig. 18-1) also ensures that the checks will be deposited to the correct bank account.

Making a Bank Deposit

Once all checks are applied to the correct patient account and endorsed for deposit, you must prepare the deposit slip (Fig. 18-2). The daily production sheet used by the dental office should provide you with a total of all the payments received for the day. Total all of the checks, cash, money orders, and traveler's checks received for payment; this total should equal the total on your day sheet. If you are using a manual peg-board system, simply detach the deposit slip from the day sheet and enclose it and the payments in a deposit envelope (Fig. 18-3). Procedure 18-1 outlines the steps involved in preparing and making a deposit.

CREDIT ACCOUNT OF:
G.S. GIRTEL PROFESSIONAL CORPORATION

LIST OF CHEQUES
CHEQUE IDENTIFICATION

1	
2	
3	
4	
5	
6	
7	
8	
9	
10	
11	
12	
13	
14	
15	
16	
CHEQUE SUBTOTAL	

DEP

FLD 2 SERIAL NUMBER

FLD 3 TOTAL NO. OF ITEMS

BUSINESS ACCOUNT DEPOSIT SLIP

CREDIT ACCOUNT OF:
G.S. GIRTEL PROFESSIONAL CORPORATION

DATE		
DAY	MONTH	YEAR

DEPOSITOR'S INITIAL'S

CASH COUNT

X2		
X5		
X10		
X20		
X50		
X100		
X		
U.S. CASH		
FLD 4 TOTAL CASH		
FLD 5 COIN		
SUBTOTAL CASH & COIN		

ITEMS	NO. OF ITEMS	AMOUNT	
SUB-TOTAL BROUGHT FORWARD			
U.S. CHEQUES			
VISA			
FLD 3 TOTAL			
U.S. EXCHANGE PLUS MINUS			
TOTAL DEPOSIT			

FLD 4 TOTAL CASH

FLD 5 COIN

TELLER

FIGURE 18-2 Manual deposit ticket.

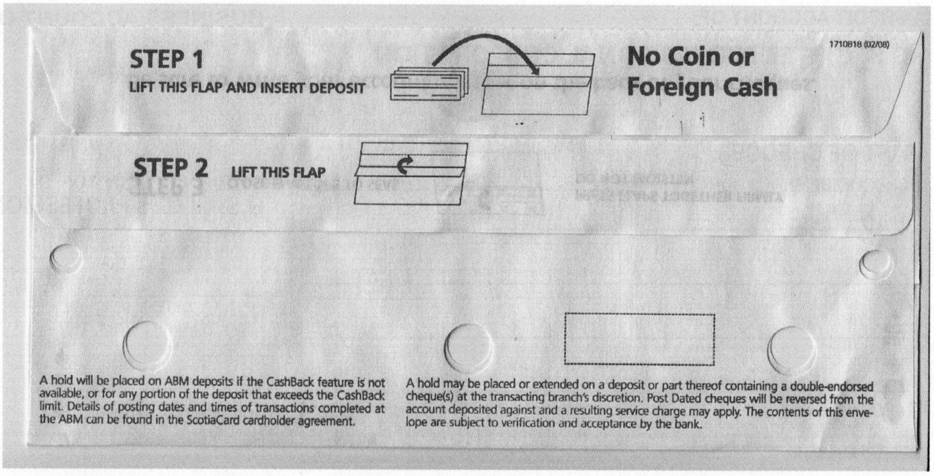

FIGURE 18-3 Deposit envelope.

You should always pay attention to the following points when preparing a bank deposit:

- Ensure the check amount exactly matches the amount you write on the deposit slip.
- Prepare the deposit in a quiet area of the office or at a time of day during which you will not be interrupted.
- The total amount of payment being deposited should be equal to the total amount of payments received in the office that day.

> **checkPOINT**
>
> 3. Name three points you should be aware of when completing the deposit.

BANK STATEMENTS AND ACCOUNT RECONCILIATION

Bank statements are a record of the transactions, such as deposits and payments by check, that have been processed on the bank account in a 1-month period.

Reviewing the bank statement every month is important to ensure that the account balance is accurate and that all transactions that have been processed are verified. Any service charges or fees that the bank has taken from the account must be

PROCEDURE 18-1 *Bank Deposit*

1. At the end of the day, gather the checks, cash, money orders, and traveler's checks, as well as any credit card payments that have been taken in throughout the day.
2. Begin by recording the date at the top of the deposit slip in the area provided for the date.
3. Using the deposit slip, begin at the first available line for recording the checks received. List the name of the person or company from whom the check is from and the amount in the spaces provided. The amount recorded on the deposit slip should exactly match the amount on the check.
4. Record the total cash amount in the space provided for currency.
5. Enter the amount of the total number of items included in the deposit. The total number of items refers to the total number of checks and other items being deposited. The bank uses this as one way of cross checking the deposit.
6. Add up the total cash, checks, and other items included in the deposit. The deposit total should be equal to the amount on the day sheet.
7. Place the checks with the deposit slip in an envelope or deposit bag. The deposit can then be taken to the bank and given to a bank teller or placed in the night deposit receptacle at the bank.

reviewed for accuracy. Additionally, all checks processed must be reviewed for accuracy, which requires a bank reconciliation.

Reconciling a bank account means making sure that the statement, the checkbook, and the monthly ledger sheet agree. That is, they should all have the same ending balance. The bank statement balance may not agree with the final balance recorded in the checkbook and the final month balance on the monthly ledger. The following points could be a reason for this discrepancy:

- Checks that were written or deposits that were made were not recorded in the checkbook or monthly ledger.
- The bank charges, or fees, were not recorded in the checkbook or monthly ledger balance.
- Deposits were made to the bank account after the statement date.
- Checks that were written were not "put through" or cleared on the account before the statement end date.

Reconciling the business checking account will provide a verification of the amount of money in the account. This verification allows you to record any fees or service charges from the bank into the ledger or accounting records for the dental office. It also provides you with information regarding outstanding checks. Reconciling the bank account is done on a monthly basis, since the bank sends a statement for a 1-month period.

Before you begin the reconciliation of the bank statement, you must gather some items that will allow you to reconcile accurately. The checkbook used to write the checks, the deposit book, which often includes a carbon copy of the deposits made, and the monthly ledger used for the month in question. Once you have all of this information, you may begin with the reconciliation. The backside of the bank statement often has an outline to follow for reconciling the bank statement. A sample reconciliation form is provided in Figure 18-4. Procedure 18-2 provides a

checkPOINT

4. What are the three reasons for a discrepancy in the bank account reconciliation?

PROCEDURE 18-2 *Bank Reconciliation*

1. Compare the deposits listed on the bank statement with the deposits shown in the ledger sheet, or, if recorded in the checkbook, compare those. Note all differences in the dollar amounts.
2. Compare each canceled check, including both check number and dollar amount, with the entry in the checkbook and on the ledger sheet. Note all the differences in the dollar amounts.
3. Mark the check number in the checkbook as having cleared by the bank. This can be done by placing a check mark beside the amount in the checkbook and on the bank statement.
4. After accounting for all checks processed through the account, those not marked in the checkbook are the checks that are outstanding. Add up the amount of all checks outstanding and write this amount in the outstanding checks line on the worksheet.
5. After accounting for all deposits processed through the account, those not marked in the checkbook are the deposits that are outstanding. Add up the amount of all deposits outstanding and write this amount in the outstanding deposits line on the worksheet.
6. Bank service charges and fees not recorded in the checkbook or ledger page should be added up and the total written in the space for service charges on the worksheet.
7. Starting with the ending balance on the bank statement, add all the outstanding deposits to this balance. Then subtract all outstanding checks.
8. Add any deposits or other credits and deduct any checks or other debits shown on the bank statement but missing in the checkbook to the transaction register of the checkbook.
9. The balance calculated from the bank statement should be verified against the account balance you have in the checkbook register. The adjusted bank statement balance should equal your adjusted checkbook balance. If you still have differences, check the previous steps to find errors.

SUNTRUST BANK
P O BOX 622227
ORLANDO FL 32862-2227

SunTrust

Account Statement

To change your address, please call 1-800-SUNTRUST (1-800-786-8787). Business clients call 1-800-752-2515.

Complete this section to balance this statement to your transaction register.

Month ______________ **Year** ______________

Bank Balance Shown on statement $ ______

Add (+) $ ______
Deposits not shown on this statement (if any).

Total (+) $ ______

Subtract (-)
Checks and other items outstanding but not paid on this statement (if any).

	$		$

Total (-) $ ______

Balance $ ______

These balances should agree

Your Transaction Register Balance $ ______

Add (+) $ ______
Other credits shown on this statement but not in transaction register.

Add (+) $ ______
Interest paid (for use in balancing interest-bearing accounts only).

Total (+) $ ______

Subtract (-) Other debits shown on this statement but not in transaction register.

Service Fees (if any) $ ______

Total (-) $ ______

Balance $ ______

In Case Of Errors Or Questions About Your Electronic Transfers:
If you think your statement or receipt is wrong or if you need more information about an electronic transfer, please contact us at the telephone number or address on this statement within 60 days of the statement on which the problem first appeared. Please give us your name and account number, describe the transaction (date, place/type, amount), and explain your concern. We will investigate and correct any error promptly. For your convenience, we will provisionally credit your account for the amount in question if we take more than 10 business days for point-of-sale transactions or foreign-initiated transfers, 5 business days for SunTrust Check Card Visa merchant transactions, or 20 business days for errors that occur within the first 30 days the account is open to complete our investigation.

FIGURE 18-4 Bank reconciliation worksheet.

step-by-step approach to bank account reconciliation, and Procedure 18-3 provides guidelines for finding errors when reconciling a bank account.

ELECTRONIC BANKING

Banking electronically, either online or through the use of an automated teller machine (ATM), has become common practice for both personal and business banking. **Electronic banking** is banking done using the computer in the dental office. The use of debit machines is one way that electronic banking is used in the dental office. When a patient makes a payment from his or her account using his or her debit card, money is taken from the patient's bank account and put into the dental office's business account. This electronic transfer of funds is used regularly in business. At the end of the business day, the dental office administrator, through a series of command

PROCEDURE 18-3 *Finding Errors When Reconciling a Bank Account*

1. Begin with the balance shown in your checkbook at the end of the previous month. To this balance, add the total deposits during the month and subtract the total amount of checks written in the month.
2. After checking your figures, the result should agree with your checkbook balance at the end of the month. If the result does not agree, you may have made an error in recording a check or deposit.
3. Add the amounts on the check stubs and compare this total with the total in the check column in the disbursements journal. If the totals do not agree, check the individual amounts to see if an error was made in your check stub record or in the related entry in the disbursements journal. Sometimes numbers may be transposed, that is, reversed.
4. Add the deposit amounts you have recorded in the checkbook. Compare that total with the monthly total in the deposit record book, if you have one. If the totals do not agree, check the individual amounts to find any errors.
5. If the checkbook and journal entries still disagree, then refigure the balances in the checkbook to make sure that the additions and subtractions are correct.

prompts on the debit machine, reconciles or deposits all funds transactions into the dental office's bank account.

Another form of electronic banking is used when the dental office administrator uses the **ATM** for daily bank deposits to the dental office account. Depositing of cash and checks can be done this way and a receipt for the deposit is provided automatically. The responsibility for this type of banking usually rests with one or two employees of the dental office and a receipt for the deposit must be provided to match to the bank account statement at the end of the month. The ATM card used by the employee will normally have limited features associated with it; that is, it will provide access to deposit funds but not withdraw funds, or view the balance of the account.

Using the computer to complete banking transactions online, or **online banking,** can also be performed from the dental office. Often, the dentist or office manager will manage this type of banking to transfer funds between accounts or pay bills.

checkPOINT

5. What are the three forms of electronic banking, and how can the dental administrator use them to more efficiently manage the dental office's finances?

Chapter Summary

There are many different accounts that may be in use in the dental office. The type of account used is strictly at the discretion of the dentist. Checking accounts and savings accounts are the most common types of accounts used. The dental office administrator is responsible for making deposits to these accounts and for accounting for checks that have been processed and those that have yet to be drawn on the account. The various types of bank fees that occur as a result of the transactions must be familiar to you to ensure accuracy of account balances. The procedures for making deposits and for reconciling the bank account or accounts are important for record keeping. Finally, a familiarity with electronic banking will allow the dental administrator to more quickly and efficiently manage the bank account or accounts for the dental office.

Review Questions

Multiple Choice

1. **An advantage to having a savings account in addition to a checking account in the dental office is that**
   a. the account balance can grow very quickly.
   b. a saving account is interest bearing.
   c. checks cannot be written on the account.
   d. only the dentist can access the savings account.

2. **Overdraft protection is**
   a. for use in cases of emergency only.
   b. available in situations where funds are not available.
   c. a form of credit extended by the bank to the business.
   d. used exclusively by businesses.

3. **Reconciliation of the bank statement is done on what basis?**
   a. Yearly, at the fiscal year end.
   b. Monthly, when the bank statement is available.
   c. Every 2 weeks with an electronic account statement.
   d. Only when a concern arises with the account.

4. **If a check is written and not recorded in the monthly ledger, this will create a**
   a. glitch in the electronic banking.
   b. discrepancy in the bank reconciliation.
   c. error in the bank deposit.
   d. a balance upset in the account.

5. **The total amount of money deposited on a daily basis should equal**
   a. the total amount of payment received in the office that day.
   b. the amount of funds electronically transferred.
   c. the total insurance check payments received.
   d. the balance on the daily bill payment listing.

6. **The ATM card used for making deposits for the dental office usually does not allow for transactions such as balance viewing and withdrawals, how is this feature beneficial to the person making the deposits?**
   a. It allows the deposits to be made easily at any time during the day.
   b. Withdrawals and balance viewing should be done by the dentist or other designated employee only.
   c. It is a security feature that protects the employee making the deposits by restricting the banking activities.
   d. It is not beneficial in any way to the person making deposits.

7. **Why is it beneficial to review the bank account statement when it arrives in the mail?**
   a. The sole purpose is to review for transaction fees.
   b. It should be expected that the account is accurate and that all the checks have cleared.
   c. Catching discrepancies early and contacting the bank immediately will rectify small errors before they become big ones.
   d. Some of the items listed on the bank statement could be transactions from a previous month.

8. **When selecting a bank account for the practice, it is important to consider fees charged per transaction by the bank because**
   a. the volume of transactions may be large or small which will affect fee amounts.
   b. most of the fees charged by the bank are charged erroneously.
   c. the cost of fees charged by the bank is always high for dental offices.
   d. the dental administrator will never have to consider fees charged when selecting an account.

9. **Which of the following should you be aware of when preparing a bank deposit?**
   a. The name on the check being deposited must be handwritten.
   b. The check amount must exactly match the amount you write on the deposit slip.
   c. Only one person in the dental office is responsible for making deposits.
   d. The office manager should review all deposits prior to these going to the bank.

10. **Bank statements are**
    a. a record of the account the bank compiles for a quarterly period of time.
    b. reviewed by the office manager prior to reconciliation by the office administrator.
    c. a record of the transactions, such as deposits and payments by check, that have been processed on the bank account in a 1-month period.
    d. made up of fees, checks, and other withdrawal transactions only.

Critical Thinking

1. You are having trouble reconciling the business checking account. What are the steps you should take to discover where the error is?
2. Another employee has asked to reconcile the bank account this month, to get some practice at performing this task. What suggestion you may make regarding this request? What concerns you may have regarding the confidentiality of this information?
3. The dentist has asked you to gather information regarding savings accounts for the practice funds. What information are you going to consider in your research?

chapter NINETEEN

Payroll

OUTLINE

OBJECTIVES

After completing this chapter, you should be able to do the following:

- Spell and define key terms
- Identify primary methods of tracking time worked by employees
- Discuss the types of payroll systems, specifically manual and computerized systems
- Explain the legalities involved in doing payroll
- Identify deductions that are federally mandated and those that are optional
- Calculate payroll and remittances
- Explain how to use an employee earnings record to track employee earnings
- Describe the W-4 form and the information found on it

KEY TERMS

- payroll
- payroll service
- time card
- time sheet
- deductions
- W-4 form
- net pay
- gross pay
- record of employment
- employee earnings record
- W-2 form

Every employee in the dental office depends on receiving a paycheck on payday to meet financial commitments in a timely manner. Computing and issuing checks for payment for work done by all employees in the office is termed **payroll.** Paychecks that are not ready for employees when promised or have errors in the amount paid can create frustration and resentment toward the employer. The dental office administrator may be responsible for issuing paychecks to employees on payday. This is an important responsibility for the office administrator. The person who is responsible for issuing payroll will also be responsible for submitting the tax withholding to the correct federal agency. For these reasons, you must understand the importance of completing the payroll accurately and in a timely manner. The focus of this chapter is to assist you in that understanding. Presented in this chapter are use of time sheets and time cards to record employees' time worked, types of payroll systems, legalities related to payroll, tax withholdings, and how to calculate payroll and remittances.

TIME SHEETS/CARDS

Before discussing different payroll systems, we will first look at how employees' time worked is tracked. Depending on the dental office you work in, you may have to complete a time card or time sheet on a daily basis and submit it to your supervisor on a specific date consistent with the pay period. The purpose of a **time card** or **time sheet** is to provide the employer with a record of the employee's hours worked for the pay period. The main difference between a time card and a time sheet is that a time sheet is usually completed by hand or typed up on a computer by the employee, whereas a time card is usually inserted into a time clock when the employee begins and ends work for the day and also at the start and end of breaks taken throughout the day. Regardless of whether a time sheet or a time card is used in the office, the following information should be found on both:

> *Administrative* TIP
>
> If handwritten time sheets are submitted by employees, make a photocopy of the time sheet. Supply the employee with the photocopy of the time sheet and keep the original copy in the employee file. This provides a good record should questions arise in the future regarding the amount of time paid.

- Employee information (name, number, position, pay rate)
- Pay period start and end date
- Start time and end time
- Breaks/lunch times taken
- Regular hour total
- Overtime hours total
- Employee signature

TYPES OF PAYROLL SYSTEMS

The withholding of taxes deducted from employee paychecks and submitted to the Internal Revenue Service (IRS) is the responsibility of the individual who makes up the payroll checks, which is often the dental administrator. A manual or computerized system of payroll can be used in the dental office. Alternatively, a payroll service may be used. A **payroll service** is an outside agency that issues all paychecks to the company's employees. A dental office with many employees may view a payroll service as advantageous because payroll for a large number of employees can take a fair amount of time to complete. A payroll service is a very cost-effective way of issuing payroll checks, since they are accurate, computerized, and aware of any changes regarding taxes immediately.

Payday in a dental office is based on an interval chosen by the dentist. It can be monthly (12 pay periods per year), biweekly (26 pay periods per year), or weekly (52 pay periods per year). Some employees may be paid a salary, whereas others are paid hourly, depending on the position of the employee. Some dental offices pay all employees the same, hourly or salary. Regardless of how the employee is paid, either a computerized or a manual system may be used.

Computerized Payroll System

A payroll software program can easily and accurately maintain payroll records. An accounting software program that allows for paying vendors and receiving payments will usually have a payroll component. However, it is not unusual to have a payroll system that is kept separate from other financial information in the practice, just because of the sensitive nature of the information. The payroll software can easily calculate deductions from employee paychecks and provide information to the employer regarding the amount to be submitted to the IRS from the employer. Because payroll can be a very time-consuming task that requires focused attention to details, a computerized system can save time and minimize mistakes.

Manual Payroll System

A common manual payroll system is the one-write system of payroll accounting, as has been discussed in Chapters 16 and 17. With this pegboard system, a payroll register is used and each employee is assigned a ledger card. The payroll register sheet is placed first on the pegboard, and the employee's ledger card is placed next and is lined up on the proper date and line. The check used is then lined up and placed on top of the ledger card, where the date, employee name, withholdings, and pay are written. The carbon strip used on the backside of the check allows the information to be recorded in three places. The payroll register allows for the payroll records to be kept separately and totaled on a regular basis. More importantly, it allows for the payroll records to be maintained in a private area, separate from other financial records.

> **checkPOINT**
>
> 1. What is the purpose of the payroll register?

LEGALITIES INVOLVED WITH PAYROLL

Regardless of whether a computerized or manual system is used, employers are required by federal law to maintain payroll records of their business. Payroll records must be kept in a secure place to ensure confidentiality of employee information. A record for each employee must be kept separately, that is, each file must have an individual file in which personal information is kept in a secure place by the employer. This file contains the necessary information for the employee's payroll for the duration of their employment with the company.

The employee file should contain the following information:

- Initial resume or job application
- Reference check form
- Pay rate
- Performance evaluations
- Completed W-4 forms

These documents must remain in the employee file and must be kept up-to-date. All information regarding pay, such as increases, must be noted in the employee file as they occur.

> **checkPOINT**
>
> 2. Why should payroll records be maintained separately from other records in the dental office?

TAX WITHHOLDINGS

Each paycheck an employee receives will be accompanied by a stub that lists details of all of the deductions taken by the employer. These **deductions** should include federal, state, and local income taxes, along with Medicare and social security. These are the minimum deductions and are legally mandated. This means that the employer, by law, must deduct and remit the deductions to the IRS. There are also deductions that are optional, which means that the employee has agreed to the deduction prior to the employer deducting them. Some of these optional deductions are as follows:

- IRA—individual retirement account contributions
- Union dues
- Employee funds (coffee fund, party fund)
- Employee loans
- Benefit plans (besides Medicare)

The legally mandated deductions are based on information that the employee supplies to the employer prior to or on the commencement of employment. Each employee must complete an Employee's Withholding Allowance Certificate, commonly known as the **W-4 form.** The information found on this form provides the employer with information regarding the category to use for withholding taxes. Failure to complete and submit this form will result in the employer deducting taxes at the highest rate available. The information found on the form includes the following: employee name address, social security number, marital status, and information regarding the number of tax exemptions the employee is eligible for. The completed form is placed in the employee's file and maintained for the duration of the employment. Changes in marital status or dependents would require completion of an updated form.

> ✓ *check*POINT
>
> 3. What does "legally mandated deductions" mean? Provide two examples of legally mandated deductions.

CANADIAN PRACTICE: TAX WITHHOLDINGS

In Canada, income taxes are paid to Revenue Canada, the counterpart to the IRS in the United States. These taxes, withheld from employee paychecks, include the federal pension plan and employment insurance, the counterparts to Social Security and Medicare in the United States. The employment insurance deduction (an unemployment tax) is 1.4 times, paid to the Canadian Pension Plan (CPP), must be deducted from the employee's paycheck, and the employer must match this amount. This means that the amount deducted from the employee's paycheck is doubled and then remitted.

In place of Social Security numbers for U.S. employees, Canadian employees have social insurance numbers that they must provide to employers and use in completing tax forms. Moreover, Canadian employees must complete a TD-1 form (the counterpart to the W-4 form in the United States) and submit it to their employers to indicate how much should be withheld from paychecks to cover taxes.

Another form, the T-4 form, must be sent out from employers to employees to inform them of their total income and taxes withheld for a 1-year period and is the counterpart to the W-2 form in the United States. The T-4 form contains the following information:

- Employment income (gross earnings)
- All CPP and employment income deductions
- Income tax deducted
- Union dues
- Charitable donations
- Pension plan amounts deducted for employer-matched pension plans
- Other taxable benefits (employer-paid benefits such as life insurance portions and employee loans)

A **record of employment** is a form used by the human resources department of the government of Canada that provides employees and the department with financial information regarding their employment. The form is required for purposes of collecting employment insurance benefits during times when the employee is without work. The form must be issued, by law, within 5 days of the employee's last working day. There are three copies when the form is complete. One copy is for the employee, one is for the employer for their records, and one copy is mailed to the human resources department of the federal government. Every employee must receive a record of employment form when he or she experiences an interruption in earnings.

CALCULATING PAYROLL AND REMITTANCES

Accurately calculating employee payroll depends on beginning with accurate information provided by the employee and careful attention to detail on the part of the dental administrator. To this end, each employee's paycheck should be calculated in its entirety before moving to the next employee's paycheck.

Taxes deducted must be paid to the IRS as they are deducted. So, if the pay period is a biweekly period, the deductions are remitted on a biweekly basis. The **net pay** or take-home pay, which is the amount of pay owed to the employee after all deductions have been taken, is calculated as follows:

Gross pay (hours worked multiplied by hourly pay rate) – total deductions = net pay

This calculation can be made using the one-write system, which allows you to write the employee's earnings information only once and record it in three places or by a computerized payroll system, which can calculate deductions for you or allow you to enter the information and maintain a record of it in the appropriate employee file.

The employer is responsible for remitting the taxes to the IRS. The IRS sends the employer a payroll remittance form each month requesting information regarding the amount of deductions withheld and other information regarding payroll, including the number of employees paid and the gross pay for all employees. The employer must ensure that the deductions are paid to the IRS by a specific date each month. Failure to meet the deadline results in a monetary penalty. It is the employer's responsibility to make sure that the following occur:

1. The correct amount of deduction is withheld
2. The correct amount of deduction is remitted
3. The remittance is done within the specified time period

In addition to the taxes withheld from employees' paychecks, the employer is also responsible for paying the Federal Unemployment Tax (FUTA) using Form 940, the Employer's Annual Federal Unemployment Tax Return. This tax is paid entirely from the employer's funds (not from taxes withheld from the employee) and is at a rate of 6.2% of taxable wages. The taxable wage base is the first $7000 paid in wages to each employee during a calendar year. Employers who pay the state unemployment tax, on a timely basis, will receive an offset credit of up to 5.4% regardless of the rate of tax they pay the state. Therefore, the net FUTA tax rate is generally 0.8% (6.2% − 5.4%), for a maximum FUTA tax of $56.00 per employee, per year (0.008 × $7000 = $56.00). Procedures 19-1 and 19-2 provide steps for manually calculating an employee paycheck and using the necessary tables.

PROCEDURE 19-1 *Manually Calculating an Employee's Paycheck*

1. To determine the employees' gross pay, calculate the gross pay by multiplying the total hours worked within the pay period by the hourly rate. You do not need to calculate gross pay for employees who are paid on a salary basis as the amount of the monthly gross pay is predetermined based on an annual amount divided equally over the number pay periods per year.
2. For employees eligible for overtime pay, calculate overtime worked by multiplying the total overtime hours by the hourly overtime rate.
3. Using the tax deduction tables, find the total deduction for federal and state, and local taxes, as well as Social Security and Medicare, for the current pay period.
4. Calculate any other employee-elected deductions for the pay period.
5. Total the deductions and subtract this number from the gross pay.
6. Write the paycheck for the final number arrived at after the deductions are subtracted.

PROCEDURE 19-2 *How to Use the Deductions Tables for Employee Payroll Deductions*

1. Always use the employee's gross pay amount when determining the amount of the deduction to withhold.
2. Ensure that the correct table is being referred to. If you are deducting for a married person, ensure that the table you are using is titled "for married persons" on the top left-hand corner.
3. Ensure that the table you are using is for the correct type of pay period. That is, if the deductions you are taking are based on a weekly, biweekly, monthly, or semimonthly pay period, double check that the correct table is being used.
4. Using the column on the left-hand side of the table, find the range of gross pay within which the employee's gross pay falls.
5. Once you have determined the range, move directly right to the amount on the table that correlates with the employee's number of deductions along the top of the table.
6. Enter this number as the deduction.

checkPOINT

4. What are net pay and gross pay?

what IF ?

What if an employee informs you that he or she does not want any tax deducted from his or her paycheck because he or she does not need to pay it? The first thing you need to ask the employee is to provide you with written documentation from the IRS that allows for this. Once you have confirmation, contact the IRS to confirm that this is a legitimate action. Inform the employee that you will be taking these steps. Explain that the employer is responsible for the deductions and submitting them and penalties will be imposed if the deductions are not taken. Always get information in writing from the employee, by way of a W-4 form, and contact the IRS if necessary.

checkPOINT

5. What is a W-2 form? What information does it contain?

The employer must pay all deductions on a regular basis. The accountant usually remits the quarterly or annual summation paid. The IRS requires a statement of total remittances throughout the year, referred to as a Form W-3, Transmittal of Wage and Tax Statements. In addition, every employee should be sent a W-2 form by no later than January 31 of the year following the tax year in question.

Employee Earnings Record

The **employee earnings record** contains information regarding an employees' pay. The information includes: gross pay, deductions, federal tax rate, salary, and the number of days worked in a pay period. The employee earnings record is an information record given to employees on payday that reflects their pay for a specific pay period. An ongoing account of pay received by the employee is included on the earnings record.

W-2 Form

At the end of the calendar year (January to December), the information regarding the deductions that each employee has paid and yearly earnings is supplied to the employee using the **W-2 form,** Wage and Tax Statement. This form must be mailed to the employee by no later than January 31 of the year following the tax year in question, so that the employee can file his or her tax return.

The W-2 form contains the following information:

- Total gross earnings from the previous year
- Total taxes withheld for state, federal, and local (if any)
- Taxable benefits
- Total net income for the year

Chapter Summary

The management of the payroll system in the dental office is a critical responsibility and is often assigned to the dental administrator. Payroll management begins with accurate tracking of actual time worked by all employees on a time sheet or time card. The payroll system itself may be a computer program or a manual system, such as the one-write system. The dentist determines the frequency of payroll in the office, and the individual responsible for issuing the paychecks must do so in a timely manner, ensuring accuracy. Withholdings from employee paychecks are determined by information supplied by the employee on Form W-4. Employee earnings are tracked by the dental office using an employee earnings record, and the dental administrator can calculate each employee's net pay by subtracting all mandatory and elected deductions from gross pay. The taxes withheld must be submitted within the timeframe specified by the IRS; otherwise the dentist is liable for financial penalties. Maintaining accurate payroll records for each employee is a legal responsibility of the dentist, and these records must provide information that matches that found on the W-2 form provided to the employee at the end of the year. Information regarding income earned and deductions withheld for a given tax year must be sent to each employee by January 31 of the following year in Form W-2.

Review Questions

Multiple Choice

1. **Which form provides employees with information regarding their pay for the entire year?**
   a. W-4
   b. W-2
   c. IRA
   d. W-3

2. **Which of the following is not considered deduction from an employee paycheck?**
   a. Federal tax
   b. Medicare
   c. State tax
   d. Employment insurance

3. **Time cards and time sheets**
   a. are methods used for keeping track of hours worked.
   b. are the best way to provide overtime information.
   c. are an outdated way of employee time recording.
   d. none of the above.

4. **A W-4 form provides**
   a. information regarding withholdings from employee paychecks.
   b. year-end tax information for employees.
   c. total deductions for the month for the employee.
   d. IRA information only.

5. **Net pay is**
   a. the total amount the employee gets paid.
   b. the total hours multiplied by pay rate.
   c. total deductions subtracted from gross pay.
   d. a and c.

6. **Which of the following is not considered a responsibility regarding monthly remittances by the employer?**
   a. The correct amount of deduction is withheld.
   b. The correct amount of deduction is remitted.
   c. The employee has approved the remittance.
   d. The remittance is done within the specified time period.

7. **If deductions are not taken and remitted by the due date every month by the employer**
   a. a jail term could be imposed by the authorities.
   b. financial penalties and fines would be added to the employer's account.
   c. the employee becomes responsible for the remittance.
   d. each employer is allowed to miss one remittance period.

8. **Keeping the original time sheet and providing a photocopy for the employee is beneficial because**
   a. the employee could be dishonest about the time worked.
   b. provides a good record should questions arise in the future regarding the amount of time paid.
   c. errors in payroll are always the result of miscalculations of hours worked.
   d. the employee needs to have a copy not the original.

9. **Payroll records must be kept in a secure place**
   a. to ensure confidentiality of employee information.
   b. to easily access the payroll records.
   c. for the dentist to review when he needs to.
   d. so that they are kept out of reach of employees.

10. **If a pay period is a biweekly pay period, deductions must be remitted**
    a. monthly.
    b. biweekly.
    c. quarterly.
    d. on demand.

Critical Thinking

1. After you have distributed the paychecks, you discover that you have erroneously calculated the amount of tax deductions from an employee's paycheck. What steps could you take to repair this error and recover the amount?

2. A new employee has been hired and wants to discuss his or her payroll deductions with you. What are you going to tell him or her regarding what types of deductions he or she can expect?

Web Site

U.S. Department of Labor, Employment & Training Administration. Unemployment Insurance Tax Topic: http://workforcesecurity.doleta.gov/unemploy/uitaxtopic.asp

part **FIVE**

Career *Considerations*

chapter TWENTY

Employment *Strategies*

OBJECTIVES

After completing this chapter, you should be able to do the following:

- Spell and define key terms
- List personal and professional attributes necessary for a successful practicum experience
- Determine the best position based on personal strengths and weaknesses
- List commonly used job search resources
- Identify necessary steps to apply for the right position
- Draft an appropriate resume and cover letter
- List guidelines for an effective interview
- Explain how to evaluate an offer and to negotiate its terms, if appropriate
- List possible reasons for not being offered the position
- Discuss the purpose of employment laws and how they impact the interviewing process

KEY TERMS

- resume
- cover letter
- practicum
- networking
- working interview

OUTLINE

Obtaining certification as a dental office administrator is an achievement that you can be proud of. The skills you have acquired through the academic and practical portions of your program are valuable to any dental office. However, the anticipation you may feel about your future may be mixed with the stress and anxiety often associated with looking for your first job in the dental industry. To help alleviate this stress and anxiety, this chapter is designed to provide you with information on how to begin your job search and how to use the new skills you have acquired to help you in obtaining that job. Specifically, this chapter covers how to use a practicum to gain valuable work experience, setting goals for employment, how to conduct a job search, preparing resumes and cover letters and applying for jobs, how to prepare for and succeed in job interviews, evaluating and negotiating the terms of an offer, and what to know about employment laws.

PRACTICUM

If the program you are enrolled in includes a work experience or practicum portion, you will need to be familiar with the etiquette required and the benefits of working as a student in the dental administration environment. A **practicum** is practical training in the industry to which you are studying to work in and involves working alongside employees of the office while under the direct supervision of one person in the office and the supervisor of your academic program. The practicum experience gives you the opportunity to apply the skills and theories you learned about in the classroom.

Practicums provide many opportunities for learning. You will witness how the position you are training for is carried out in the dental office and apply your knowledge to real-life experiences. You may spend your work experience time in a specialist's office or a general dentist practice. This can provide you with a chance to develop your preference for a certain type of office. As your professional skills and confidence develop through the work experience, your desire for wanting to excel in the position will show. Most importantly, the practicum portion should give you a first-hand look at how the dental office administrator position is a big part of the dental team and the impact this position has on the team.

As a student in a dental office, remember first and foremost that you are a guest in the office. To assume that the office will hire you when your work experience is completed would be erroneous on your part. The dental office is providing you with an opportunity to gain work experience that you can include on your resume and use as a reference for future employers. You must consider that this dental office can assist you in a positive job search experience. You should view your work experience as an opportunity to grow professionally and a time for you to show that you are an asset to the profession. There are three main areas that you should pay particular attention to while you are on your work experience:

- Dependability
- Professionalism

> **checkPOINT**
>
> 1. What are the two main areas you should pay attention to on your work experience?

We will now consider each of these areas in detail.

Dependability when you are a student in the dental office is a sign that you are a reliable and feel that the experience you are gaining is important. Dependability involves being on time, being considerate of the other staff members, and showing concern for the patients in the dental office. Being prepared well in advance of your work experience will create a smooth experience for you and the office you work in. Preparation for your work experience involves knowing how you are going to get to the office on time, having daycare in place for your children, if applicable, and having financial coverage or support for the amount of time you will be at the work experience site and not able to attend your regular job, if you have one. By making sure that all areas of your life are attended to for you to achieve your goal, you will likely have a successful work experience.

Arriving on time each day is important. Do not wait until the first morning of your work experience to find a route to the office. Practice once or twice using different routes to determine the quickest route possible. You should also consider whether you will be traveling during rush hour, as this can make a difference in the time you arrive at the office. Part of the responsibility of the dental office administrator is to prepare the office prior to patients' arrival. For this reason, being on time consistently sends a message to your supervisor that you are a person who can be relied on.

Professionalism is a term that encompasses your attitude, confidence, and desire to help patients and to work as a team with other staff members. If you are rushed in the morning before arriving at work, you may show up in a frazzled state at the office. This may be difficult to hide, especially when you are trying to focus on helping a patient. A dental office administrator who is anxious or stressed may project that energy toward patients and other staff members. Dealing effectively with patients is the main role of the dental office administrator. When you are a student in a dental office you may not feel perfectly confident to handle some situations. Your professionalism in these situations is very important. Asking your supervisor to deal directly with such situations and observing carefully will help you in developing skills. Letting a patient know that you are a student and that your authority is limited will go a long way toward you gaining respect and confidence.

Your flexibility and adaptability are standards by which professionalism is also judged. If you are requested to assist in another area of the office, such as with the insurance clerk or observing a procedure in the operatory, you should gladly accept these assignments. If you refuse or show apprehension you could jeopardize a positive reference and practicum experience. However, you should not perform duties that are outside your scope of practice, such as those involving clinical procedures. If you are asked to perform clinical procedures, you should inform your supervisor immediately. The flexibility of all staff members in many areas of the dental office is what contributes to a team that functions well together. Flexibility is a testament to your professionalism and a desirable trait in a dental office administrator.

FINDING THE RIGHT JOB

As you begin your search for meaningful employment, you must make a decision regarding the type of office you wish to work in and know what you need from a job before beginning your search. Tips on conducting a job search are provided in Box 20-1. You should consider components such as amount of pay, hours,

BOX 20-1 *Job Search Tips*

- *Sending a poorly written resume.* Avoid having your resume end up in the garbage. Have friends or family read your resume over for spelling and grammar. The same goes for your cover letter. Make sure both resume and cover letter are error-free.
- *Not stating why you are the right candidate for the job.* Take the time to carefully define why the position matches your skills and experience. Learn about the organization and personalize your cover letter to reflect why you are the perfect person for the position.
- *Not following directions.* Make sure to pay attention to directions in the job advertisement. If the job listing instructs you to fax the application in, do not drop it off in person. Job descriptions are written with specific instructions for a reason.
- *Applying for jobs you are not qualified for.* Do not apply for jobs that are out of your range of experience. You either will be disappointed because you are not getting call backs or prospective employers will be annoyed during the interview when it becomes evident that you are not qualified for the position.
- *Applying to jobs you do not really want.* Before starting your job hunt, think about what you want from a job. Do not waste your time applying for a job you do not want.
- *Pretending to be perfect.* Recognize your weaknesses. A well-known interview question is, "What do you think your weaknesses are?" Be prepared to answer it intelligently with a response that puts a positive spin on things.
- *Not trying hard enough.* Looking for a full-time job is a full-time job in itself. It involves making phone calls, sending out resumes, and following up on leads.
- *Forgetting your manners.* Always send a thank you note or a polite e-mail after meeting with an interviewer. Your manners and etiquette say a lot about you as a potential employee.

benefits, and the size of the practice before beginning your search. Instead of sending out a number of resumes to as many dental offices as you can and hoping to get any job that is available, set a goal. You can set a goal by deciding on what type of office you want to work in and knowing the position you want to perform. You also must identify your own strengths and weaknesses, so that you can know how best to market your skills to prospective employers. These topics are covered below.

Setting Goals for Employment

When deciding on the type of dental office in which you wish to work, take into account your experiences at the office at which you are a patient and the office at which you did your practicum, your experience working with colleagues in the industry, and any interest you have in a specific area of dentistry. You may come in contact with employees in the dental office who are not hired as permanent or part-time employees of the office, but are contract employees. Contract employees are individuals who work in the dental office but are not employees of the dental office, that is, they are responsible for paying their own taxes and withholdings to the IRS and the dental office is not involved with ensuring that this happens. The independent contractor employee is paid directly by the dental office and decides when to work in the office as needed. The independent contractor is not eligible for benefits provided to employees of the dental office.

Use the following points as a guide in making your decision about your employment goal:

- Type of dentistry (general or specialty)
- Size of office (number of dentists)
- Ideal hours
- Proximity to home
- Atmosphere of office
- Amount of responsibility
- Opportunity for advancement

A few of these points are covered in more detail below.

Type of Office

If you are unsure about the type of office you wish to work in, do some research in the area of dentistry you are most interested in or talk to friends and family about their experiences. Working in a specialist area of dentistry such as orthodontic or endodontic offices, you will have greater exposure to the specific area of dentistry that the dentist practices. This will provide you with a more in-depth knowledge of the area and exposure to general dentistry practices will be minimal. Although some specialist offices continue to provide dental cleanings for patients, the practice is generally focused on the specific specialty. The administrative functions remain the same regardless of being in a general dental practice or a specialist's office.

As you increase your experience level in the administrative sector of the dental industry, you will gain exposure to the clinical aspects. This exposure may prompt you to acquire a clinical background in dentistry as a dental assistant, dental hygienist, or dentist. Gaining clinical certification will also assist you if you choose to move into other areas of dentistry, such as teaching in dental-assisting programs, working in insurance firms, and working with dental product development companies. As a dental office administrator, your experience will provide you with knowledge and background required to work in insurance companies processing claims, sales positions with dental product companies, or lecturing and teaching within a dental consulting firm to aid in the development of successful dental office administrators.

Size of Office

In addition to dental specialty and setting, another factor to consider is the number dentists in the practice. Some students may prefer to work in an office with more than one dentist because it is busy and provides exposure to many different types of patients and procedures. Other students may prefer a dental office that is smaller, with perhaps only one dentist. As a general rule, the smaller the office, the greater the responsibilities for the dental office administrator. A larger office may have more positions for different areas, such as treatment coordinator or office manager, meaning that the dental administrator position has less responsibility in those areas.

Ideal Hours

You should consider the hours in which you are not only willing to work, but can realistically commit to working. If you have commitments outside of regular workday hours, such as a family that you must be available for, or other work, or school commitments, you should carefully consider your availability time. In other words, if the office hours of the dental practice you wish to work in are Monday to Friday from 7 AM to 3 PM, but you are unable to be at the office until 7:30 AM, committing to working these hours may put you in a position where you are arriving late for work, and may put you in a position where you are dismissed. Try to find an office where the hours are more suitable to your commitments, or adjust your commitments to accommodate your work schedule.

Atmosphere of Office

The office atmosphere you are in on a daily basis can greatly affect your mood. Consider if you are the type of person who can thrive in a fast-paced environment or if you prefer a slower, quieter atmosphere. Larger practices tend to have more patients attending the office on a daily basis, and therefore more employees must accomplish more tasks. A smaller office will have fewer people attending and fewer employees to accomplish tasks. A smaller office dose not necessarily equate to a lower stress level, just a smaller volume of tasks to be completed on a daily basis and usually a quieter atmosphere.

Opportunity for Advancement

Early on your career you may be looking to see where you can advance to in the administrative sector of the dental industry. Depending on the size of the dental office, there are many positions to advance to, such as office manager, treatment coordinator, scheduling coordinator, and clinical positions. Working in a smaller office does not imply that these positions will not be available to you in the future, since, as the office grows, a need for these positions may become available.

Assessing Your Strengths and Weaknesses

Once you have made decisions regarding where you wish to work and what your ideal job would be, you can begin to prepare to sell yourself to your potential employer. Selling yourself means that you will need to present your qualifications of the position and convince the employer that you are the best person for the job. Usually you will need to provide them with information that sets you apart from all the other applicants, that is, something about you that is unique and that will provide benefit to the employer.

To discover what your strengths and weaknesses are, you should engage in the process of self-reflection. Make a list of your strong points and a list of the areas you wish to improve. If you need help getting started, ask someone who is honest with you to provide you with one point for each area. This is a good exercise to engage in since interviewers often ask applicants for their opinion on what their strengths and weaknesses are.

Use your strengths to sell yourself to your potential employer. For example, if you are a sympathetic person, this is a point that you could raise in an interview. Sympathy with patients may be necessary from time to time, and a genuinely sympathetic person will be more effective in helping patients. However, when presenting your strengths, be sure to provide concrete examples from your life that demonstrate the trait. For instance, an example of sympathy might be that you volunteer with your local hospice care or visit the elderly in nursing homes.

You can also use your weaknesses to sell yourself. Remember, nobody is perfect and if you represent yourself as someone who is perfect, the interviewer will see this as your weakness. The best way to handle a weakness is to acknowledge it but to provide an example to the interviewer about how you working to improve it. For example, if you are a person who avoids conflict, stress that you are aware of this weakness and are working toward improving it. Then provide an example of how you are working to improve it, such as phoning your landlord for the third time about some repairs that still need to be made in your apartment. The first step in improving weaknesses is recognizing that you have one.

> **checkPOINT**
>
> 2. How can assessing your strengths and weaknesses help prepare you for an interview?

Job Search Resources

There are several effective resources to use when pursuing employment. These include networking, the Internet, newspaper advertisements, yellow pages, and employment agencies, each of which is discussed below.

Networking

Networking is the development of relationships that can produce employment leads and is an excellent way to learn of job opportunities. The dental industry can be a small industry or large industry, depending on where you live. A small town may only have a few dental offices, whereas a larger city may have hundreds or thousands. Regardless of where you live, it is important for you to develop contacts in the industry. You can start your networking process through the people you work with during your practicum. These people can be lifelong contacts for you if you act professionally toward them and maintain a positive attitude.

Besides people in the industry, you can also network through your friends and family. So, when you are looking for a job, make sure you tell as many people as possible. Many people find employment through a friend or referral.

Advertisements

Another excellent source for job leads are advertisements. Advertisements can be found in the classified section of your local newspaper and usually specify the qualifications of the individual sought. An address, phone number, or fax number may be provided. Employers using this method may also limit the information they provide because they may wish to meet with the applicant before interviewing. Make sure that you follow the instructions provided in the advertisement. That is, if the advertisement states "no phone calls," do not phone, even if you know exactly where the dental office is or who the contact person is.

Yellow Pages

The yellow pages of your phone book are also a good source to consult. Turn to the section on dentists or dental offices and select the dental offices that are situated in the area in which you would most prefer to work. Telephone each dental office and ask if they are looking to hire new employees, or tailor a cover letter and resume addressed to the contact person at the dental office (we will look at this in detail next).

Internet

More and more, the Internet is becoming a powerful resource for job seekers, particularly through web sites that specialize in bringing employers and job seekers together. The web site usually lists the various advertisements placed by employers and will keep the name of the employer confidential. This is done so that employer can contact applicants directly without the applicant being able to enquire directly to the employer regarding the position. Some of these web sites are listed at the end of this chapter.

Moreover, many dental offices have their own web sites, which job seekers can peruse for information on the office. For instance, a web site might identify the specialty of the practice, location, office hours, staff names and contact information, and services provided. Additionally, a web site may even provide information on open positions within the dental office.

Finally, professional organization web sites, such as that of the American Dental Association (ADA), are also good resources for the job seeker. Besides information on member dental practices, the ADA web site also provides job listings for dental team members.

Employment Agency

An **employment agency** can provide short-term or temporary work for people searching for full-time positions. These agencies are also a good place to work part-time in the dental industry and maintain skills, without making a firm commitment to one office. People who require a certain amount of flexibility in their lives on a regular basis, which a full-time job cannot provide, may find the idea of working temporarily quite desirable. Assignments range from days to weeks in some offices. On occasion, an employer will ask for temporary help as a way of meeting potential employees for certain positions, and if the right individual is found, he or she can be hired permanently. A placement fee is often paid to the employment agency.

> **checkPOINT**
>
> 3. What are the most common resources used for job searches?

APPLYING FOR THE JOB

Once you have identified one or more job opportunities that you would like to pursue, you must prepare a professional-looking resume and cover letter and complete the job application form. These topics are discussed below.

Preparing Your Resume

A **resume** is a document listing one's work-related skills, employment history, educational credentials, and other qualifications for employment. Most employers will request that job applicants submit a resume via fax, mail, or e-mail in application for any position.

When preparing a resume, keep in mind that it represents you. If it is sloppy—that is, wrinkled, folded, torn, smudged, or possessing spelling and grammar errors—the potential employer will likely see this as a reflection of your carelessness or inattention to detail and not consider you for the position. Much of the dental office administrator position involves paying attention to details. If you submit a resume with flaws, you are sending the message that you may not be able to perform the position effectively. Your resume is the first impression you make on a potential employer and the difference between getting called for an interview and not getting a response.

There are many resources available for those who are job seeking to develop a resume. Tips on how to create a resume are available on the Internet at sites such as the resumebuilder.com, monster.com, and job search at about.com. Some companies will even create a professional-looking resume for you for a fee. Alternatively, you can purchase software that provides resume templates and that can even create your resume based on the information you provide.

Resumes can have many different formats. Two types of resume formats are presented in this chapter. These are functional and chronological. A functional

BOX 20-2
Resume Writing Tips

- Keep your resume to one page.
- Include information pertaining to education, employment, and skills.
- List any affiliations with professional organizations.
- Be honest.
- Use a 12-point font with black ink on white or beige paper. Using colored paper may send the message that you are not professional.
- Do not include your references with your resume; state that references will be available on request. Make sure that you have permission from the people you have listed to use them as references.
- Do not list your hobbies and personal interests that are not related to the position you are applying.
- Make sure you proofread your resume or have someone proofread it for you.
- Do not fold your resume. Deliver or mail your resume in an 8.5 in. × 11 in. envelope to ensure it stays flat and neat.

legal TIP

One important aspect of developing a resume is to be honest. Providing false information on your resume is a misrepresentation of yourself and, if hired, could later cost you the job, if discovered.

resume is one that emphasizes the skills and qualifications of the applicant. A chronological resume, on the other hand, emphasizes the employment history of the applicant and is organized based on the date of the employment.

Box 20-2 provides you with resume writing tips to keep in mind as you develop your resume.

Your resume should include information that is pertinent in order for you to be considered for the position. This information includes your career objective, work experience, and education.

Career Objective

This section of your resume defines the position you are seeking. In other words, if you are applying for a dental administration position, the career objective should reflect this by clearly stating that you are seeking a position where you will utilize your dental administrative skills and education.

Work Experience

Include at least two names of past employers and your present employer. Provide dates of employment and the title of the position you held. Since you may have limited experience in your field early in your career, and as a new graduate, you should consider including your practicum experience in this category and be prepared to provide the name of the person who directly supervised your practicum work. References should be provided on request to the potential employer. Provide at least two references, although most employers may request three references. Always contact your references before providing his or her name to ensure that you have permission to do so.

Education

Begin this section by listing your most recent education first. All colleges and universities attended should be listed in this area. If you have any certifications that may be pertinent to the position, such as First Aid or cardiopulmonary resuscitation (CPR), these should be listed in a separate section elsewhere on the resume.

Preparing the Cover Letter

In addition to your resume, you must always prepare a **cover letter**. Submitting a resume for a position is not helpful to an employer if you do not provide information as to what position you are looking for. Your cover letter should outline who you are, what position you are applying for, and why you would be a desirable candidate for the position. You may even highlight your qualifications in this letter.

Your letter should be addressed to the appropriate contact person at the office. If you are not sure about the person's title, do not use one. For example, if the contact name is Pat Smith, do not assume that you would address your letter Mr. Pat Smith. Pat could be the shortened form of Patricia. If you know for sure that the person is male or female and you are sure of the honorific to use, then do so. Otherwise, using the salutation: Dear Pat Smith, would be acceptable.

Three areas should be addressed in your cover letter:

1. The position for which you are applying (state this in the first paragraph).
2. Highlights of your skills and an explanation of how they pertain to the position.
3. A request for an interview (state that you will call to follow-up with them in a couple of weeks).

Your cover letter should not exceed one page and should be typed using the same paper as your resume, using the same font size and style. Your name, address, and phone number should appear in a prominent place on the cover letter. At the top of the page on the right-hand side is most common, although other styles are also used. Your computer software program may provide samples of cover letter styles to follow.

The cover letter you provide to a potential employer should provide the following information: the reason you are providing the letter, information regarding your qualifications for the position, and what you hope to achieve by providing the letter.

Your cover letter should clearly state why you are providing the letter. That is, if you are applying for a position, state that you are applying and where you found the advertisement. The body of the letter should describe in more detail why you qualify for the position. If you have a diploma or certification in the area of dental administration, or work experience as an administrator, you should state this in this section. Discuss your years of experience, or specific courses you took that pertain to the position. The final paragraph of the letter should state that you would like to have an interview with the potential employer. You can either request that the person call you to arrange or state that you will contact the office to set up a suitable interview time. Follow through with any statements you make regarding this, that is, if you write that you will call to set up an appointment, provide a day on which you will do this and make sure to call on that day.

Completing the Application

Some dental offices require that you complete a job application form. Even if you provide a resume, completing an application may be a formality that the office requires of all employees. Be prepared to do this, even if you have a resume ready.

Not all application forms are the same layout, although they do ask for the same information, such as work experience, education, and personal information such as address, birth date, and Social Security number. Although the personal information is not necessary for interviewing purposes, it is necessary once you are hired. Read through the application before completing it, this will help you organize your thoughts and gather any information you may need, such as previous employment information. If there are areas on the form that do not pertain to you, draw a line through the section or write "not applicable" in that area. Answer all areas honestly and make sure that your responses are consistent with the information found on your resume. Oftentimes employers will ask for a copy of your resume in addition to the completed job application.

THE INTERVIEW

The next step in acquiring a position is the interview. The interview is the employer's opportunity to learn more about you and your suitability for the position and your opportunity to learn more about the employer and the position. Often, employers have a two-interview process. The first interview usually involves talking with one person in the organization and is used to screen out the most promising candidates for a position. If you meet the employer's criteria for a position, you will be invited back for a second interview. The second interview usually involves one or more people from the organization who are in the position to decide whether you get the job.

Below are guidelines on preparing for an interview, interview etiquette, and following up on an interview.

Interview Preparation

Before participating in an interview with a prospective employer, it is wise to prepare for it so that you can make the best possible impression. First, try to find out as much as possible about the dental office you are interviewing with. Ask friends or family if they are familiar with the dental office and drive by the office one evening so you can have an idea of where it is and how long it may take you to drive there. Visit the office's web site, if available.

Another way to prepare for the interview is to anticipate what questions you may be asked and develop responses to them and to formulate questions that you would like to ask the employer. Some interviewers use a formal approach to the interview process, in which they systematically ask specific questions related to the position. Other interviewers may use an informal approach, in which they use a conversational style to the interview. It may seem as if you and the interviewer are "just talking," but the interviewer is getting an idea of your personality and how well you will interact with patients and other employees. Therefore, remember that every conversation you have while in the office is part of the interview and may be used to evaluate you. Box 20-3 provides potential questions that an interviewer may ask. Additionally, do a search on the Internet for common interview questions; you can usually find these at employment agency web sites, such as about.com and search for "interview questions."

Once you have found some questions that you may expect to encounter in the interview, practice answering them with a friend or family member in a mock interview. If you have an employment counselor, he or she may have additional resources for you to use in preparing for the interview. Note, too, that some questions are illegal for employers to ask candidates during an interview. These are discussed in the "Employment Laws" section.

BOX 20-3
Interview Questions

1. What are your strengths?
2. What are your weaknesses?
3. Why do you want this position?
4. Why did you leave your last job?
5. What salary are you expecting?
6. Can you tell me about a time when you handled a stressful situation well?
7. What did you like least about your last job?
8. What did you like the best about your last job?
9. What does confidentiality in the dental office mean to you?

Finally, think of some questions you would like to have answered by the employer. Interviewers typically ask if you have any questions for them at the end of the interview, and you should be prepared to ask one or two. Write your questions down on a note pad, which you should bring with you. Some sample questions to ask are as follows:

- What characteristics are you looking for in an employee?
- What tasks would I be spending most of my time doing in this position?
- Are there opportunities for future advancement?
- How long is the probation period for the position?
- Does the office close for holidays at any time? Would there be one or two employees in the office at that time?
- What type of benefits do you offer?

If the interviewer provides answers to your questions during the interview, make note of these answers at the time. Inform the interviewer that all of your questions were answered throughout the course of the interview, if that is case.

Interview Etiquette

Besides the points already made above, it is also important to remember proper etiquette before and during an interview. Dress appropriately for the interview. Wear neutral or dark colors for both top and bottom of your outfit. Both skirts and pants are appropriate for a job interview; decide which one you will be more comfortable wearing. Do not wear jeans or exercise clothing to a job interview. Ask a friend or family member for their opinion on the outfit you have chosen if you are unsure as to its appropriateness. You should appear neat and professional. You should pay attention to personal hygiene as well. Remember, you will likely be in a room or office with the door closed; wearing a lot of perfume or cologne or being unbathed will be evident and could be offensive. Do not smoke or eat strong-odored foods prior to the interview. Remember to brush your teeth and floss before the interview. If you are applying for a job in a dental office, you must have clean teeth!

Arrive 10 minutes prior to the interview. If your children or friends accompany you to the office, ask them to wait in the waiting room. Bring the following items:

- A copy of your resume and cover letter. Always have another copy available to present to the interviewer.
- A note pad and a pen. Record information you are given regarding the position that you may not remember at a later time.
- A page of your references. If your resume states "references are available upon request," have them available to present to the interviewer.

checkPOINT

4. What should you definitely do prior to the interview in a dental office?

Throughout the interview you may have the opportunity to discuss your clinical experience in the dental office. Be honest with the employer, if you do not have a lot of clinical experience, or exposure to the clinical side of dentistry, be clear about this. Emphasize your willingness to learn and your enthusiasm for this area. Do not attempt to use clinical terminology that you are not fully familiar with, as you may be using it out of context!

Working Interviews

Some employers may request that you come in for a working interview. A **working interview** is when a potential employee spends 2–4 hours in the position working. Some employers will pay you for the few hours spent working, but it is not a guarantee. The employer will observe your interactions with staff members and patients to make a judgment regarding your skills and how you may fit in. This also gives you the opportunity to really see if you can "see yourself" in this position, in the particular office.

Use the following tips to prepare for your working interview:

- Arrive early to locate items and information you will need throughout the day.
- Dress appropriately for the position.
- Bring your lunch and snacks to eat, do not assume you will be able to leave the premises for food.
- Ask questions! If you are not sure of a policy that must be followed, do not assume and ask someone who may know.

Follow Up

The day of the interview, or the next day, mail, e-mail, or hand deliver a letter of thanks to each person you interviewed with at the office. Providing a follow-up letter to the interview is polite and provides you with an opportunity to let the employer know how interested you are in the position and restate your qualifications. It also provides you with the opportunity to supply additional information to the interviewer that may not have been addressed at the interview.

BEYOND THE INTERVIEW

Being offered a position in the office you want to work in can be very exciting. Before accepting, however, you should carefully evaluate the pay and benefits offered and be prepared to negotiate, if needed, to ensure fair compensation.

Unfortunately, there may be a time when you are not offered the position after an interview, and you may be concerned as to why you did not get the job when you felt you were the best candidate. There are many reasons you may not be offered a job, including the following:

- Poor appearance
- Poorly written resume
- Late arrival to the interview
- Improper humor or comments made
- Negative talk of past employers
- Poor hygiene or emphasized perfume or makeup
- Emphasis on wages or time off

Alternatively, sometimes your qualifications are equal to those of other candidates and the reason may be that another candidate seemed to fit better with the personalities in the office. You should look upon each interview as an experience from which you can gain knowledge. You will be better prepared for the future interviews if you contemplate the questions asked of you and how you may answer them differently or in more depth in future interviews. This is particularly true if you are not offered a position. Asking for feedback from the potential employer about the reasons for not being offered the position should be done with care. Employers often have difficult decisions to make when choosing between qualified candidates. Offer to have your resume remain on file for the employer should the position become available in the future.

Terminating your employment relationship should be done following the process and policies in place in the dental office. Use the following guidelines if you are unclear or there are no policies in place for termination:

- Provide your employer with 2 weeks written notice of termination.
- Include a reason for your termination.
- Do not discuss with others your leaving your position before discussing it with your employer.

- Do not discuss your previous employer or employees with your new or potential employer.

EMPLOYMENT LAWS

As you go about applying and interviewing for positions, you should keep in mind that there are federal laws governing hiring and terminating employees to which employers must adhere. These laws help prevent discrimination and promote the equal treatment of all prospective and current employees. Specifically, you cannot be denied a position based on any of the following reasons:

- Race
- Color
- Nationality
- Sex
- Age
- Religion
- Disability
- Sexual orientation
- Marital status

Illegal interview questions include the following:

- Are you married?
- How old are you?
- What religion do you practice?
- What disability do you have?

checkPOINT

5. What do federal employment laws do for employees?

These laws also protect employees against sexual harassment, receiving equal pay for equal work, and discrimination in the workplace. Know how to contact the federal agency Equal Employment Opportunity Commission (EOCC) involved in the administration of these rules should you ever experience harassment or discrimination in any way while on the job.

Chapter Summary

The practicum or work experience portion of your program is the transition from student to employee. Making sure that the practicum experience you have is a positive and successful one will help ensure employment for you in the future. Your practicum placement is your first reference for the dental industry.

In searching for jobs, set appropriate goals to ensure that you find a job that meets your needs and that is a good fit for you. Make use of such resources as networking, advertisements, the yellow pages, the Internet, and employment agencies when looking for jobs.

Once you have found a position you would like to apply for, carefully prepare a resume and cover letter and complete all required application documents for the position. Prepare ahead of time for the interview by learning as much as you can about the dental office, practicing answering common interview questions, formulating some questions of your own to ask the interviewer, and practicing proper interview etiquette. Be familiar with all employment laws to protect your employment-related rights.

After the interview, promptly send a thank you note to each person you interviewed with. If you receive an offer for employment, carefully evaluate it and be prepared to negotiate its terms, if appropriate. Negotiating your employment terms can be as simple as stating that you would like to discuss the area of concern further.

For example, if you are offered a rate of pay that is lower than you anticipated, discuss when you would be eligible for a higher rate of pay, or if the employer is willing to commit to paying you the desired rate after a certain period of time.

If you are not offered the position, try to determine why you did not receive it and make changes to your approach, if needed. When you find the position you have always wanted, work hard to keep it! The rewards will come with time, and satisfaction comes from hard work, as does recognition.

Review Questions

Multiple Choice

1. **A practicum in the dental office is intended to provide you with the opportunity to**
   a. experience working as a dental administrator while you learn.
   b. evaluate the other staff member's performance.
   c. assess the productivity of the practice.
   d. realize your goals as a dental administrator.

2. **Preparation for a job interview includes**
   a. reviewing interview questions you may have for the employer.
   b. gathering information about the employees.
   c. understanding the clinical terminology completely.
   d. knowing who the direct competitor is for the office.

3. **When asked what your weaknesses are in a job interview, the best response would be**
   a. denial of any weaknesses.
   b. acknowledgement of weaknesses and admitting that you need help with improvement.
   c. acknowledgement of weaknesses and admitting that you working to improve it.
   d. denial of weaknesses and awareness that you do not require any help.

4. **One important aspect of developing a resume is**
   a. to include your future goals.
   b. to be honest.
   c. to omit information.
   d. to add false information.

5. **Which of the following is not considered a reliable job search source?**
   a. Yellow pages
   b. Previous employer
   c. Internet
   d. All of the above

6. **Which section of your resume defines the position you are seeking?**
   a. Introduction
   b. Work experience
   c. Career objective
   d. Personal goals

7. **Which of the following responses is the most appropriate response for the question "What is the main role of the dental office administrator"?**
   a. Answering the phone.
   b. Dealing effectively with patients.
   c. Fielding complaints.
   d. Collecting money.

8. **The body of a cover letter should describe**
   a. your career goals.
   b. why you qualify for the position.
   c. your drive to succeed in the dental industry.
   d. a description of your education only.

9. **Which of the following is not an example of an illegal interview question?**
   a. Are you married?
   b. When are you available to work?
   c. How many children do you have?
   d. What is the name of your church?

10. **The development of relationships that can produce employment leads is referred to as**
    a. employment.
    b. networking.
    c. dependability.
    d. professionalism.

Critical Thinking

1. During a job interview, the employer asks you whether or not you practice any religion. How are you going to respond?

2. You have been offered the position you have always dreamed of. The only catch is that the rate of pay is much less than anticipated. Are you going to turn the position down? Will you negotiate for an increase in the near future based on performance? Discuss this with two or three other students and come up with a written response/negotiation.

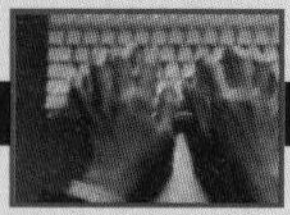

Hands-On Activity

1. Create a resume that reflects your experience and education today. Then, create your future resume, one that represents the experience and education you would like to gain over the next 5 years. Look for positions that can help you get that experience.
2. Create a cover letter and resume based on a job advertisement in the classified ads. Invite another student to review your cover letter and look for ways to improve or add to your information.
3. Look for two dental employment agencies in your area using the Internet or yellow pages. Make a list of the information that you need to supply to apply.

Web Sites

U.S. Equal Employment
www.eeoc.gov

Canada Equal Employment
www.hrsdc.gc.ca

Appendix

Answers to Checkpoint and *Review Questions*

CHAPTER 1

Answers to Checkpoint Questions

1. Maintaining the reception area, answering incoming telephone calls, greeting patients, ensuring patient chart completeness, and scheduling appointments.
2. Effectiveness in communicating with dental professionals, the ability to act calmly and precisely in stressful and emergency situations, attention to detail, honesty at all times with patients and coworkers, respect for patient confidentiality.
3. Remaining calm in emergency situations is important for the safety and security of the patients and staff members in the office. In emergency situations, it is crucial that the situation is addressed immediately. Remaining calm avoids placing undue stress on others.
4. This is a position of great responsibility and importance. Patient relationships, first impressions, and smoothly running schedules are dependent on the actions of the dental office administrator.
5. A well-lit area, warm colors, comfortable furniture.
6. Maintaining a neat desk, positive attitude, and efficient manner.
7. Pediatric specialist.
8. Oral hygiene instruction and patient education, taking radiographs and using intra-oral cameras, placing pit and fissure sealants on teeth, administering local anesthesia for hygiene or dental treatment (in some states), working in the educational setting to provide oral hygiene education.
9. Help dentists by preparing instruments, setting up instruments and equipment, and recording patient information accurately, as well as providing assistance to patients.

10. Managing payroll, dealing with insurance companies, handling difficult patients, managing account concerns, motivating employees.
11. Sterilization assistant assists in the sterilization area, office assistant assists in the business area.

Answers to Review Questions

1. a	6. c
2. d	7. a
3. c	8. b
4. b	9. c
5. c	10. b

CHAPTER 2

Answers to Checkpoint Questions

1. An agreement that is entered into between two or more parties and that has the following three components: (1) an offer, (2) an acceptance, and (3) consideration.
2. Expressed contracts consist of specific details and are expressed verbally or in writing. The responsibilities of each party involved are made explicit, to alleviate misunderstandings. An implied contract, on the other hand, is a type of contract in which the circumstances imply that parties have reached an agreement, even though they have not done so expressly.
3. Follow this process when a patient requests to change dentists: (1) document the request in the patient's chart, (2) advise the patient of any incomplete treatment plans, and (3) offer to forward patient information to a dental office of their choice.
4. Negligence refers to performing an act that a reasonable healthcare worker would not have done or omission of an act that a reasonable and prudent healthcare worker would have done.
5. HIPAA is the federal law that provides standards regarding the security and privacy of patients' health information.
6. It is acceptable to discuss patient information with other staff members, in private areas, to facilitate patient treatment or with the patient to collect information.
7. The privacy rule is a set of HIPAA privacy regulations that mandate how patients' protected health information is held or transmitted by a covered entity or its business associate in any form or media, whether electronic, paper, or oral.
8. Information included in the notice of privacy practices includes the following: (1) how the patient information is to be disclosed and used, (2) what entity is disclosing or receiving the information, (3) expiration of the acknowledgment, (4) patient's right to revoke authorization.
9. The "minimum necessary" standard refers to the practice of only using and disclosing the minimum of patient information necessary.
10. The four responsibilities of the privacy officer are as follows:
    - To develop privacy policies and procedures.
    - To ensure availability of privacy policies to patients through the accurate display of these policies.
    - To create forms and documents needed to accurately collect and retain personal health information.

- To serve as a contact for patients and third parties regarding protection and retention of health information and addresses complaints in this regard.

11. What is important to remember regarding the protection of personal health information is that the dental office staff members are to make every reasonable effort to protect the privacy of patients, and this is done by following the privacy policies in place.
12. HIPAA privacy regulations apply to all forms of communication in the dental office—written, verbal, and electronic. Security regulations apply specifically to electronic communication or electronic-protected health information.
13. Nonmaleficence refers to the dentist's duty to refrain from harming the patient, and beneficence is the dentist's duty to promote the patient's welfare.
14. These will vary based on the listing in Box 2-10.

Answers to Review Questions

1. a
2. b
3. b
4. d
5. b
6. b
7. a
8. c
9. b
10. c

CHAPTER 3

Answers to Checkpoint Questions

1. Any of the following: direct, indirect, cross-contamination, bloodborne, parenteral, and airborne transmission.
2. With infection control procedures in place and staff members being conscious of the steps required to avoid this happening, the instance of infectious disease transmission is minimized.
3. OSHA establishes guidelines regarding worker safety that includes disposal if hazardous materials. CDC controls and monitors the incidence disease and provides guideline regarding the safety and prevention of transmission of disease in the dental office.
4. Safety procedures used before and during treatment for each patient to prevent the transmission of infectious diseases.
5. Any of following: face mask, eyewear, latex or nonlatex medical gloves, and uniform (scrubs/lab coat).
6. Hand washing.
7. Refers to biological hazards. These are items that are contaminated with blood and saliva during treatment and that pose a risk to humans or the environment.
8. Product information: name of the product and manufacturers' and suppliers' names, addresses, and emergency phone numbers; hazardous ingredients, physical data, fire or explosion hazard data, and reactivity data; information on the chemical instability of a product and the substances it may react with; toxicological properties: health effects; preventive measures and first-aid measures; preparation information: who is responsible for preparation and the date of preparation of the MSDS.

Answers to Review Questions

1. a	6. c
2. c	7. d
3. b	8. d
4. b	9. a
5. c	10. d

CHAPTER 4

Answers to Checkpoint Questions

1. Speech, mastication, esthetics.
2. Enamel, dentin, cementum, and pulp.
3. An opening at the apex of the root of the tooth.
4. When both primary and permanent teeth are present at the same time.
5. The maxillary and mandibular arches.
6. Incisors, canines, premolars, and molars.
7. International, Palmer Notation, and Universal.
8. Incisal, lingual, facial or labial, mesial, and distal.

Answers to Review Questions

1. c	6. b
2. d	7. b
3. b	8. b
4. b	9. b
5. b	10. d

CHAPTER 5

Answers to Checkpoint Questions

1. Understanding the hierarchy of needs and how they affect a person's motivations can provide some perspective when communicating with patients.
2. Communication is a process that requires a sender, a receiver, and a message that is intended. During the transfer of the message, external components can distort themessage, which can prevent the receiver from receiving the message as it was intended.
3. Any description of vocabulary, conciseness, inflection, timing, and meaning.
4. Examples include body language that involves a variety of different behaviors, such as facial expression, eye contact, posture, proximity, and gestures.
5. Allowing your mood to be demonstrated to coworkers and patients through actions such as slamming doors, being short with responses, or having a scowl on your face, can be perceived as a negative attitude.
6. Five techniques of effective communication are reflecting, paraphrasing, open-ended questions, summarizing, and clarification.
7. If you are wearing stained or ripped clothing, the message you will send to patients is that you are not concerned with your personal appearance and that your supervisor is not concerned either.
8. Preconceived notions, receiver's past experiences, fatigue or poor health.
9. Nonverbal language may be misinterpreted by those from cultures other than your own.
10. Discrimination is the act of making a distinction between people on the basis of some aspects such as class, race, color, sexual orientation, or disability and allowing it to influence your interactions.

11. Keeping your relationships with your colleagues amicable and professional is important for the longevity of the working relationships and positive atmosphere in the office.

Answers to Review Questions

1. b	6. d
2. b	7. d
3. b	8. c
4. d	9. c
5. a	10. d

CHAPTER 6

Answers to Checkpoint Questions

1. The telephone is the main lifeline to the dental practice. The person answering the telephone makes the first impression of the dental office on the caller.
2. Managing the voice mailbox by clearing out messages frequently to create room for new messages to be left, as well as returning patient phone messages within the promised timeframe, maintains positive relationships and sends nonverbal messages to patients that their calls are important.
3. Examples include saying please and thank you, positive feedback, and addressing the person you are speaking to directly. This helps to build positive relationships and shows respect.
4. Voice tone and inflection convey emotion and assist in letting the patient know you are concerned and willing to help.
5. The patient should be given full attention and not be made to feel as if he or she is not important. Providing a quiet area to speak with the patient on the phone and not answering other phone calls while speaking with him or her lets him or her know you are focused on him or her.
6. Nod and smile at the patient as he or she enters the office. You can also ask the caller to hold momentarily, greet the patient, inform him or her you are completing a call and assure him or her you will be with him or her soon, and return to the call.
7. Personal calls should be restricted to emergency calls only on the office phone. There may be one line of the multiline phone that staff members will have available to them.
8. Technical difficulties, background noise, and impairments to speech and hearing are all barriers to effective telephone communication.
9. Ask the patient to explain the reason he or she is upset. Speak calmly and never raise your voice. Assure the patient that you want to help him or her.

Answers to Review Questions

1. d	6. c
2. c	7. b
3. a	8. d
4. c	9. b
5. c	10. c

CHAPTER 7

Answers to Checkpoint Questions

1. Knowing the distinction between sentences assists in the correct usage in writing correspondence.
2. Read the sentence and determine if you can place a period somewhere in the sentence to develop two sentences.
3. Not paying attention to the language you are using creates a negative impression of the dental office and the staff.
4. Letterhead, heading, inside address, salutation, body, closing, signature line, and enclosure.
5. "Encls." is typed to indicate that there is something included with the letter.
6. Identify the purpose, organize the facts, know your audience, choose a template, and proof the copy.
7. To mark a special occasion such as birthday, or anniversary, or to recognize a loss.
8. First class mail.
9. Packages and parcels are sent via standard mail.
10. Prevents information regarding the contents from being identified.
11. Postal delivery, courier, facsimile, and electronic mail.

Answers to Review Questions

1. d
2. b
3. a
4. b
5. d
6. c
7. b
8. b
9. b
10. b

CHAPTER 8

Answers to Checkpoint Questions

1. Patient charts must be complete, legible, accurate, and easily retrievable.
2. A general rule of thumb to follow regarding what information to include in the patient chart is as follows: if it has to do with the patient, document it or copy and place it in the patient chart.
3. Being aware of the patient's history regarding dental treatment and the barriers they may have had can help to anticipate future concerns for treatment.
4. If the dentist is aware of the patient's medical condition, the preparation and approach used for the procedure can be changed to avoid a negative outcome.
5. Infection of the heart's inner lining or valves, which can destroy the valves.
6. It is important to understand the guidelines in this area since the patient will often tell the office administrator about medical conditions and your role will be to educate the patient on the necessity for prophylactic antibiotics.
7. This form provides an illustrated representation of the dental treatment a patient has or will receive. Charting is essential to record the presence of health and/or disease in a form that can be used now and later.
8. A treatment plan is an itemized and prioritized list of the dental treatment that a patient requires to achieve optimal oral health. The breakdown would provide a description of the treatment and the cost of the treatment.

9. The following patient communications should be recorded: instructions for the patient from the dentist or hygienist, information you receive from the patient regarding the follow-up treatment, any e-mails or phone messages from patients.
10. Discuss and clarify any or all of the following:
    - How the incident may have been prevented?
    - How future incidents can be more effectively addressed?
    - What areas of the office most incidents occur in?
    - What topics, treatments, or situations most often lead to incidents occurring?
    - How to avoid future incidents?

Answers to Review Questions

1. b	6. a
2. a	7. c
3. b	8. c
4. a	9. d
5. b	10. b

CHAPTER 9

Answers to Checkpoint Questions

1. Dressing professionally, smiling when speaking with patients, addressing the patient promptly, not making personal calls in front of the patient, giving verbal cues to the patient that you are aware he or she has entered the office, keeping the front desk area clean and organized.
2. The goal of the dental administrator is to create a positive image of the office for the patient to facilitate an enjoyable dental experience and a lasting relationship.
3. Patients are in the schedule and willing to be contacted if an earlier appointment becomes available. Also, the goal of effectively maintaining the daily schedule, and the level of production, is much more easily achieved since patients do not have to be encouraged to set appointments after he or she have left the practice.
4. A letter regarding treatment completed is a gentle and effective way of maintaining contact with patients, particularly if it has been some time since they have been into the dental office.
5. Appointment reminder cards and mailed reminder postcards.
6. Patient retention marketing refers to the marketing that is done within the dental practice to retain patients. Marketing done outside of the dental office with a goal of attracting new patients to the clinic is new patient marketing.

Answers to Review Questions

1. b	6. b
2. b	7. b
3. a	8. d
4. d	9. b
5. d	10. a

CHAPTER 10

Answers to Checkpoint Questions

1. A manual appointment system consists of an appointment book, which when open, typically displays either 1 day or 1 week of appointments. The appointment book holds enough room for scheduling appointments for an entire year. Each page in the appointment book is divided into the number of columns necessary for either each practitioner in the office or each operatory in the office.
2. Computerized appointment scheduling systems can save a lot of time for dental office staff. Entering information into the daily schedule such as lunch, break, and office hours only has to be done once in the computerized system, whereas the manual system requires daily manual entry of this information.
3. Patients who are coming into the practice to see the hygienist are coming in for varied reasons: dental prophylaxis, treatment follow up, or periodontal issues or treatment.
4. Patients may be double booked in the following situations: when scheduling a patient who requires a procedure such as a denture reline, in which the patient must wait in the operatory for a certain period of time; when scheduling an emergency procedure in which the patient is asked to wait for radiographs to be developed; when scheduling a patient who is having an in-office whitening procedure done and the patient must remain in the operatory for a period of time.
5. Any three of these questions:
   - What is the reason for the appointment?
   - How long has the patient been experiencing symptoms of pain (sudden or for a period of time)?
   - What day and time is the patient looking to make an appointment for?
   - Does the patient depend on transportation assistance?
   - Does the patient need to see more than one staff member (dentist and hygienist)?
   - If the patient has dental insurance, will this visit be covered by the insurance?
   - If involved in a work-related accident, does the patient have the appropriate documentation or contact information for the dentist to complete?
6. Questions to ask of a patient calling for an emergency appointment include the following: Are you experiencing any discomfort? What tooth do you think it is?

   Can you describe the discomfort for me? Is there any swelling? When did the discomfort start? Are you taking any pain relievers? How often? Do they seem to be working? Can you come in today?
7. You should first ask if he or she would like to reschedule the appointment. The information should be written on the daily appointment schedule and then in the patient's chart.
8. The use of a general explanation is often recommended. Give the patient as much notice as possible. Give the patient the next available appointment time, or one of his or her choice.

Answers to Review Questions

1. c
2. b
3. b
4. b
5. c
6. b
7. b
8. c
9. c
10. b

CHAPTER 11

Answers to Checkpoint Questions

1. A policy in the dental office refers to the recommended guidelines concerning a specific area of practice. A procedure is an outline of a step-by-step process that must be followed for the accurate performance of a particular task.
2. The policy and procedure manual is a source of information for all employees regarding task procedures and employer expectations.
3. The purpose of the organizational chart is to depict the chain of command and the interrelationships between staff members, in order to promote effective communication among departments and employees.
4. The mission statement illustrates the purpose of the company. It describes and depicts the main goal of the company and summarizes actions to meet those goals.
5. Examples of emergencies in the dental office include the following: a patient losing consciousness, fire occurring in any area of the office, a patient having trouble breathing, a person in the office choking, and allergic reactions.
6. Consult with the dentist regarding preferences in any of the specific sections of the manual, before starting. Use guidelines provided by the dental regulatory bodies and licensing agencies as a model in developing policies. Include outside regulations and agencies, such as HIPAA and OSHA, to provide policies that ensure compliance in these areas. Create scripts and forms for employees to use to accurately complete tasks as required. Select a central area where all staff members will have access to the manual and it will be kept secure.
7. The morning meeting is designed to improve the overall efficiency and consistency of communication among staff members regarding the patient flow in the dental office.
8. A job description provides employees a written outline of their duties and expectations of the job. Job descriptions also assist in hiring and evaluating employees.
9. The disciplinary process consists of the following: having one-on-one meetings with the employee to discuss performance concerns, issuing a verbal warning first, recording performance concerns and relevant interactions with the employee, and issuing three written warnings before terminating the employee.
10. Providing the employee with a written warning to improve performance is documentation of failure to improve and, hence, grounds for termination.

Answers to Review Questions

1. d	6. c
2. b	7. c
3. a	8. c
4. c	9. b
5. b	10. d

CHAPTER 12

Answers to Checkpoint Questions

1. The following four steps should be followed to ensure accurate and efficient filing: conditioning, indexing, sorting, and storing.

2. The numerical filing system uses numbers to place items in order, and the alphabetical filing system uses the names of patients to file alphabetically.
3. Active patients are those who attend the dental office for regular care appointments and have been seen in the past 2–4 years. Inactive patient are those who have not been into the dental office for 5 or more years.
4. All requests should be in written form and should include name, address, date of birth, and Social Security number.

Answers to Review Questions

1. b	6. d
2. a	7. b
3. b	8. c
4. a	9. c
5. c	10. a

CHAPTER 13

Answers to Checkpoint Questions

1. Disposable items are those items that are used once and then thrown away. Gloves, masks, rubber dams, fluoride trays, and cotton-tipped applicators are examples of disposable items.
2. Capital supplies are large equipment that is purchased to carry out duties required in the dental office.
3. The criteria that dictate when to order and how much of an item should be ordered are as follows: expiration dates, storage space availability, frequency of usage, and product promotions.
4. Dental supply companies can be given an order through a salesperson, Web site, or telephone call.
5. A description of the goods is provided in the middle portion of the invoice.
6. A manual inventory system involves hand-writing entries on a card or page to track supplies and is maintained by one or two people.
7. A computerized inventory system is a system of inventory maintenance using a computer software program that tracks inventory and creates alerts for reordering items when they become low in supply.

Answers to Review Questions

1. b	6. d
2. b	7. c
3. c	8. a
4. c	9. a
5. c	10. d

CHAPTER 14

Answers to Checkpoint Questions

1. A computer system consists of essential peripherals and optional peripherals, along with the CPU.
2. Essential peripherals are peripheral items that are required to use the computer system. Examples of essential peripherals are the monitor, keyboard, and mouse.

3. Optional peripherals are peripherals that are not necessary to operate the computer but extend the capabilities of the computer. These include network cards and modems, printers, scanners, external hard drives and backup devices, speakers, and digital and x-ray cameras.
4. Features of a dental imaging system that benefit the dentist include the following: linking images to the patient's chart and managing them by allowing categorization of images; the ability to make notes directly on the image, as well as to add or subtract colors to the image for educational purposes; the use of patient's images to explain and describe treatment and provide a rendition of the image showing what it would look like after treatment; automatic image protection, which prevents irreversible altering of the image.
5. Dental software programs can provide patients with a three-dimensional animation of their own teeth to explain and have them understand the treatment they require.
6. A cookie is a small file that is placed on the hard drive of your computer and that contains information that can control your computer in certain aspects. Keeping the Internet security system on at all times should deny the acceptance of cookies on your computer.
7. Being specific in the terms that you enter to begin your search is necessary to gather information quickly and accurately.

Answers to Review Questions

1. b
2. a
3. c
4. d
5. c
6. d
7. c
8. b
9. a
10. d

CHAPTER 15

Answers to Checkpoint Questions

1. Most dental insurance plans provide coverage for both preventive and major treatments. Generally, patients must assume a larger portion of the costs for major procedures, such as crown and bridge placement, than for preventive procedures.
2. Eligibility means that some services will be covered by the insurance plan and others may not, depending on certain criteria set out within the plan.
3. Fee-for-service means that the patient pays the dental provider for the treatment rendered and then submits a dental claim form directly to the insurance company for reimbursement.
4. A schedule of benefits is a defined list of benefits that are reimbursed to the dentist for a specified amount.
5. Obtaining the correct insurance information from patients is necessary to ensure that claims can be filed accurately and payment received in a timely manner.
6. The birthday rule refers only to dependents (children) of parents having dental insurance: the insurance plan of the parent whose birthday occurs first in a calendar year is the primary plan.

Answers to Review Questions

1. a
2. b
3. b
4. c
5. a
6. b
7. a
8. a
9. b
10. d

CHAPTER 16

Answers to Checkpoint Questions

1. Bookkeeping is the recording of all financial transactions undertaken by the dental office.
2. An adjustment that is made to reduce the patient's balance is called a credit adjustment.
3. At the end of each month, specific tasks must be completed to keep the records of the business accurate. Examples of month-end procedures are processing statements for outstanding accounts, reconciling bank accounts, and managing accounts receivable by contacting outstanding accounts or sending them to collection agencies.
4. The form of payment should be noted on the same line as the description on the ledger card or receipt by writing "cash" or "check" and then recording the amount in the credits column.
5. The journal sheet provides information regarding accounts receivable on a daily basis. As the charges and payments change with each transaction, the accounts receivable total also changes.
6. Information found on the charge and receipt forms includes patient's name, account balance, list of treatment received at the appointment, and future appointment times.
7. The ledger card is the primary financial record regarding the patient's account.
8. The single most important aspect of collecting payment from patients and maintaining accounts receivables is informing the patient about his or her financial responsibility before starting treatment.

Answers to Review Questions

1. b
2. b
3. b
4. c
5. d
6. b
7. b
8. b
9. c
10. d

CHAPTER 17

Answers to Checkpoint Questions

1. Overhead expenses are the usual expenses or costs involved in running a business. All of the costs that are paid out to various suppliers and vendors fall under the category of accounts payable.
2. The difference between overhead expenses and other expenses is that overhead expenses generally occur on a continual basis. Without the services covered by these expenses, the business would not operate.
3. Paying with a credit card can be done quickly and easily over the telephone or online, or the credit card number can be kept on file by the vendor and the account balance can be paid in full every month, and a receipt sent to the dental office. A credit card is also useful for vendors who will not ship supplies without prepayment of the goods.
4. A check is generally valid for 6 months after the date of issue, after which it is considered stale-dated. A check that is written for a future date is considered a postdated check.
5. Each time money is disbursed from petty cash, a petty cash voucher corresponding to the amount of cash disburse must be placed in the petty cash

account. The voucher represents money spent and should have a store receipt attached to it as proof that the reimbursement was legitimate.

6. The main advantage of using the computer system for accounts payable record keeping is that it is more likely to ensure the accuracy of the mathematical computations and the completeness of the checks.

Answers to Review Questions

1. c	6. c
2. b	7. b
3. c	8. a
4. a	9. a
5. b	10. c

CHAPTER 18

Answers to Checkpoint Questions

1. Savings accounts are interest bearing and provide easy access to funds. A disadvantage is that checks cannot be written on them.
2. Overdraft protection is a service provided by the bank in which the bank covers checks written on the account in the event that there are not enough funds to cover them.
3. Ensure that the check amount exactly matches the amount you write on the deposit slip, prepare the deposit in a quiet area of the office or at a time of day during which you will not be interrupted, and the total amount of payment being deposited should be equal to the total amount of payments received in the office that day.
4. Reasons for discrepancies include the following: checks that were written or deposits that were made were not recorded in the checkbook or monthly ledger; the bank charges, or fees, were not recorded in the checkbook or monthly ledger balance; deposits made to the bank account after the statement date; checks that were written were not "put through" or cleared on the account before the statement end date.
5. Three forms of electronic banking include electronic transfer of funds via telephone, ATM banking, and online banking. Each of these methods helps save time when completing banking transactions.

Answers to Review Questions

1. b	6. a
2. b	7. c
3. b	8. a
4. b	9. b
5. a	10. c

CHAPTER 19

Answers to Checkpoint Questions

1. The payroll register allows for the payroll records to be kept separately and totaled on a regular basis. More importantly, it allows for the payroll records to be maintained in a private area, separate from other financial records.

2. Payroll records must be kept in a secure place to ensure the confidentiality of employee information. A record for each employee must be kept separately that contains the necessary information for payroll for the duration of employment with the company.
3. This means that the employer, by law, must deduct and remit the deductions to the IRS. Examples of mandatory deductions include federal, state, and local income taxes and Social Security and Medicare taxes.
4. The net pay or take-home pay is the amount of pay owed to the employee after all deductions have been taken. Gross pay is the total hours worked multiplied by the hourly pay rate.
5. The W-2 form is a document sent by the employer to the employee at the end of the calendar year (January to December) that contains information regarding the deductions that each employee has paid and his or her yearly earnings. Specifically, the W-2 form contains the employee's name; address; Social Security number; total gross earnings; total state, federal, and local (if applicable) taxes withheld; taxable benefits; and total net income.

Answers to Review Questions

1. b	6. c
2. d	7. b
3. a	8. b
4. a	9. a
5. c	10. b

CHAPTER 20

Answers to Checkpoint Questions

1. The two main areas to pay attention during your work experience are dependability and professionalism.
2. The employer is looking for that unique quality that sets you apart. To discover what your strengths and weaknesses are, you should engage in the process of self-reflection.
3. The most common forms of resources used for job searches are networking, advertisements, yellow pages, the Internet, and employment agencies.
4. Remember to brush your teeth and floss before the interview. If you are applying for a job in a dental office, you must have clean teeth!
5. Federal laws that regulate the standards by which employers adhere to regarding hiring and terminating employees protect employees against sexual harassment and discrimination in the workplace.

Answers to Review Questions

1. a	6. c
2. a	7. b
3. c	8. b
4. b	9. b
5. b	10. b

Glossary

abandonment: a unilateral discontinuation of services without reasonable notice provided to the patient after treatment has been started but before it is completed

accounts payable: all of the costs that are paid out to various suppliers and vendors

accounts receivable: money owed to the practice

active listening: listening while giving your full attention to the person with whom you are communicating

active patients: patients who attend the dental office for regular care appointments and have been seen in the past 2–4 years, with the time frame varying between practices

administrative safeguards: practices designed to provide accountability of covered entities in ensuring confidentiality of protected health information and the integrity of the data transmitted

administrative supplies: supplies that are used to carry out administrative tasks and duties to facilitate patient care

aged accounts receivable listing: a record for each patient that lists the patient's name, balance owed, and number of days the account has been unpaid

airborne transmission: transmission of disease via contact with droplets containing microorganisms that can remain in the air for long periods of time

alphabetical filing system: a system in which files are kept in alphabetical order by the patient's last name

Americans with Disabilities Act of 1990: a civil rights law that prohibits discrimination based on a person's disability

anterior: toward the front of the mouth

apical foramen: a small opening at the base of a tooth's root

assignment of benefits: an approach in which patients assigns their insurance benefits to the dental office in payment of the treatment received; the patient usually pays for the portion of treatment that is not paid for by the insurance carrier at the time of the appointment

attitude: one's outlook and how one chooses to express it

automated teller machine (ATM): a machine that may be used to withdraw funds from or deposit funds to an account

backordered item: an item that is not in stock at the time it is ordered and, thus, will be shipped at a later date

bank draft: a check issued by a bank on its own account for a customer for payment to a third party

bank statement: a record of the transactions, such as deposits and payments by check, that have been processed on the bank account in a 1-month period

banking fees: fees charged to the business by the bank for providing banking services

benefit booklet: a document provided by the insurance company to the insured listing the benefits provided in the plan

bias: a personal preference that influences your behavior

biohazardous waste: items that are contaminated with blood and saliva during treatment and pose a risk to humans or the environment

birthday rule: a rule related to coordination of benefits that applies to cases in which dependents (children) of parents who both have dental insurance; in such cases, the insurance plan of the parent whose birthday occurs first in a calendar year is the primary plan

bloodborne transmission: spread of an infectious disease by contamination of the blood

body: the portion of the letter that conveys the message

bookkeeping: the recording of all financial transactions undertaken by the dental office

breach of confidentiality: disclosure of confidential patient information to an outside or third party, particularly to persons who do not have legal access to the patient's chart

budget: an estimation of the expenses for the business for a certain time period

buffer times: times that are blocked off on the schedule as if they were patient bookings but these are used for emergency appointments and various office activities

business bank account: a bank account used for financial transactions of the business, such as deposits received and checks written for accounts payable and payroll

capital supplies: large, expensive equipment needed to carry out duties required in the dental office that are included in the inventory list but are not replaced on a regular basis, such as dental chairs and stools

capitation: a system in which the insurance company pays providers a fixed per capita rate per member regardless of the treatment provided

carrier: the insurance company that carries the dental plan and that is responsible for paying the dental claims and collecting the premiums

cashier's check: a check issued by a bank on its own account for a customer for payment to a third party

cementoenamel junction (CEJ): the point at which the cementum covering the root of the tooth meets the enamel covering the crown of the tooth

cementum: tissue that covers the root of the tooth and consists of about 55% inorganic material

central processing unit (CPU): the minute circuitry imprinted on silicon chips housed within the computer's case that processes computer language data and instructs the operation of the computer

certified check: a check issued by a bank on its own account for a customer for payment to a third party

certified dental assistant (CDA): a healthcare professional in the dental office whose responsibilities include providing assistance to the dentist in clinical procedures and other tasks; a professional credential similar to registered dental assistant

certified dental technician (CDT): a dental healthcare professional who makes and repairs dental restorations and appliances based on written instructions from the dentist, typically in a dental laboratory

channel of communication: the method of sending a message

checking account: a bank account on which checks are written on the basis of the amount of money held in the account; deposits are made into the account and checks are written for payment of bills and payroll

chronological filing system: a system in which files are organized by date

civil law: law in which a private party, such as a patient, files a lawsuit and becomes the plaintiff; the defendant, such as a dentist, is not incarcerated; usually resolved by the plaintiff, or patient, being reimbursed for any losses he or she endured

clarification: a technique of communication in which you ask follow-up questions to ensure that you understand a client's message

clinical chart form: a form that provides an illustrated representation of the dental treatment a patient has or will receive

clinical crown: the surface of the crown; the part that is visible and accessible during routine dental examination

clinical supplies: supplies used for clinical procedures in the dental office

closing: the complimentary words that appear at the end of a letter (i.e., "Sincerely yours," "Best regards," and "Respectfully"), along with the signature line of the sender

code of ethics: a guideline of professional conduct dentists adhere to in their practice of dentistry

code of professional conduct: an outline of the type of behavior, or conduct, that is required of dentists on the basis of the principle in question

coinsurance: the amount is a percentage of the expenses that the patient is financially responsible for

communication: the act of sending and receiving information through verbal and nonverbal forms

complex sentence: a single independent clause and one or more dependent clauses

compound sentence: two or more independent clauses joined together

compound-complex sentence: two or more independent clauses and one or more dependent clauses

computer system: the combination of the essential peripherals and optional peripherals along with the central processing unit

computerized appointment management system: a computer scheduling program that is used for setting up and tracking appointments

computerized inventory system: a system of inventory maintenance using a computer software program that tracks inventory and creates alerts for reordering items when they become low in supply

conciseness: use of as few words as are needed to convey a message

conditioning: the preparation of documents being filed, such as taping up torn pages, removing paper clips and staples, and making sure that any document that is part of a patient's chart has the patient's name on it where it is visible

confidential: private

consent: the patient's agreement to being treated prior to treatment being performed

consultation area: a separate office or other space within the clinic where dental team members can consult privately with one another or with patients

contract: an agreement that is entered into between two or more parties

cookie: a small file that is placed on the hard drive of your computer by a remote site and that contains information that can identify or control your computer

coordination of benefits: the process of determining which insurance plan will pay which portion of medical expenses when the patient is covered by more than one plan

counter check: a bank check given to customers who have run out of checks or whose checks are not yet available

cover letter: a letter submitted together with a resume to prospective employers that outlines who you are, what position you are applying for, and why you would be a desirable candidate for the position

covered entity: any dentist who transmits patient information electronically

credit adjustment: an adjustment that reduces the patient's balance

credit balance: an overpayment or a payment made in advance of treatment, resulting in a credit on the patient's account

credit memo: a credit on the account noted on a supplier's statement, reflecting items returned to the supplier

creditworthiness: the ability of a patient to pay his or her accounts on time as agreed, as based on past payment performance of the patient

criminal law: law in which the litigation is always filed by the government, who is called the prosecution; punishment for violating criminal law involves either incarceration, fines paid to the government, or execution

cross-contamination: transmission of microorganisms from one source to another, whether the transmission is from one person to another, as in direct transmission, or through the use of an intermediary object, as in indirect transmission

crown: the part of the tooth that is above the gumline

customary fee: a fee that is charged for the same service by similar dental providers in the same geographic area

day sheet: a record of charges and receipts that have occurred throughout the day

DDS: Doctor of Dental Surgery

debit adjustment: an adjustment that adds to the patient's balance

deciduous dentition: primary teeth, which fall out and are replaced by permanent teeth

declarative sentence: a sentence that makes a statement and is typically punctuated with a period

deductible: a set dollar amount that the plan member must pay in qualified expenses over the course of a year before coverage from the insurance company is applied

deductions: amounts of money regularly deducted from an employee's paycheck, including federal, state, and local income taxes, along with Medicare and social security

defamation: written or spoken injury to a person or organization's reputation

dental health maintenance organizations (DHMO): organizations of dental providers who provides dental treatment to members of the dental plan

dental indemnity insurance: a fee-for-service insurance plan, in which the patient pays the dental provider for the treatment rendered and then submits a dental claim directly to the insurance company for reimbursement

dental insurance: coverage by contract whereby one party (insurance company) pays all or some portion of dental expenses accrued by the other party (patient) in exchange for regular payments by the second party (premium)

dental office administrator: the person who manages the daily flow of the dental office through control and maintenance of the front office and administrative functions in the dental office

dental office manager: the team member who is responsible for the overall smooth operation of the day-to-day business of the dental office

dental operatories: treatment rooms within the dental clinic

dental preferred provider organization (DPPO): a dental benefit program in which providers have a contract with a third party, such as an insurance carrier or self-insured employer, with a purpose of providing members with services at prenegotiated reduced rates

dental specialist: a dentist who has received additional formal education and post-graduate training in an area of dental specialty

dental specialty: a field of study and practice within dentistry that has been recognized by the American Dental Association

dentin: the main tissue surrounding the pulp; a yellow material that lies below the enamel and cementum and gives teeth their bulk

dentinal fibril: fibers lying within the dentinal tubules that assist the dentin in providing nourishment to the tooth and transmitting pain stimuli

dentinal tubules: microscopic S-shaped tubes in the dentin that extend from the pulp canal to the enamel of the crown and the cementum of the root

dentinoenamel junction (DEJ): the surface of the enamel that joins to the dentin

dentist: a healthcare professional who practices the examination, diagnosis, treatment, planning, or care of conditions within the human oral cavity or its adjacent tissues and structures

dentistry: the examination, diagnosis, treatment, planning, or care of conditions within the human oral cavity or its adjacent tissues and structures

dependent: a family member of the subscriber, such as a spouse or child

desktop: a computer system that consists of a monitor, which rests on a desktop, a case housing the central processing unit and various disk drives, a keyboard, and a mouse

diastema: a gap between the central incisors

direct reimbursement plan: an insurance plan in which the plan member pays the dental provider directly for the fees that are charged, and the employer reimburses the employee a percentage of the fees paid, based on the plan specifications

direct transmission: transmission of infection via direct contact with body fluids, such as blood and saliva

discount: a lower-than-normal rate charged for services, such as family discounts or seniors' discounts

discrimination: the act of making a distinction between people on the basis of some aspects such as class, race, color, sexual orientation, or disability

disposable items: items that are used once and then thrown away, such as gloves, masks, rubber dams, fluoride trays, and cotton-tipped applicators

DMD: Doctor of Dental Medicine

double booking: intentionally scheduling two patients at the same time to see the dentist

dovetailing: a scheduling strategy in which either the first or last 15 to 30 minutes of the patient's appointment with a dentist involves duties or procedures that can be managed by the dental assistant

edentulous: without teeth

electronic banking: banking done using the computer in the dental office

electronic data interchange (EDI): the electronic interchange of business information using a standardized format that allows the dental office to send information (dental claims) to the insurance carrier through electronic means rather than mailing the claim

eligibility: a set of criteria established with an insurance plan that determine which services will be covered, for whom, and when

emergency patients: patients who come to the office because they are experiencing oral pain or have broken a tooth which requires immediate intervention by the dentist

empathy: the accurate recognition of emotions of others and the ability to communicate your understanding to them

employee earnings record: a record containing information on an employee's pay, including gross pay, deductions, federal tax rate, salary, and the number of days worked in a pay period

employee evaluation: an assessment of the on-the-job performance of an employee conducted by a manager on the basis of annual goals; typically involves a written evaluation and a meeting of the manager with the employee to discuss the evaluation

employment agency: a company that provides short-term or temporary work for people searching for full-time positions

enamel: the hard, outer tissue that covers the crown of the tooth

enclosure: any items included with the letter, such as other documents or photos

endorsed: signed on the back

environment: the surroundings in which the communication occurs

exclamatory sentence: an emphatic declarative sentence, typically marked with an exclamation point

exfoliation: the shedding and replacement of primary teeth by permanent teeth

expiration date: a date listed on a perishable item by which time the item should be used before it becomes ineffective

explanation of benefits (EOB): a document that provides information regarding how much is being paid on a claim, who is receiving the payment, as well as any deductible or copayment information

expressed contracts: contracts expressed verbally or in writing

eye contact: a nonverbal cue in communication involving looking at the eyes of the person with whom one is communicating

facial expression: use of facial features in the process of communication

feedback: information that the receiver returns to the sender providing the sender with a confirmation that the intended message was received or that the message was distorted somehow

fiscal year: a 12-month period of time that is set up by the practice's accountant to serve as the time frame for the yearly accounting of the practice

fixed fee: a set fee that an insurance company will reimburse for a specific service performed by the dental provider

fraud: an act of deception committed for personal gain

geographical filing system: a system in which files are organized by the geographical locations of the patients such as country, state, province, territory, or even location within a city or county

gestures: actions used in communication

Good Samaritan Act: a law designed to ensure that caregivers are immune from liability in an emergency situation, as long as the care is provided in a way that a reasonable and prudent person would provide in the same situation; does not apply to emergency situations that occur within the dental office, only to emergency acts outside of the formal practice of the dental office

gross pay: the amount of pay owed to an employee before any deductions have been taken; calculated by hours worked multiplied by hourly pay rate

group: the employer or organization that provides the dental plan

group member: the person who has coverage in his or her name under the group dental plan

heading: the portion of the letter at the top of the page, typically including the address of the person sending the letter and the date the letter is written

health and dental history form: a form used to collect information regarding a patient's medical and dental history

Health Insurance Portability and Accountability Act (HIPAA): a federal law that provides standards regarding the security and privacy of patients' health information

imperative sentence: a sentence that issues a command

implied contract: a contract in which the circumstances imply that parties have reached an agreement, even though they have not done so expressly

inactive patients: patients who have not been into the dental office for 5 or more years, with the time frame varying from practice to practice

incident report: a report that documents incidences of patient or staff injury or medical emergency, negative behavior, or other unusual events of concern, completed by a staff member who was involved in or who witnessed the incident

indexing: separating documents by type when filing

indirect transmission: transmission of infection via contact with a surface or an instrument that is contaminated by infectious microorganisms

individual practice association: a collective organization of dentists and dental associations that contracts to provide dental treatment to specific plan member populations

individually identifiable health information: information that pertains to a patient's health or healthcare and can be used to identify the patient

infection control: all procedures in both the clinical and administrative areas of the dental office that are to protect patients and dental team members from exposure to infectious agents

infectious disease: a disease that is contagious or can be spread from one person to another in some way

infective endocarditis: an infection of the heart's inner lining or valves that can destroy the heart valves

inflection: tone or pitch of voice, used in the process of communication

inside address: the name and address of the receiver of the letter

insured: a type of insurance plan in which the employer or other organization pays a portion of the monthly premiums to an insurance company on behalf of the employee or group member

International Numbering System (Federation Dentaire Internationale, or FDI): a tooth numbering system that assigns each primary and permanent tooth a two-digit number

Internet security system: a program that protects a computer from harmful viruses and intruders

interpersonal variables: factors related to the sender or receiver that greatly influence the communication process

interrogative sentence: a sentence that asks a question and is punctuated with a question mark

inventory: all the items held available in stock for any area of the dental office, including all clinical and administrative items

invoice: a legal document given to the customer or client, listing goods or services provided, along with prices and terms of sale

job description: a written outline of the specific duties and responsibilities related to a given position

journal sheet: a record of charges and receipts that have occurred throughout the day

laboratory: an area in the dental office where clinical staff perform functions such as pouring up impressions and developing diagnostic models

laptop: a small, portable computer with integrated monitor that opens like a notebook

law: a system or body of rules of conduct in society enforced through a set of institutions

ledger card: the written record of financial transactions for each patient

letterhead: special paper used by businesses for letter correspondence that has the preprinted name and address of the business and other contact information located at the top, and sometimes the bottom, of the page

litigation: a lawsuit that is in progress; for example, when a suit has been filed against the dentist

malpractice: an action by a professional that has brought harm to a client or patient

managed care: a system of healthcare that controls costs by placing limits on physicians' fees and by restricting the patient's choice of physicians

mandibular arch: lower dental arch

manual appointment scheduling system: an appointment book that displays either 1 day or 1 week of appointments per two-page spread, typically for a full year, and on which appointments may be manually recorded

manual inventory system: an inventory system in which entries are handwritten on a card or page to track supplies

margins: spaces left on the right and left sides and top and bottom of a letter

maxillary arch: upper dental arch

meaning: the information that is intended to be conveyed in a message

Medicaid: a program jointly funded by the State and the Federal governments that provides additional coverage for health and dental services for low-income families

Medicare is a government-funded program that provides health and dental coverage for senior citizens

message: the information being communicated

midline: an imaginary line that separates the right and left sides of the body

midsagittal plane: the reference plane that runs longitudinally (up and down) and separates the right and left sides of the body

minimum necessary: a standard that dictates that only the patient information that is necessary should be used and disclosed, and no more

mission statement: a statement of the goals, philosophy, and purpose of a business

mitigation: the responsibility of a covered entity to alleviate by every reasonable effort any harm resulting from the covered entity's violation of the privacy rule in its handling of a patient's information

mixed dentition: the combination of primary and permanent teeth present in the oral cavity at the same time during a 6-year period

money order: a check sold by a post office for payment by a third party for a customer

monitor: the visual display screen used with the computer

monthly fee: a fee charged by the bank to the business on a monthly basis, based on a certain number of transactions in the account within the month or on maintaining a minimum dollar amount in the account

morning meetings: a daily staff meeting held before the office is open to review the schedule and discuss areas where team members can assist one another in managing the flow of patients

negligence: performing an act that a reasonable and prudent person (in this case, a dental professional) would not have done or omission of an act that a reasonable and prudent person would have done

net pay: the amount of pay owed to the employee after all deductions have been taken

network: a network of providers, including dentists and dental specialists, under contract to the dental health maintenance organization

networking: the development of relationships that can produce employment leads

new patient marketing: any type of marketing done outside of the dental office that has the goal of attracting new patients to the clinic, such as a sign displayed outside the building indicating where the dental office is located, a phone book listing, or an advertisement in a newspaper

nonregulated waste: common garbage or trash, including paper products, disposable items, and plastic and paper wrap

nonverbal communication: communication without spoken words

numerical filing system: a system in which files are kept in numerical order by unique six-digit numbers assigned to each patient

occupational exposure: any reasonably anticipated skin, eye, or mucous membrane contact with blood or infectious materials that may result from the performance of duties

office policy and procedure manual: a document that is written by an owner or a manager of the dental office and provides the office policies and recommended procedures to be followed

one-write accounting system: a manual system of account management that uses a pegboard and carbon forms, on which transactions are recorded

online banking: use of a computer to complete banking transactions online

open-ended question: a question that cannot be answered with a "yes" or "no" response

order check: a check that is payable only to the named payee and that is the most common form of check, usually contains the language "Pay to the order of"

organizational chart: a diagram showing the hierarchical relationship between positions within an organization

overdraft protection: a bank account feature that allows for checks written on the account to be covered in the event that there are not enough funds in the account to cover them

overhead: expenses in running the business

overhead expenses: the usual and ongoing expenses involved in running a business

Palmer Notation System: a tooth numbering system that uses brackets to represent the quadrant of the tooth, with the tooth number appearing inside the bracket

paperless office: an office in which patient records are entirely electronic

paraphrasing: rephrasing in your own words what someone has said to you

parenteral: related to the piercing of the skin or the mucous membrane

pathogens: organisms that cause disease

patient chart: a legal document that contains the dental and medical history of the patient, along with demographic information

patient recare system: a proactive method of scheduling future appointments with patients and reminding the patients of these appointments; also known as a recall system

patient retention marketing: marketing that is done within the dental practice to retain patients

payee: the person to whom a check is written

payroll: the computing and issuing of checks for payment for work done by all employees in the office

payroll service: an outside agency that issues all paychecks to the company's employees

periodontal disease: an infection of the tissues that support the teeth

peripheral: a type of computer hardware that is connected to a computer to expand the range of functions the computer can perform

permanent teeth: adult dentition

personal protective equipment: items the healthcare worker wears to prevent being infected by pathogens, including face masks, eyewear, medical gloves, and uniforms

personal representative: a person who is legally authorized to make healthcare decisions on the patient's behalf

petty cash: an amount of cash kept on hand in the office to pay for small purchases

physical safeguards: practices designed to protect the privacy of protected health information (PHI) in the immediate work areas where such information may be visible to unauthorized persons, such as the cabinets or shelving units where patient files are stored, the front desk, where computer monitors may be visible and where the central processing unit may be located, and fax machines, where PHI may be received

policy: the recommended guidelines concerning a specific area of practice

postal money order: a check sold by a post office for payment by a third party for a customer

postdated check: a check that is written for a future date

posterior: toward the back of the mouth

posture: a nonverbal cue in communication involving the position of the sender's body

practicum: an opportunity for practical training in the industry to which one is studying, in which one works alongside employees of the office while under the direct supervision of one person in the office and the supervisor of an academic program

predetermination of benefits: an itemized estimation of cost for dental treatment that a patient requires

preventive dental care: regular, routine care that focuses on preventing future disease rather than treating existing conditions, such as examinations, radiographs, and dental cleanings

primary dentition: the first set of teeth that a human possesses

Privacy officer: a person assigned by a covered entity in compliance with HIPAA legislation to be responsible for the implementation of HIPAA policies and procedures and to ensure their compliance with HIPAA legislation

privacy practices notice: notice provided to patients regarding their legal rights to their health information and the organization's legal duties regarding protecting this information

Privacy rule: collective HIPAA privacy regulations that have been established to mandate how patients' protected health information is held or transmitted by a covered entity or its business associate, in any form or media, whether electronic, paper, or oral

procedure: an outline of a step-by-step process that must be followed for the accurate performance of a particular task

professional: one who treats patients and colleagues with respect at all times and shows pride and competence in the work one does through the way one dresses, talks, and acts

professional associations: organizations that provide support, recruitment, and retention for dental professionals and that are dedicated to the advancement of the profession and the promotion of oral health

professionalism: the practice of treating patients and colleagues with respect at all times and showing pride in the work that one does through the way one dresses, talks, and acts

progress notes: the section of a patient chart in which a narrative documentation of patient care and communication may be recorded chronologically

proof of posting: the balance of transactions at the end of the day

prophylactic antibiotics: an antibiotic regimen administered to a patient before and after a dental procedure to help prevent infection

protected health information (PHI): individually identifiable health information, which is information that pertains to a patient's health or healthcare and can be used to identify the patient

provider: the dentist who provides treatment

provider identification number: a number assigned to each dentist to identify him or her to the insurance company and that is included on the dental claim form

proximity: the degree of nearness to something or someone

pulp: a soft tissue that contains the nerves and blood supply of the tooth

reactivation letter: a letter to a patient who has not been in the dental practice for a long time

reasonable fee: a fee that is greater than what is usually charged by the dental provider because of exceptional circumstances but is considered to be reasonable by the insurance company if it is justified by the dental provider

receiver: the person who decodes the message in communication

record of employment: a form used by the human resources department of the government of Canada that provides employees and the department with financial information regarding their employment

reference check: the act of contacting a job applicant's past employers to verify employment experience and work ethic displayed by the applicant

reflecting: a communication technique in which one repeats back to the person with whom one is communicating part of what the person has already said

registered dental assistant (RDA): a healthcare professional in the dental office whose responsibilities include providing assistance to the dentist in clinical procedures and other tasks; a professional credential similar to certified dental assistant

registered dental hygienist (RDH): a licensed dental professional who specializes in providing services that focus on the prevention of oral health problems and disease

regulated waste: biohazardous waste or medical waste, including blood or saliva, sharps contaminated with blood or saliva, and tissues (either hard or soft) that have been removed from the patient

resorption: the wearing away or absorption of the root of the primary teeth caused by pressure from the permanent teeth erupting

resume: a document listing one's work-related skills, employment history, educational credentials, and other qualifications for employment

reusable items: items that can be sterilized or disinfected and, thus, can be reused, such as dental mirrors, explorers or scalers, and curing lights

root: the portion of the tooth that is not normally visible and that lies below the gumline in the mouth

salutation: a greeting to the receiver of the letter

savings account: a bank account that earns interest at a higher rate than what is typically offered with a checking account and that is usually used to set aside money for future capital expenses or transfer money not being used

search engine: a Web site that uses software that allows you to enter a search term and then lists all the sites that match your search term

secondary insurance: an insurance plan to which the patient is not the primary subscriber (i.e., a spouse's plan); this plan will be tapped only after the primary insurance has been used

secondary teeth: adult dentition

security rule: the security regulations pertaining to collecting, maintaining, using, or transmitting protected health information with which covered entities must comply

self-funded: a type of insurance plan in which the employer collects premiums and, instead of providing the insurance company with the funds, invests the funds; all dental claims are then processed and paid by the employer on the employees' behalf

sender: the person who encodes the message in communication

sharps: instruments used for cutting or that have pointed ends, such as scalpel blades and needles

signature line: the space left for the signature of the sender of the letter, along with the printed name of the sender

simple sentence: an independent clause without any dependent clauses

sorting: putting a group of records into order before filing them

stale-dated check: a check that has a date more than 6 months old

standard of care: the degree of care and skill that would be exercised under similar circumstances by reasonable and prudent members of the same profession

standard precautions: safety procedures used before and during treatment for each patient to prevent the transmission of infectious diseases

statement: a listing of all the invoices that have been billed to the dental office from a supply company within a 30-day period, as well as any outstanding invoices from earlier periods

statutory law: law that is upheld and written by a governing authority

stereotyping: the process of characterizing a whole group of people on the basis of a single or a few representative examples

sterilization area: an area within the clinic that houses equipment used to sterilize and prepare dental instruments for reuse

storing: filing records into the proper filing system

subject filing system: a system in which files are organized first by subject and then by alphabetical order of subjects

subject line: a word or phrase that briefly describes the purpose or content of the letter

subscriber: the person who has coverage in his or her name under the group dental plan

succedaneous teeth: teeth that succeed or follow the primary teeth, occupying the space they previously had; permanent teeth

summarizing: a technique in which you verbally review information with the patient that he or she has provided

tablet PC: a small, flat computer that consists primarily of a touch-sensitive monitor that may be written on with a stylus

team member: one who consistently assists one's colleagues in achieving common goals

technical safeguards: practices designed to protect the privacy and integrity of information that is transmitted electronically

telecommunications device for the deaf (TDD): a telephone typewriter, used to send typed messages through an electrical communications channel over the telephone to an operator, who translates the message to speech for the receiver and then translates the receiver's response back to text for the caller

telecommunications relay service: an operator service that allows people with hearing and speech disabilities to place calls to regular telephones using a telecommunications device for the deaf

teller's check: a check issued by a bank but drawn on an account with another bank

time card: a record of the employee's hours worked for the pay period

time sheet: a record of the employee's hours worked for the pay period

timing: a factor in effective communication that pertains to the appropriate time to send a message

transaction fee: a fee charged to the business by the bank for each transaction in the business account

traveler's check: a type of check that is purchased by the payer from a bank or other financial institution, that is available in fixed denominations, and that is generally treated as cash

treatment plan: an itemized and prioritized list of the dental treatments that a patient requires to achieve optimal oral health

units of time: standard increments of time (i.e., 15 minutes) that are used to indicate amount of time required or allotted for treatment

Universal Numbering System: the tooth numbering system most often used in the United States

usual fee: a fee normally charged by the dental provider for the service

usual, customary, and reasonable (UCR) fee: a method of reimbursement in which the insurance company agrees to reimburse fees at a rates that are considered usual, customary, and reasonable

verbal communication: the act of conveying messages through the use of words or language

virus: a small file that may be transferred to your computer system with the intent to sabotage or annoy

vocabulary: the means by which verbal communication is expressed

W-2 form: a tax document mailed to the employee from the employer at the end of the calendar year containing information regarding the deductions that the employee has paid and yearly earnings; also known as the Wage and Tax Statement

W-4 form: a tax document completed by the employee that determines how much tax is withheld taxes; also known as the Employee's Withholding Allowance Certificate

walk-in patients: patients who show up at the dental office without a scheduled appointment

wisdom teeth: third molars, which may never fully erupt or erupt later, in the teen to early adult years

working interview: an employment interview in which the candidate either works or observes others working in the dental office for a few hours or a full day

Workplace Hazardous Materials Information System (WHMIS): a classification system established by the Canadian Center for Occupational Health and Safety that groups chemicals that have similar properties

Index